Multivariate Methods in Epidemiology

Monographs in Epidemiology and Biostatistics
Edited by Jennifer L. Kelsey, Michael G. Marmot,
Paul D. Stolley, Martin P. Vessey

2. CASE CONTROL STUDIES
Design, Conduct, Analysis
James J. Schlesselman   1982

3. EPIDEMIOLOGY OF
MUSCULOSKELETAL
DISORDERS
Jennifer L. Kelsey   1982

8. CLINICAL TRIALS
Design, Conduct, and Analysis
Curtis L. Meinert   1986

12. STATISTICAL METHODS IN
EPIDEMIOLOGY
Harold A. Kahn and
Christopher T. Sempos   1989

13. RESEARCH METHODS IN
OCCUPATIONAL
EPIDEMIOLOGY
Harvey Checkoway,
Neil E. Pearce, Douglas J.
Crawford-Brown   1989

18. THE DRUG ETIOLOGY OF
AGRANULOCYTOSIS AND
APLASTIC ANEMIA
David W. Kaufman,
Judith P. Kelly, Micha Levy,
Samuel Shapiro   1991

19. SCREENING IN CHRONIC
DISEASE
Second Edition
Alan S. Morrison   1992

20. EPIDEMIOLOGY AND
CONTROL OF NEURAL
TUBE DEFECTS
J. Mack Elwood, Julian Little,
J. Harold Elwood   1992

21. PRINCIPLES OF EXPOSURE
MEASUREMENT IN
EPIDEMIOLOGY
Bruce K. Armstrong, Emily White,
Rodolfo Saracci   1992

22. FUNDAMENTALS OF
GENETIC EPIDEMIOLOGY
Muin J. Khoury, Terri H. Beaty,
Bernice H. Cohen   1993

23. AIDS EPIDEMIOLOGY
A Quantitative Approach
Ron Brookmeyer and
Mitchell H. Gail   1994

25. STATISTICAL ANALYSIS OF
EPIDEMIOLOGIC DATA
Second Edition
Steven Selvin   1996

26. METHODS IN
OBSERVATIONAL
EPIDEMIOLOGY
Second Edition
Jennifer L. Kelsey, Alice S.
Whittemore, Alfred S. Evans,
W. Douglas Thompson   1996

27. CLINICAL EPIDEMIOLOGY
The Study of the Outcome of Illness
Second Edition
Noel S. Weiss   1996

28. MODERN APPLIED
BIOSTATISTICAL METHODS
Using S-Plus
Steve Selvin   1998

29. DESIGN AND ANALYSIS OF
GROUP-RANDOMIZED
TRIALS
David M. Murray   1998

30. NUTRITIONAL
EPIDEMIOLOGY
Second Edition
Walter Willett   1998

31. META-ANALYSIS, DECISION
ANALYSIS, AND COST-
EFFECTIVENESS ANALYSIS
Methods for Quantitative Synthesis
in Medicine
Second Edition
Diana B. Petitti   2000

32. MULTIVARIATE METHODS
IN EPIDEMIOLOGY
Theodore R. Holford   2002

33. TEXTBOOK OF CANCER
EPIDEMIOLOGY
Hans-Olov Adami, David Hunter,
Dimitrios Trichopoulos   2002

MONOGRAPHS IN EPIDEMIOLOGY AND BIOSTATISTICS
VOLUME 32

Multivariate Methods in Epidemiology

THEODORE R. HOLFORD
Department of Epidemiology and Public Health
Yale University School of Medicine

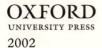
2002

OXFORD
UNIVERSITY PRESS

Oxford   New York
Auckland   Bangkok   Buenos Aires   Cape Town   Chennai
Dar es Salaam   Delhi   Hong Kong   Istanbul   Karachi   Kolkata
Kuala Lumpur   Madrid   Melbourne   Mexico City   Mumbai   Nairobi
São Paulo   Shanghai   Singapore   Taipei   Tokyo   Toronto

and an associated company in Berlin

Copyright © 2002 by Oxford University Press, Inc.

Published by Oxford University Press, Inc.
198 Madison Avenue, New York, New York, 10016
http://www.oup-usa.org

Oxford is a registered trademark of Oxford University Press

Library of Congress Cataloging-in-Publication Data
Holford, Theodore R.
Multivariate methods in epidemiology / by Theodore R. Holford.
p. cm. — (Monographs in epidemiology and biostatistics ; v. 32)
Includes bibliographical references and index.
ISBN 0-19-512440-5
1. Epidemiology—Statistical methods.
2. Multivariate analysis.
I. Title. II. Series.
RA652.2.M3 H654 2002   614.4'07'27—dc21   2001050091

9 8 7 6 5 4 3 2 1

Printed in the United States of America
on acid-free paper

*To
Maryellen*

Preface

Epidemiology provides the scientific basis for much of public health practice, and the current revolution in health care and disease prevention indicates that the demand for valuable results from this field will continue to grow. Sound epidemiologic research requires a solid statistical basis for both study design and data analysis. Hence, it should come as no surprise that epidemiology has provided modern statistics with some of its deepest problems. As knowledge about the underlying causes of diseases increases, we often see that they have multiple causes, so that it is generally not possible to limit conclusions to a single factor. We also need to consider the possibility that other factors may confound a particular association or modify its estimated effect. Therefore, a multivariate approach to data analysis is usually an essential part of epidemiologic research.

The multivariate methods considered in this book involve the simultaneous analysis of the association between multiple attributes of an individual and the risk of a disease. The underlying framework is one in which a single response is associated with multiple regressor variables. Some reserve the term *multivariate methods* for techniques that deal with more than one response in a single analysis, which is not the main focus of this book. The definition of *variate* in the *Oxford English Dictionary* does not distinguish attributes of an individual that are identified with the response from those that predict that response. It is multiples of the latter that are the primary focus in the following chapters, although some of the log-linear models would fall into even the narrow definition of multivariate methods.

This text is directed to students interested in applying multivariate methods to the analysis of epidemiologic data. It draws from material I have offered in a course in the Department of Epidemiology and Public Health entitled "Topics in Statistical Epidemiology," which is required of all biostatistics students and all doctoral students in epidemiology at Yale University. Applications and the interpretation of results are emphasized, so the techniques are demonstrated with examples from epidemiologic studies. These examples include setting up a problem for analysis using the SAS® statistical package, and then interpreting the resulting output. Some may prefer to use alternative software, but the rationale for setting up the problem, as well as the resulting output, should be recognizable from what is shown here, even though details of syntax may vary.

This book is intended to serve as a textbook for readers who are seeking to address the practical questions of how to approach data analysis. On a first reading, these readers may be willing to take much of the theory for granted. Others may not wish to use any method without first developing some understanding of its basis, however. I have tried to strike a balance between the two types of readers by providing an informal rationale for the underlying assumptions for a method of analysis in each chapter, along with a more detailed rationale of the theory in a corresponding appendix. The chapters are meant to stand alone if one is willing to take the more detailed rationale for granted. However, a reader with the background and inclination to learn why a particular formula is appropriate can do so by studying the appendix with the title "Theory on" followed by the corresponding chapter title.

The assumed background of readers depends on the extent to which they wish to deal with the theoretical material. A reader who only wishes to understand how to apply the methods and interpret the results will require a previous course in applied statistics, including an understanding of the use of regression methods for building quantitative descriptions of data. The mathematical knowledge required for this level of understanding of the material is basic algebra. Alternatively, a reader who wishes to tackle the theoretical sections should have completed a calculus-level course on statistical inference.

The range of statistical techniques currently used by epidemiologists includes chi-square methods, as well as generalized linear model applications. Both approaches are described, but some of the computationally simpler techniques, such as the Mantel–Haenszel methods, are motivated from the standpoint of score statistics for generalized linear models. Thus, the reader will be able to appreciate that this is just one of several approaches to likelihood-based inference that could be used. The advantage of this motivation is that it ties together the different methods that are currently used in the field, and it will help readers see that the various techniques are essentially cut from a similar piece of theoretical cloth.

This book is organized into four parts. Part I introduces ways of thinking quantitatively about the disease process. Part II explores some of the computationally direct methods that have long been a part of classical epidemiological data analysis. Separate chapters deal with the analysis of proportions, rates, and semiparametric approaches to time to failure data. Formal model fitting is considered in much more detail in Part III, which considers not only the analysis of proportions, but also parametric and semiparametric approaches to the analysis of hazard rates. Part IV deals with special problems that arise when one incorporates aspects of the study design into the analysis, along with approaches to designing a study that will be the right size for addressing the study aims. In addition, Chapter 12 describes some of the new directions that show considerable promise for extending the statistical tools that are becoming more widely available to epidemiologists.

Statistical epidemiology has become one of the most active areas of biostatistical research, with a correspondingly huge literature. In supplying references to the methods discussed in each chapter, I have not tried to be exhaustive but have instead concentrated on those that have been key in motivating a particular line of analysis.

It is impossible to remember all of the sources for one's ideas, but Colin White stands out—both for his patient guidance in my early thinking about statistical epidemiology and for his encouragement in pursuing approaches to data analysis that includes a thoughtful consideration of the underlying biology. Robert Hardy helped me appreciate mathematical approaches for formulating the processes that lead to the development of disease. In addition, I am grateful for the insight provided by the outstanding epidemiologists that I have been privileged to collaborate with because they have insisted that the techniques being applied to their studies address the interesting questions, not just those that could be easily answered with an obvious analysis. The collaborations that have been especially useful in developing the ideas presented here have involved my work with Michael Bracken, Jennifer Kelsey, Brian Leaderer, and Tongzhang Zheng. Finally, I would like to thank the students in my course on Topics in Statistical Epidemiology for helping me hone some of my ideas and for providing editorial assistance in early drafts of some of these chapters.

New Haven, Connecticut   T. R. H.

Contents

Part I Concepts and Definitions

1. Associations between Exposure and Disease, 3

   Strategies for Studying Disease in a Population, 4
      Individuals Followed for Equal Times, 4
      Individuals Followed for Varying Times, 5
      Studies of Cases and Controls, 6
      Vital Statistics and Disease Registries, 8
   Rationale for Multivariate Methods, 9
   Statistical Approaches to Data Analysis, 10
   How to Use This Book, 11

2. Models for Disease, 15

   Models for the Disease Process, 15
      Stochastic Models, 17
      Basic Disease Model, 19
      Outcomes for Analysis, 20
      Theoretical Relationship among Outcomes, 21
   Models for the Effect of Factors, 22
      Models for Rates, 23
      Models for Risks, 31
   Summary, 34

Part II Non-Regression Methods

3. Analysis of Proportions, 39

   Studies That Yield Proportion Responses, 39
   Cross-Sectional Studies, 40
   Cohort Studies, 41
   Case-Control Studies, 42
   A Single Binary Risk Factor, 43
   Likelihood-Based Inference, 47
   Wald Test, 48
   Score Test: Pearson Chi-Square, 48
   Likelihood Ratio Test, 51
   Exact Test, 51
   Interval Estimates of the Odds Ratio, 54
   Logit Method, 54
   Cornfield's Method, 55
   Exact Method, 56
   More Than Two Levels of Exposure, 58
   Nominal Categories, 58
   Ordered Categories, 62
   Stratified Analysis, 63
   Cochran and Mantel–Haenszel Tests, 65
   Mantel–Haenszel Estimator for the Odds Ratio, 68
   Testing for Homogeneity of the Odds Ratio, 70
   Stratified Analysis of Trends, 73
   Summary, 74
   Exercises, 75

4. Analysis of Rates, 81

   Rates as an Outcome, 82
   Censored Observations with Constant Hazard, 82
   Population Rates, 85
   Standardized Ratios, 86
   Comparing Nominal Groups, 88
   Score Test for Trend, 94
   Stratification, 95
   Summary Rates, 97
   Summary, 103
   Exercises, 104

5. Analysis of Time to Failure, 109

Estimating Survival Curves, 109
  Actuarial Estimate, 110
  Piecewise Exponential Estimate, 113
  Product Limit Estimate, 115
Graphical Displays, 119
  Diagnostic for Constant Hazard, 119
  Diagnostic for Weibull Hazard, 121
  Diagnostic for Proportional Hazards, 124
Tests for Comparing Hazards, 126
  Piecewise Constant Hazards, 127
  Log-Rank Test, 129
  Stratified Log-Rank Test, 132
Types of Incomplete Data, 133
  Right Censoring, 133
  Left Censoring, 134
  Interval Censoring, 135
Summary, 135
Exercises, 136

Part III Regression Methods

6. Regression Models for Proportions, 141

Generalized Linear Model for Proportions, 142
  Linear Logistic Model, 144
  Log-Linear Hazard Model, 145
  Probit Model, 146
Fitting Binary Response Models, 147
  Fitting the Linear Logistic Model, 147
  Fitting Alternatives to the Logistic Model, 151
  Problems in Model Fitting, 156
Summary, 159
Exercises, 160

7. Defining Regressor Variables, 163

Categorical Variables, 163
  0 1 Coding, 165
  −1 0 1 Coding, 169

Deviations from the Model, 172
Threshold and Other Models for Trend, 176
Interactions and Parallelism, 182
Testing Linear Hypotheses, 186
Wald Tests for Linear Hypotheses, 189
Likelihood Ratio Tests for Linear Hypotheses, 192
Power Transformations of Continuous Regressor Variables, 195
Summary, 200
Exercises, 202

8. Parametric Models for Hazard Functions, 205

Constant Hazard Model, 206
Log-Linear Model for Rates, 206
Generalized Linear Model, 207
Alternatives to Log-Linear Models, 212
Models for Standardized Ratios, 215
Weibull Hazard Model, 218
Other Parametric Models, 220
Gamma Failure Times, 220
Log-Normal Failure Time, 221
Gompertz–Makeham Model, 222
Extreme-Value Distribution, 222
Extra Poisson Variation, 223
Summary, 224
Exercises, 225

9. Proportional Hazards Regression, 227

Piecewise Constant Hazards Model, 228
Proportional Piecewise Constant Hazards, 228
Testing for Constant Hazards, 230
Alternatives to Proportional Hazards, 233
Nonparametric Proportional Hazards, 235
Evaluating the Fit of a Proportional Hazards Model, 239
Time-Dependent Covariates, 240
Effects That Vary with Time, 241
Exposures That Vary with Time, 245
Summary, 247
Exercises, 249

Part IV Study Design and New Directions

10. Analysis of Matched Studies, 253

Designing Matched Studies, 254
  Matched Pairs, 254
  Many-to-One Matching, 255
  Frequency Matching, 256
  Caliper Matching, 256
  Strategies for Analysis, 257
Case-Control Studies with Matched Pairs, 258
  McNemar's Test and Its Extensions, 258
  Logistic Regression Method I, 262
  Logistic Regression Method II, 265
Case-Control Studies with More Than One Control per Case, 268
Cohort Studies with Matched Pairs, 272
Summary, 276
Exercises, 277

11. Power and Sample Size Requirements, 281

Estimation, 281
  Proportions, 282
  Rates, 283
  Association Measure, 285
Two-Group Hypothesis Tests, 286
  Proportion Comparisons, 288
  Rate Comparisons, 289
  Survival Curves, 291
  Matched Pairs, 292
General Hypothesis Tests, 295
  Steps for Calculating the Noncentrality Parameter, 298
  Testing for Trend, 298
  Covariate Adjustment, 305
  Interactions, 308
Simulation, 309
Summary, 310
Exercises, 311

12. Extending Regression Models, 315

Classification and Regression Trees (CART), 316
　Growing Trees, 317
　Trees for Binary Responses, 320
　CART for Survival Data, 325
Splines, 326
　Linear Splines, 326
　Polynomial Splines, 327
　GAMS and MARS, 329
Missing Observations, 330
Variance Components, 332
Errors in Variables, 333
Collinearity, 335
Summary, 339

Appendix 1. Theory on Models for Disease, 343

Constant Rates in Time, 345
Idealized Model for Rates Changing over Time, 346
Observed Effects of Age on Rates, 347
Relationship between Models for Rates and Proportions, 347

Appendix 2. Theory on Analysis of Proportions, 351

Likelihood for the Linear Logistic Model, 351
Wald Statistic for a 2×2 Table, 353
Likelihood Ratio Statistic for a 2×2 Table, 354
Score Statistics for an $I \times 2$ Table, 355
Score Statistics for Combining $I \times 2$ Tables, 357

Appendix 3. Theory on Analysis of Rates, 361

Likelihood Formation, 361
　Time to Failure Models, 361
　Counts of Failures, 362
　Comparisons to Standard Rates, 363
Estimation, 363
Score Test for Nominal Categories, 364
Score Test Controlling for Strata, 366

Appendix 4. Theory on Analysis of Time to Failure, 369

Actuarial Estimate, 369
Product Limit Estimate, 372

Two-Sample Score Test for Piecewise Constant Hazards, 372
Log-Rank Test, 374

Appendix 5. Theory on Regression Models for Proportions, 377

Distribution for Binary Responses, 377
Functions of the Linear Predictor, 379
Using Results to Conduct Inference, 380

Appendix 6. Theory on Parametric Models for Hazard Functions, 385

Poisson Regression, 385
Weibull Hazards, 387
Alternatives to Log-Linear Hazard Models, 390

Appendix 7. Theory on Proportional Hazards Regression, 393

Appendix 8. Theory on Analysis of Matched Studies, 397

Conditional Likelihood for Case-Control Study, 397
Matched Pairs for Case-Control Studies, 398
N-to-One Matching in Case-Control Studies, 399
Conditional Likelihood for Cohort Studies, 399

Index, 403

I

CONCEPTS AND DEFINITIONS

1

Associations between Exposure and Disease

Epidemiology is the search for the root causes of disease. As in any scientific endeavor, the thoughtful investigator must exercise care in separating cause from effect. The fact that disease often results from not single but multiple causes only makes the study more intriguing because the interplay among the factors can have unexpected implications for their effect on the outcome. One must also be concerned about some of the fundamentals of the philosophy of science when trying to establish causal relationships, which usually requires the use of innovative techniques that are often unique to the study of a particular disease.

A weaker objective for the epidemiologist is the study of factors that are associated with disease. We can begin to appreciate the distinction between causes and associations by understanding that changing the level of a cause of disease will usually produce a change in risk. Therefore, causes are associated with disease risk. However, the converse does not always hold, in that changing the level of a factor that is merely associated with disease may not change the risk. We can appreciate this distinction by considering an example given by Miettinen and Cook (1) in which one considers the association between match-carrying behavior and risk of lung cancer. Our current understanding of the etiology of lung cancer is that cigarette smoking is the leading cause of the disease, and a smoker will obviously be more likely to carry matches than most other people. Thus, if we were to look for an association between match carrying and lung cancer, we would probably find one. We know that by quitting cigarette smoking, an individual can lower risk of lung cancer. However, a smoker who continued the habit but stopped carrying matches, perhaps using a lighter instead, in all likelihood would not reduce lung cancer risk because the causal exposure remained. Clearly, one must work much harder to establish the causal effects that underlie observed associations. This additional effort often requires that one bring together different elements of research into a coherent theory that will explain what is observed in a population.

In this text, we shall explore a variety of ways to analyze the association between multiple factors and disease risk. Although these techniques are an essential part of the study of the causes of disease, to arrive at an understanding of cause, one must not only perform an analysis that is technically correct but also design a study that will eliminate the possibility of associations resulting from artifact and bias.

To begin thinking about the process of formulating a question about an association, let us first consider some of the study designs that might be used to address a particular question. We shall then consider the rationale for studying more than one factor at a time. Finally, we will discuss the quantitative framework that can guide our approach to formulating studies of disease etiology.

Strategies for Studying Disease in a Population

The difficulty in discerning the difference between associations that are causal and those that are spurious has led to the use of a variety of design strategies. Choosing a particular design is an art that often requires a delicate balancing of the most definitive approach to addressing a question with what is feasible in terms of cost and ethics. The first rule of any analysis is that it must reflect the study design, so let us first consider some of the approaches that have been especially useful in epidemiological studies.

Individuals followed for equal times

Martin and Bracken (2) report the results of a study on the association between exposure to secondhand cigarette smoke by the mother and the risk of giving birth to a low birth weight baby. A group of pregnant women was identified, and because there is preliminary reason to think that exposures early in pregnancy are especially relevant, an effort was made to identify mothers early in their pregnancy. To avoid the difficulty of separating possible effects of sidestream smoke from those of directly smoking cigarettes, this study was limited to nonsmoking mothers. The essential nature of the data collection required the measurement of exposure to secondhand cigarette smoke by interviewing the mothers to determine the amount of time spent in a smoky environment, as well as the level of smokiness.

Determining exposure to cigarette smoke by interviews is not easy; some people are extremely sensitive and complain vociferously about the slightest whiff of smoke that may go unnoticed by another person. Perhaps some become so used to a smoky environment that they systematically downplay the severity of their exposure relative to those who are accustomed to a smoke-free environment, thus systematically introducing error into the exposure assessment. One might also try to develop an objective measure of exposure, perhaps by using a biomarker, such as a biochemical byproduct of nicotine metabolism that can be measured from urine. The problem here is that metabolic rates can vary among individuals, and the rates themselves can also be affected by pregnancy. Another alternative measure of exposure would make use of a monitor that could either be placed in the home for a few days or worn by the subject so that exposure outside the home will also be tallied. Whether one can be certain that a women would actually wear a utilitarian-looking monitor to a fancy dinner in which many guests smoked is a potential problem for such an exposure measure. Hence, none of these measures is perfect, even those that we might consider to be "objective," and none of them is actually measuring the level of exposure to the fetus, which could be the most relevant exposure for a causative agent.

Subjects in Martin and Bracken's study (2) were followed until the end of pregnancy, when the birth weight was recorded and it was noted whether birth weight was low by a standard criterion, thus identifying the final outcome of interest. While the gestation time does vary somewhat, it often makes sense to regard the overall pregnancy as an event in itself, ignoring time. Hence, the outcome of interest in this study was whether the baby had a normal or a low birth weight. The results of such a binary outcome study would be reported in terms of the proportion with the condition of interest, and then all the analyses would focus on this binary response.

Individuals followed for varying times

The Physician's Health Study (3) was established to study the effect of regularly taking either 325 mg of aspirin on the risk of cardiovascular disease death or 50 mg of beta carotene on the risk of cancer death. Long-term effects of these drugs were of interest, so it was essential to recruit a population who would be easy to follow and likely to comply with a regular program of treatment. In this instance the choice was male physicians between the ages of 40 and 84 who resided in the United States in 1982. Using a membership list from the American Medical Association, a total of 261,248 subjects were invited to participate in the study. Of these, 112,528 responded to the invitation, and 59,285 were willing to be enrolled in the study. However, some of the subjects had a history of heart disease and cancer, so they were excluded from the next phase of the study. After removing the men who did not meet all of the entry criteria, the 33,223 who remained participated in an 18-week run-in period, which required that they take the aspirin and beta carotene and record their compliance. Subjects who were not able to maintain the required regimen were once again excluded from the primary study. Ultimately, 22,071 physicians were randomly assigned to one of four treatment groups:

1. Active aspirin and active beta carotene
2. Aspirin placebo and active beta carotene
3. Active aspirin and placebo beta carotene
4. Aspirin placebo and beta carotene placebo.

Because subjects were assigned to one of these groups at random, each group would tend to be balanced with respect to any risk factor for cardiovascular disease or cancer. This would be true not only for known risk factors but also for those that were not known at the time of the study. Hence, the evidence from such a controlled experiment is often the strongest evidence that can be provided by epidemiological research.

To enroll such a large group of carefully selected subjects required a considerable effort, so it obviously took place over a period of time. The result was that when it came time to report the results of the study, some subjects were enrolled earlier than others, and thus had a longer period of follow-up. In the Physicians' Health Study, it turned out that aspirin had a strong effect on reducing the risk of cardiovascular mortality, so much so that the investigators stopped this part of the study early so that those who were taking aspirin placebo could take advantage of the results and begin taking active aspirin to decrease their risk of cardiovascular death. When the final report on the aspirin results was prepared, the average length of follow-up was 60.2 months, but this varied from 45.8 to 77.0 months (4). All things being equal, a subject followed for 77.0 months would have approximately $77.0/45.8 = 1.7$ times the risk of death from a particular cause than a person followed for 45.8 months, and the method of analysis should reflect this. The analysis would obviously focus on whether the subject died of cardiovascular disease during the course of follow-up, but the variability in the follow-up requires the consideration of a two-part outcome: a binary indicator of cardiovascular death and the length of time the subject was followed.

Studies of cases and controls

To learn about the association between exposure to PCBs and risk of breast cancer, a study was conducted in which the exposure history of breast cancer cases was compared to a group of women without breast cancer. Because the concentrations typically found in the environment are extremely low, individuals are usually not aware that they have been exposed, so it becomes impossible to employ interviews in such a study. Zheng et al. (5) conducted such a study by recruiting women before breast surgery and obtaining samples of breast adipose tissue, which were then chemically analyzed. Many PCBs are extremely stable in that they do not react with the body's biochemical processes that normally eliminate many harmful agents. Thus, the levels in a person tend to cumulate over time, and because PCBs are fat soluble, they are stored in fat or adipose tissue. For breast cancer, the levels that build up in that part of the body are especially relevant should any of the PCBs be carcinogenic because breast tissue is the site at which the disease itself develops. By analyzing the PCB concentration in breast adipose tissue, the investigators believed that they had a quantity that was closely related to the cumulative exposure to PCBs in the breast, thus providing a biomarker for PCB exposure.

In this study, many practical issues arose because of the invasive medical procedure required to obtain the tissue samples. For most breast cancer cases it was not difficult to obtain a sample that was large enough for chemical analysis because the surgical removal of the tumor that is required for treatment usually requires that enough of the surrounding tissue is also removed, and this can then be used for chemical analyses. However, there were many other practical problems that required considerable care in collecting samples for analysis. It was essential that fresh tissue samples be used, and not samples that may have been preserved in paraffin blocks because of the possibility that the preservation process might have contaminated the sample with PCBs. When surgeons remove tissue, it is usually placed in a container of formalin, which preserves it for subsequent analysis by a pathologist. However, for this study the investigators were concerned about whether the formalin would dissolve some of the PCBs in the tissue, so that the measured level would be lower than what had actually been present in the tissue. There was also concern about whether the ink that surgeons use to mark guidelines for what is to be cut also contained PCBs, so that too much ink would contaminate the sample for the purposes of this study. Because the effective conduct of this study depended on so much control of factors in the surgery itself, it was conducted in Yale–New Haven Hospital, which is a research hospital in which the staff can more readily be acclimated to the special needs of a study like this.

If the collection of data from cases seemed complex, controls introduced even more thoughtful consideration. Randomly selecting individuals from the population was out of the question because it would be unethical to subject them to the invasive procedure required to obtain a comparable sample of breast adipose tissue. Instead, women were recruited from among those treated with breast surgery at the same hospital. Many of these subjects had received biopsies, but the pathologist had determined that no malignancy was present. If the condition that required the biopsy was also caused by exposure to PCBs, or if that condition was an early step in a process that ultimately would lead to a malignancy, then the exposure levels in the controls might be more similar to those seen in the cancer cases and would result in an underestimate of the association.

We can see from this example that while an essential part of this study involved the comparison of exposure in cases and controls, considerable effort was essential to minimize artifactual factors. One important factor was age, because these exposures accumulate as a person goes throughout life, and yet increasing cancer risk it also part of the aging process. Hence, women with the highest exposure will tend to be older, so it becomes essential that we consider both factors at the same time. As we shall see, this might be accomplished by designing our study in a way that balances the age distribution in the two groups, or we might adjust for age along with various other factors during the analysis at the end of the study.

Vital statistics and disease registries

Governmental agencies collect and report a variety of data on health indicators that are important for monitoring the health of a population and planning for the best allocation of health resources. Cancer registries, like the Connecticut Tumor Registry, have been especially useful for the study of disease trends for this leading cause of mortality in the U.S. Figure 1–1 shows age-specific lung cancer incidence rates among women for various groups of calendar years, which are connected by solid lines. The graph illustrates the fact that there are two time elements that need to be considered at the same time, age (A) and year of diagnosis, which is often referred to as calendar period (P). A curious feature of this graph is that while the rates generally increase with age, a result of the effect of aging on cancer risk, in the oldest ages the rates tend to reach a plateau or even decline. Another way of looking at these trends with age is to follow birth cohorts (C)—that is, groups of individuals born around the same time— as they go through life, and this is shown by the broken lines in Figure 1–1. Now we can see that the peak or plateau with age has disappeared, thus providing a summary of trends that are consistent with the underlying biology of aging.

The pattern in Figure 1–1 is also consistent with what is now known about the etiology of lung cancer, which is primarily caused by cigarette smoking. Most individuals who smoke begin the habit in their late teens or early twenties, thus giving rise to generational differences in smoking

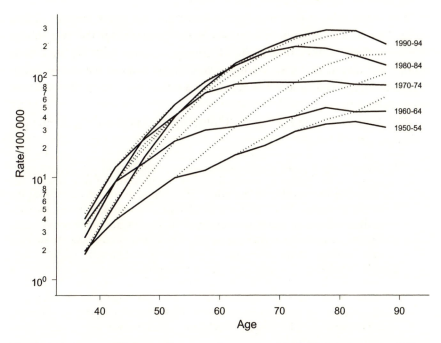

Figure 1–1 Age-specific mortality rates for women in California by year of diagnosis (*solid lines*) and year of birth (*dotted lines*). [Data from public use files of the National Cancer Institute].

rates. Birth cohort is simply a representation of generational effects, and the increase in lung cancer incidence for more recent generations can be attributed to a greater proportion of women who smoke cigarettes.

In this example we can begin to appreciate the interplay between the particular form for an analysis and the interpretation of results. The indicators of time are actually interrelated by $C = P - A$, so that by knowing two of them we can immediately find the third. This implies that there are not really three distinct time indicators, but two. Hence, an analysis of these factors requires that we find a description that provides a sensible way of bringing together these elements of time.

Rationale for Multivariate Methods

A common thread in these examples of epidemiological studies arises from the importance of an interplay among various factors. Most diseases are multifactorial, especially the chronic diseases. But even when a disease results from a known infective agent, we must come to grips with an array of different factors if we are to understand the best ways for controlling them. The AIDS epidemic, for instance, has pointed out the complexity of the cultural factors that facilitate transmission of HIV, so that even though the causative agent is known, one needs to jointly consider more than one factor at a time when trying to develop a public health strategy for attacking it.

The reasons for conducting a multivariate analysis for an epidemiological study are as follow:

1. *Adjustment for confounding*—addressing the question of whether an association is the result of an imbalance in the distribution of a known risk factor. In the context of the study of PCBs and breast cancer risk, we would be interested in the extent to which an association between the biomarker indicating cumulative exposure is due to the tendency of older women to have the higher exposures. Therefore, conducting an analysis that adjusts or controls for age would be a critical element of our study.
2. *Effect modification*—addressing the question of whether an effect is the same for all subgroups of the population. This actually implies that the nature of an effect is more complex, in that the magnitude changes with the level of another factor. Are PCBs more harmful to younger women, for instance? In addition, it usually depends on the way we choose to summarize an association.
3. *Exposure–response characterization*—describing the interplay among the various factors that affect disease risk in ways that are readily interpreted by other investigators.

Statistical Approaches to Data Analysis

A sometimes bewildering array of statistical tools are now available to epidemiologists, and many of these can be easily applied by using widely available statistical packages. Some of these techniques involve calculations that are not difficult to apply with a hand calculator, while others are greatly aided by the availability of a spreadsheet. Still other methods require specially prepared software, because the complexity of the numerical algorithms are much too complex to attempt with even a fairly sophisticated spreadsheet. Fortunately, some common threads underlie all of these methods, but the numerically simpler methods often make more restrictive assumptions about the mathematical form for the effect of a factor of interest. In this text, we will study statistical methods used in epidemiology by starting with those that are computationally simpler and then build to the more complex approaches that may be required for the analysis of multiple factors.

As we shall see in greater detail later, the likelihood or the probability that gave rise to a particular set of data from a study can motivate many of our current techniques. The likelihood can be used to provide an expression for an optimal estimate of a parameter, and its precision. It can also provide an approximate test of significance, whether using any of three approaches. It is the choice of these approaches that can have the greatest impact on whether it is feasible to do the calculations by hand, by spreadsheet, or by specially prepared software. Hence, for a given set of assumptions, one could propose three different tests that are all equivalent in large samples, so why not use the one that is easiest to compute? One of the aims of this text is to instill an appreciation for the way in which many of the most commonly used methods have arisen by adding branches of complexity to a relatively basic set of initial assumptions.

The application of a particular statistical technique is not an end in itself but merely a tool used to address a question of scientific interest. Hence, when choosing a tool, the investigator needs to keep in mind the following:

1. *The question of interest.* The results of the study must address the question posed when the study aims were initially developed. This requires careful planning from the very beginning of a study, and it may be too late if the issue is first considered at the analysis phase.
2. *The study design.* It is always necessary to reflect the study design in the method of analysis. Failure to do so may result in either biased estimates of the parameters of interest or incorrect estimates of precision.
3. *The assumptions underlying the technique.* The distributional assumptions about the random mechanism that gave rise to a set of data must be realistic. Thus, it is essential to look for violations of these assumptions so that one arrives at a valid description of the results.

How to Use This Book

While the emphasis of this text is on practical ways of using current methods of data analysis, I have tried to include background material for the methods, so that the interested reader can gain an appreciation for the rationale behind a particular method of analysis. Each chapter provides an intuitive description of methods for approaching the analysis of data from a particular study design. It is assumed that the reader has a working familiarity of applied regression and categorical data analysis.

While intuitive descriptions of statistical methodology might be sufficient for interpreting the substantive results of data analysis, one really needs a deeper discussion of the rationale for the formulae to extend or modify their applicability. A more detailed discussion of the theory underlying the presentation in each chapter is provided in a series of appendices. For a full appreciation of this material, the reader will need an understanding of the fundamentals of probability and the basics of statistical inference. For a first reading, some readers may wish to take the theoretical details for granted, thus concentrating on the material in the body of the text. Others will not want to use a formula if its origins are unfamiliar, in which case they will find further detail behind the techniques in an appendix that corresponds to the chapter.

This text is arranged into four parts. Part I provides an introduction. Chapter 2 includes definitions of some of the terms to be used throughout, as well as a framework for using statistical methodology in epidemiological science. Part II discusses methods that do not require the fitting of regression models to the data. These rely instead on basic summary measures and significance tests, each of which is computationally fairly easy to apply by using either a hand calculator or a spreadsheet program. Part III describes regression methods of data analysis for epidemiological studies. Because each type of study design has corresponding methodology in both analytic paradigms, there is a correspondence between the methods of analysis. Table 1–1 provides a summary of the types of methods that can be appropriately applied to the analysis of data from a particular type of study. Chapter 7 discusses the rationale for specifying regressor variables, so that one can address research questions of interest. These concepts can be applied to any of the modeling approaches discussed in this section. Separate chapters are devoted to outcomes that are proportions, rates, and time to failure data. Part IV introduces extensions to some of the regression methods by introducing methods of analysis that do not require a highly parameterized mathematical formulation for the exposure–disease associ-

Table 1–1. Summary of statistical techniques by data type

Data type	Non-regression methods		Regression methods	
	Chapter	Technique	Chapter	Technique
Proportions	3		6	
Cohort or		Chi-square		Logistic
Case-control		Trend		Generalized linear
studies		Mantel–Haenszel		models
Rates	4		8	
Count data or		Chi-square		Poisson regression
Failure rates		Trend		Parametric survival
		Stratification		models
		Summary rates		
Time to failure	5		9	
		Survival curves		Proportional hazards
		Log-rank test		model
Matching	10		10	
Case-control		McNemar		Conditional logistic
or Cohort				regression
studies				

ation. An advantage of these methods is that they can allow the form for the exposure–response relationship to emerge from the data and not from a set of strong assumptions. It is likely that these methods will become more commonly employed, sometimes being used in their own right and at other times providing justification for a particular formulation that may have been used in a regression model. In this part of the text, we also discuss some issues of study design, particularly the question of samples size and whether a study is large enough to be meaningful.

In applied statistics, one often learns through practice. Examples of the approaches to setting up data for analysis and interpreting the results are provided in the body of the text. For consistency, the SAS (6) package was used in most of these examples, but there are now a variety of other statistical software packages that could also be similarly employed for these analyses. At the end of each chapter, problems have been posed for the reader to try out the methods discussed. Some of these require larger data sets that can be obtained at the website, http://gisserver.yale.edu/holford/examples.

References

1. Miettinen OS, Cook EF. Confounding: essence and detection. *American Journal of Epidemiology* 1981;114:593–603.
2. Martin TR, Bracken MB. Association of low birth weight with passive smoke exposure in pregnancy. *American Journal of Epidemiology* 1986;124:633–642.
3. Steering Committee of the Physicians' Health Study Research Group. Preliminary report: findings from the aspirin component of the ongoing Physicians' Health Study. *New England Journal of Medicine* 1988;318:262–264.
4. Steering Committee of the Physicians' Health Study Research Group. Final report on the aspirin component of the ongoing Physicians' Health Study. *New England Journal of Medicine* 1989;321:126–135.
5. Zheng T, Holford TR, Tessari J, Mayne ST, Owens PH, Ward B, Carter D, Boyle P, Dubrow R, Archibeque-Engle S, Zahm SH. Breast cancer risk associated with congeners of polychlorinated biphenyls. *American Journal of Epidemiology* 2000;152:50–58.
6. SAS Institute. *SAS/STAT User's Guide* (Version 6). Cary, NC: SAS Institute, 1989.

2

Models for Disease

Diseases afflict people in a variety of ways and for a variety of reasons. Hence, it is not surprising that epidemiologists who investigate risk factors often adopt different designs for their studies. This book considers the problem of data analysis for epidemiological data. While the design of studies may be quite varied, the statistical methods used in their analysis are often closely related.

To make a quantitative summary for an association in a set of data it is often advantageous to have a concrete idea of the form for the relationship. The mathematical equation or model for the association between disease and a risk factor is necessarily tentative and is put forward as a guide for the calculations. Keep in mind that a model may be inadequate as a description for a particular disease process. Statistical theory yields an estimate of a parameter or a significance test assuming a particular model is true, but at the same time the data may reveal that the description provided by the model is unrealistic. A good analysis of data will not only consist of using an appropriate estimator or the correct significance test but will also consider the agreement between data and the underlying model that gives rise to a particular form of analysis.

When considering models for disease it is convenient to visualize the model in two parts: (1) a description of the disease process and a specification of how potential risk factors affect that process. The former deals with events that occur in an individual's lifetime which ultimately leads to a diagnosis of disease. The latter describes the way in which a person's work environment, diet, lifestyle habits, genes, and other factors determine risk of developing the disease.

Models for the Disease Process

The disease process describes events as they occur in an individual's life from a well-defined point in time, such as birth or the beginning of employment at a factory. A general representation of that process, described by Armitage and Doll (1), is shown in Figure 2–1. At some point a person is first exposed to a factor that is thought to possibly change the risk for disease. The body changes after this exposure initiates the disease process, but the changes may be so imperceptible that there is no known way of detecting them medically. However, this is only the first step, and under appropriate conditions, these changes will eventually lead to a change that can be observed—first pathologically and then clinically.

To obtain a good theoretical understanding of the disease process, it would be ideal to know the point in time at which the disease is initiated. This would enable us to study the way in which factors affect the preinduction period (the time from first exposure until the initiation of disease). Similarly, it would be desirable to study the induction period (the time between the beginning of the disease process and the clinical manifestation of the disease). Unfortunately, it is generally not possible to know when a disease may first be observed pathologically in a subject. This may be because of limits in the technology used to detect a disease, but very often there are also ethical limits from risks inherent in the medical procedures themselves. Hence, one cannot study either the larval stage (between initiation and pathologic appearance of the disease) or the developmental stage (from pathologic to clinical appearance of disease). In fact, it is not possible in general to determine any of the periods indicated on the left of the diagram shown in Figure 2–1, except in unusual circumstances.

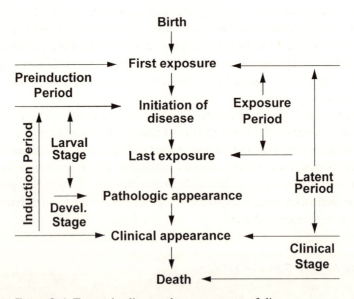

Figure 2–1 Events leading to the appearance of disease.

While practical limitations exist when studying the occurrence of disease, other information that is of general interest can be obtained. For example, the exposure period can usually be measured, and the latent period (the time from first exposure up to the clinical appearance of the disease) can also be determined in most cases. In addition, one can study subjects after the clinical appearance of disease, in the clinical stage of the disease. The time periods that can often be analyzed are given to the right of the diagram in Figure 2–1, and a major consideration of this book will involve ways of either directly analyzing these times or designing and analyzing a study that takes them into consideration.

Stochastic models

An important feature to incorporate into a model is the element of chance. In medicine, as in most life sciences, one cannot state with a chemist's certainty that if A is added to B then a reaction will result in C. For instance, it is known that cigarette smoking is an important cause of lung cancer, and yet there are examples of 95-year-olds who have smoked for a lifetime with no apparent adverse effects. If the occurrence of lung cancer is regarded as a chance event, then the effect of smoking is to increase one's chance of acquiring the disease, but for a particular individual it may still be far from certain that the disease will be acquired.

To understand the stochastic element in the disease process, consider a disease that has a well-understood life cycle, an infection by the organism *Schistosoma mansoni*. This organism infects large numbers of people in northern Africa by entering the body through the skin of those who come in contact with water infected with schistosome cercariae. A remarkable transformation takes place in the organism between the entry into the host and the clinical diagnosis of infection by observing schistosome eggs in the stool, and some of these steps in the development of this disease are shown in Figure 2–2. The first stochastic element in the process involves the contact between the cercariae and an individual. A person may enter water that contains the organism, but none may become attached to the skin because the concentration at that point is low or the water may be flowing swiftly, making it difficult for the cercariae to take hold. After boring through the skin and entering the bloodstream, the parasite migrates to the liver where it matures, but in the meantime it must survive any assaults from the immune system (2).

An interesting aspect of this disease is that at this stage in the life cycle there are both male and female schistosomes, and they must form pairs in order for the cycle to be complete; the pairing process requires that the males and females somehow find each other in the labyrinth of blood ves-

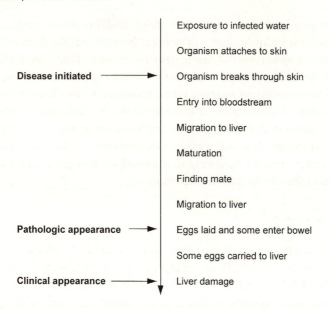

Figure 2–2 Events leading to liver fibrosis in *Schistosoma mansoni*.

sels that lead to the liver. Ultimately, a schistosome pair resides in the lumen of the bowel, where they live on the nutrients. At this stage, the female begins laying eggs; some eggs break through to be passed out with the feces, which is necessary for completion of the life cycle, but others are carried by the blood to the liver, where they may eventually cause liver disease. Once again, the stochastic aspect of the disease can be important because the destination of the eggs can depend on the position of the pair in the blood vessels. In addition, both the severity of disease and the ability to detect eggs will depend on the number of eggs laid, which can vary considerably from pair to pair.

It is clear that from the time a person comes in contact with water infested with *S. mansoni* cercariae and the initiation of the disease by the organism breaking through the skin, a number of events must transpire, which from the standpoint of mathematical modeling can be viewed as random occurrences. Each of the subsequent steps are also governed to some extent by the laws of chance, and to describe these in a precise mathematical way can be extremely challenging. As knowledge of a particular disease process increases, it quickly becomes apparent that the steps referred to in Figure 2–1 are often made up of many small steps, each with its own stochastic element.

To describe the development of a disease like schistosomiasis in mathematical terms is an extremely difficult task, even though the exercise can be useful for ultimately understanding it (3). However, a model for schistosomiasis will be unique and will directly apply to few if any other diseases. For many chronic diseases, like cancer and heart disease, much less is known about the biology underlying the disease process, making it impossible to formulate an accurate mathematical model. An alternative to a detailed model is a simplified model for disease that is sufficiently general to be of use in many situations. While the simplification may result in a lack of the specificity necessary to obtain ultimate understanding of a disease process, it can provide a wide range of methods that can be used to learn about the etiology of different diseases.

Basic disease model

Rather than using a detailed model that only applies to a specific disease, we consider a more general model of disease. Assume that three states exist for an individual:

1. Healthy—person has never acquired the disease in question
2. Diseased—person has acquired the disease at least once
3. Dead or no longer under active follow-up.

The diseased state, defined in this way, does not allow a person to return to the healthy state; the possible pathways are shown in Figure 2–3.

Sometimes an individual may die from a cause other than the disease under study, which removes the subject from further observation with respect to the disease of interest, and the information on time to disease occurrence is incomplete. For these individuals it is only possible to specify the length of time that a person lived without acquiring the disease. Such a person is said to be *right censored* with regard to information on time to development of the disease in question. This means we do not know if and when the disease would have occurred had the person lived.

The preceding definitions necessarily require the development of disease to be a well-defined event that occurs once in time; although this may

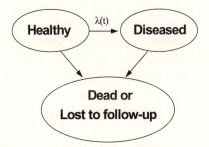

Figure 2–3 Simple model for disease process.

be an idealization, it is usually possible to satisfy the conditions by carefully defining the disease. The most straightforward realization of this process is when one is studying death from any cause where individuals clearly do not leave the state once they have entered it. In addition, subjects may be removed from observation due to their being lost to follow-up or to the study ending while they are still alive. The states in such a survival study are shown in Figure 2–4, which may be compared to our simple disease model in Figure 2–3. We can see the equivalence of the analytical problems in that survival studies are simply a special case of our simple disease model, the only difference being that the rate of going from dead to lost to follow-up is zero. Hence, there is a direct analogy between many of the methods described in this book and the analytic techniques used for failure-time data, as described next.

Outcomes for analysis

To quantitatively describe the transition from the healthy to the diseased state, we can formulate the problem in terms of *rates* (intensity of disease occurrences in time), *risks* (probability of failure after a specified period of time), and, *time to failure* (distribution of time to failure).

When studying putative risk factors for a particular disease, we can formulate the analysis to make statistical inferences on the way in which that factor affects the outcome of interest. It is also important to realize that there are direct mathematical relationships among these three quantities, so that when one specifies a model for one of them, the other two can be derived from it. These relationships follow directly from the definitions, as shown in Appendix 1, so that a study that determines the effect of a factor on the disease rate can be used directly to state its effect on the disease risk in a specified period of time.

Rates. We shall represent the rate of occurrence for a particular outcome by $\lambda(t)$, which describes the rate of transition from the healthy to the dis-

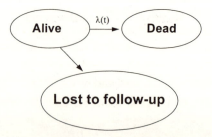

Figure 2–4 Survival model.

eased state or from alive to dead, depending on the study. Such quantities are called *hazard functions*, or instantaneous transition intensities. A synonym used in discussions of disease is the *incidence rate*, and for survival studies this quantity is sometimes referred to as the *mortality rate* or the *force of mortality*. The hazard may vary with time, t, because of factors such as the age of the subject or the accumulation of exposure over time. To account for this possible time-dependence, we specify the hazard as a function of time, t, which may represent age or time in the study.

Risks. Disease risk represents the probability that a disease occurs after a specified period of follow-up, t. When mortality is the outcome, we consider instead the risk of death, or its complement, the *survival function*, $\mathscr{F}(t)$, which is the probability that a person under active follow-up is still alive or healthy at t. If T is a random variable representing the actual time that the outcome event occurs, then $\mathscr{F}(t)$ represents the probability that T is greater than t, provided the individual is not lost or withdrawn from active follow-up for some other reason.

Time. Perhaps the method of analysis that is most directly analogous to standard regression is to consider time itself as the outcome, with the factors under study as possibly affecting the mean time to occurrence of disease or death. In standard regression analysis, the unexplained error in the data is assumed to have a normal distribution, which results in a response that can take any value, including those that are negative, and thus is inappropriate for failure times that are necessarily positive. In this case, model specification becomes a question of defining the probability density function for the time to occurrence of disease or death.

Theoretical relationship among outcomes

An important feature of rates, risks, and failure times is that they are mathematically interrelated: if any one of them is known, the other two can be mathematically derived from it, as is discussed in greater depth in Appendix 1. Hence, an analysis that shows an association between exposure and any one of these outcomes will automatically establish the existence of an association with the other two. In addition, we will come across situations where the form for a relationship is sometimes more easily derived for one outcome than another. These interrelationships will then enable us to establish the form for a quantity that is not so easily determined. An example of this arises for the constant rate assumption, $\lambda(t) \equiv \lambda$. It is not particularly easy to estimate a rate that varies with time without making a strong assumption about the form for that relationship. However, we shall see in Chapter 5 that the survival function is quite easy to obtain. If the rate is constant over time, then the survival function is given by

$$\mathcal{F}(t) = \exp\{-\lambda t\}$$

(see Appendix 1). This expression implies that if we were to construct a graph of $\mathcal{F}(t)$ on t, using a log-scale for the vertical axis, then we would have a straight line with slope $-\lambda$. Suppose we have an estimate of the log survival function that was obtained without any parametric restrictions, and we plot its relationship with t. If the result is very nearly a straight line, then we could conclude that the data are consistent with the constant rate assumption. This technique can provide us with a useful diagnostic tool for determining the adequacy of a particular set of assumptions.

Models for the Effect of Factors

In a study of disease etiology, the investigator obtains information on a number of variables that are thought to be potential risk factors. These would be expected to show their effect by modifying one of the fundamental quantities, such as the hazard function or the survival function. In this section several potential models are presented for doing this.

The way in which an investigator goes about formulating a model depends on the extent of knowledge about the disease process. Returning to the schistosomiasis example, one's knowledge of the life cycle of the parasite, shown in Figure 2–5, may be useful in trying to understand how a factor might affect incidence. If one begins the cycle with a person infected with *S. mansoni*, the parasite passes out of the host by eggs shed in the stool. If there is improper sanitation, some of these eggs find their way into a stream, where they hatch to form miracidia which swim about in the wa-

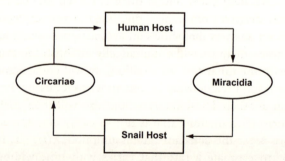

Figure 2–5 The life cycle of *Schistosoma mansoni*.

ter. A tiny fraction of these miracidia find an appropriate intermediate host, which is a particular species of snail in which the organism goes through yet another transformation, and the number of organisms multiply considerably. The organism that passes out the snail is called a cercariae, which is another free-swimming form of the parasite that is now capable of infecting a person by attaching itself to the skin, and entering the bloodstream (2).

It is clear from an understanding of the life cycle that many factors may influence the occurrence of schistosomiasis in a population, and the way in which they affect the process depends on the particular point in the cycle that is involved. For example, swimming or washing habits, perhaps measured in minutes per day, would affect the opportunity of the cercariae to attach to the skin, the point immediately before a person is infected. Alternatively, the use of molluscicides to decimate the snail population and the improvement of sanitation facilities would reduce the cercariae population in the water by interrupting the cycle at an earlier stage, thus reducing disease transmission. It is not surprising that the functional relationship between such factors and the diagnosis of the disease become very complex because of the many steps involved in the process. Several investigators (3, 4) have done interesting and important mathematical work in describing the disease process for schistosomiasis, but one thing that becomes immediately clear when studying this work is the complexity of the mathematics that results from each attempt to make the model more "realistic" in terms of the known biology. It is also clear that any results from such modeling for schistosomiasis does not immediately apply to another disease, even another infectious disease. Hence, this method is of limited value as a general approach to the problem of analyzing the possible effect of multiple factors on the disease process.

This book takes a pragmatic approach to the problem of selecting a model. The choice of a model is tentatively put forward, and it is used as a possible way in which to describe the influence of factors on the disease process. Statistical inference using these models will be considered in later chapters where the adequacy of fit, referred to as the *goodness of fit*, of a particular model is an important part of the overall data analysis. However, let us first consider several models that might be used to introduce an effect due to risk factors.

Models for rates

An investigation into disease etiology is carried out through the collection of data on a series of factors that are being studied for their possible association with risk of developing disease. In a later chapter we will discuss the specification of $\mathbf{X}$, but for now suppose there are p of these variables, represented by the row vector, $\mathbf{X} = (X_1, X_2, \ldots, X_p)$, and the hazard, which may affect the disease mortality rate, $\lambda(t;\mathbf{X})$. In this section, a number of forms for $\lambda(t;\mathbf{X})$ are described, along with their implications.

Proportional hazards. The first step one might take in formulating a model is to use the proportional hazards model suggested by Cox (5); that is, the rates are given by

$$\lambda(t;\mathbf{X}) = \lambda_0(t) \cdot h(\mathbf{X})$$

where the functions $\lambda_0(\cdot)$ and $h(\cdot)$ are as yet unspecified. In this model, the regressor variables identify different risk groups in a populations, and their rates are assumed to be proportional to each other.

As an example, suppose there are two groups of subjects who are characterized by the regressor variables $\mathbf{X}_1$ and $\mathbf{X}_2$. We can express the hazard function for the second group in terms of the hazard for the first by

$$\lambda(t;X_2) = \lambda_0(t) \cdot h(X_1) \cdot \left[\frac{h(X_2)}{h(X_1)} \right]$$

$$= \left[\frac{h(X_2)}{h(X_1)} \right] \cdot \lambda(t;X_1)$$

$$= R(X_2, X_1) \cdot \lambda(t;X_1)$$

The quantity, $R(X_2, X_1) = [h(\mathbf{X}_2)/h(\mathbf{X}_1)]$, represents the proportional change in the hazard function, and under the proportional hazards model it does not depend on time, t. In this book, the ratio of two hazard functions is called the *hazard ratio*. The proportional hazards model implies that the hazard ratio may be represented as a single number that is not a function of time, t.

Another implication of the proportional hazards model is that there is an additive effect for time and the regression components if one takes the log of the hazard function

$$\log \lambda(t;\mathbf{X}) = \log \lambda_0(t) + \log h(\mathbf{X})$$

(In this text "log" refers to the natural logarithm or log to the base e, sometime denoted by "ln.") This relationship means that if one were to graph the log hazards for different risk groups against t, one would expect to see a series of parallel lines, as shown in Figure 2–6. The distance between these lines is the log of the hazard ratio, $\log R(\mathbf{X}_2, \mathbf{X}_1)$.

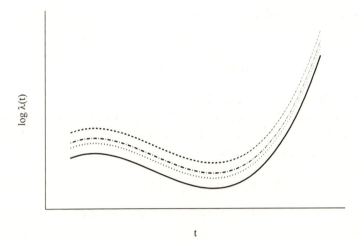

Figure 2–6 The log hazard for various risk groups under the proportional hazards model.

In order to carry out the analysis of data it will be necessary to be more explicit about the function $h(\cdot)$. There are many possible choices for $h(\cdot)$, but two that are of particular interest are the log-linear hazard and the proportionally linear hazard.

Log-linear hazards. The most common choice for $h(\cdot)$, indeed the one first used by Cox (1972), expresses the proportional hazards model in a log-linear form:

$$\log h(\mathbf{X}) = X_1\beta_1 + X_2\beta_2 + \cdots + X_p\beta_p \tag{2.1}$$

where $\beta_1, \beta_2, \ldots, \beta_p$ are regression parameters. If the parameters are written as a column vector,

$$\beta = \begin{bmatrix} \beta_1 \\ \beta_2 \\ \vdots \\ \beta_p \end{bmatrix}$$

then one can use matrix notation for equation (2.1):

$$\log H(\mathbf{X}) = \mathbf{X}\boldsymbol{\beta}$$

so that the proportional hazards model becomes

$$\lambda(t;\mathbf{X}) = \lambda_0(t) \exp\{\mathbf{X}\boldsymbol{\beta}\} \tag{2.2}$$

We call this the log-linear hazards model, because the log of the hazard function,

$$\log \lambda(t; \mathbf{X}) = \log \lambda_0(t) + \mathbf{X}\boldsymbol{\beta}$$

is a linear function of the covariates.

To understand the interpretation of the regression parameters, suppose that there are just two groups of subjects. We represent them in the model by introducing an indicator variable:

$$X = 0 \quad \text{if group 1 (factor absent)}$$
$$= 1 \quad \text{if group 2 (factor present)}$$

The hazard ratio for group 2 compared with group 1, or for $X = 1$ compared with $X = 0$, is

$$R(1,0) = \frac{\lambda(t; 1)}{\lambda(t; 0)}$$

$$= \left[\frac{\lambda_0(t) \exp\{1 \cdot \beta\}}{\lambda_0(t) \exp\{0 \cdot \beta\}} \right]$$

$$= \exp\{\beta\}$$

Hence, the parameters for simple binary variables can be interpreted as the log of the hazard ratio.

Sometimes the measurement of a factor is not just in terms of exposed or unexposed, but consists of a measure that can take any in a range of values, for example, the exposure dose for a factor. In order for the concept of hazard ratio to have meaning here, we must choose a reference value, X_0, and other values are then compared to it. Under the log-linear hazard model, the hazard ratio for X_1 compared to X_0 is

$$R(X_1, X_0) = \exp\{\beta(X_1 - X_0)\}$$

A graph, plotting log $R(X_1, X_0)$ against X_1 will be a straight line, intersecting the abscissa at X_0, as shown in Figure 2–7. In practice, one would need to investigate whether the relationship was actually linear and consider an alternative model if it was not.

Finally, this model allows for the inclusion of more than one regressor variable, which has the following implications for the inclusion of two factors. If one has two binary factors, A and B, then there are a four possible

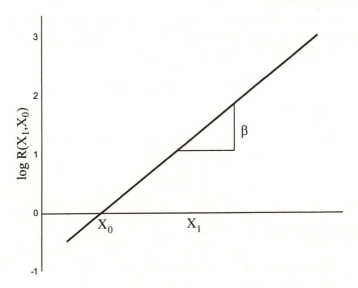

Figure 2–7 Plot of the log relative risk against X_1 for the log-linear hazards model.

risk groups, as shown in Table 2–1. These can be represented in a regression model by three regressor variables:

$$X_1 = 0 \qquad \text{if level 1 of A}$$
$$= 1 \qquad \text{if level 2 of A}$$
$$X_2 = 0 \qquad \text{if level 1 of B}$$
$$= 1 \qquad \text{if level 2 of B}$$
$$X_3 = X_1 X_2 = 1 \qquad \text{if level 2 of A and level 2 of B}$$
$$= 0 \qquad \text{otherwise}$$

Writing each group's variables as a row yields a design matrix, with each of four rows representing all possible combinations of the three variables.

Table 2–1. Regressor variables and hazard ratios for two binary factors under the log-linear and the proportional linear models

Factors		Hazard ratio	Design matrix			Hazard ratio, $R(\mathbf{X},0)$	
A	B		X_1	X_2	X_3	Log-linear	Proportional linear
1	1	1	0	0	0	1	1
	2	10	0	1	0	$\exp\{\beta_2\}$	$1 + \beta_2^*$
2	1	8	1	0	0	$\exp\{\beta_1\}$	$1 + \beta_1^*$
	2	50	1	1	1	$\exp\{\beta_1 + \beta_2 + \beta_{12}\}$	$1 + \beta_1^* + \beta_2^* + \beta_{12}^*$

The hazard ratio associated with this model can be found by comparing the hazard with the reference group, which we will consider as exposure level 1 for both A and B. This is found by

$$R(\mathbf{X}, 0) = \exp\{(\mathbf{X} - 0)\boldsymbol{\beta}\}$$

where

$$\boldsymbol{\beta} = \begin{bmatrix} \beta_1 \\ \beta_2 \\ \beta_{12} \end{bmatrix}$$

The corresponding hazard ratios are shown in Table 2–1. The interpretation of the parameters is as follows:

$\exp\{\beta_1\}$ hazard ratio for A at level 1 of B

$\exp\{\beta_2\}$ hazard ratio for B at level 1 of A

$\exp\{\beta_{12}\} = \dfrac{R[(1\ 1\ 1),(0\ 1\ 0)]}{R[(1\ 0\ 0),(0\ 0\ 0)]}$ ratio of hazard ratio for A in level 2 of B, to hazard ratio for A in level 1 of B

The term β_{12} is often called the *interaction* or *effect modification parameter*, and it represents the change in the risk of A with the level of B. If this parameter is 0, then the effect of A is not changed by the level of B. Under this condition, the implication of the model is that the hazard ratios are multiplicative; that is, the hazard ratio when both A and B are at level 2 is the product of the hazard ratios when only one of them is at level 2. Choosing regressor variables to represent categories can become fairly complex, and this is considered in much more detail in Chapter 7.

Proportional linear hazard. The choice of a proportional hazards model with a log-linear dependence on the regressor variables is necessarily an arbitrary one that may not be valid for particular sets of data. Another model that is sometimes considered is one in which the covariate portion of the model, $h(\cdot)$, is a linear function of the regressor variables (6). This can be written as

$$H^*(\mathbf{X}) = 1 + \mathbf{X}\boldsymbol{\beta}^*$$

where $\boldsymbol{\beta}^*$ is used to distinguish these regression parameters from the log-linear parameters used in equation 2.1. Hence, the hazard function becomes

$$\lambda(t, \mathbf{X}) = \lambda_0(t) \cdot [1 + \mathbf{X}\boldsymbol{\beta}^*] \tag{2.3}$$

The intercept value chosen is 1 instead of an arbitrary constant because $\lambda_0(t)$ is unspecified, thus yielding a redundancy in the model. For example, a hazard given by

$$\lambda(t,\mathbf{X}) = \lambda_0(t) \cdot [\alpha + \mathbf{X}\boldsymbol{\beta}^*]$$
$$= \alpha \cdot \lambda_0(t) \cdot [1 + \mathbf{X}(\boldsymbol{\beta}^*/\alpha)]$$

which has the same form as equation 2.3, except that the parameters have now changed by the factor $1/\alpha$.

The hazard ratio under the additive model, if one has a single binary factor under study, is $R(1,0) = 1 + \beta^*$, so that the parameter β^* represents the deviation of the hazard ratio from 1, or $\beta^* = R(1,0) - 1$. Such a model has been proposed for the relative risk by Rothman (7, 8) although his justification is different from this one.

If there is a single factor, X, under consideration which can take any in a range of values, then the hazard is a linear function of X for a given t, as shown in Figure 2–8. Unlike the log-linear model, there is now no restriction forcing the hazard to be positive. This leaves open the possibility of clearly inadmissible values of the hazard function, as shown in the figure. For example, if $\beta^* > 0$, the hazard is negative when $X < -1/\beta^*$. Likewise, if $\beta^* < 0$, the hazard is negative for $X > -1/\beta^*$. By saying the hazard is inadmissible, we mean that a value which is undoubtedly closer to the truth is found by using the trivial estimate, 0, because the hazard cannot

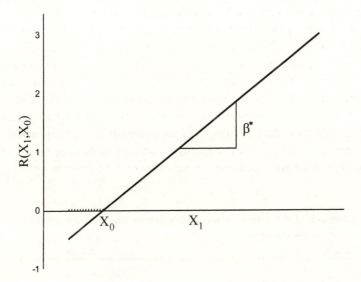

Figure 2–8 Plot of the relative risk against X_1 for the proportionally additive hazards model.

be negative by definition. It is feasible to fit models that have the shape of a hockey stick; such models are specified by forcing the hazard to be a number near zero instead of a negative value over a particular range, but this procedure can complicate the estimation process considerably. In this sense, there are clear advantages for the log-linear model because it is admissible over the entire range of X.

When considering the joint behavior of the two binary factors, A and B, as shown in Table 2–1, one can find the corresponding hazard ratios for the four categories. In general, the parameters for the additive model are not the same as those for the multiplicative model. This is especially clear from consideration of the interaction terms, β_{12}^* and β_{12}. If the hazard ratios for each group are 1, 10, 8, and 50, respectively, then the model parameters are as shown in Table 2–2. Clearly, parameters like those for the interaction may even change sign, depending on the model. This can cause interpretational problems because some investigators may choose to interpret interactions as an indication of synergy or antagonism, depending on whether the coefficient is positive or negative, respectively. In this example, the multiplicative model results in $\beta_{12} < 0$, which would indicate antagonism, while for the additive model, $\beta_{12}^* > 0$, which would imply synergy.

While we can usually agree that factors are antagonistic if the log hazard ratio for B is positive for $A = 1$ but negative for $A = 2$, we often cannot base our conclusion on the regression parameters alone. This is because their sign may depend on the arbitrary choice of the model. Nevertheless, in this instance one can clearly describe the hazard ratio using either model, and the ultimate public health decisions on the impact of a factor should be based on a model that provides a good description of the data. When one model suggests that the interaction is zero, there is some advantage to using that scale in the interest of reducing the number of parameters to be estimated, thus giving a more parsimonious summary of the data. Situations in which the conclusions are very different for alternative models, which describe the data equally well, are generally those in which the data are somewhat weak, so that we might consider collecting more relevant data before reaching a definitive conclusion on which scale is best.

Table 2–2. Parameters for the multiplicative and additive models for specified hazard ratios

Multiplicative	Additive
$\beta_1 = \log 8 = 2.08$	$\beta_1^* = 8 - 1 = 7$
$\beta_2 = \log 10 = 2.30$	$\beta_2^* = 10 - 1 = 9$
$\beta_{12} = \log(50/8 \cdot 10) = -0.47$	$\beta_{12}^* = 50 - [1 + 7 + 9] = 33$

Models for risks

An alternative to models for the hazard function are models for risk, or the probability of disease after a specified period of time. Such a binary response can be represented by the response variable:

$$Y = 1 \qquad \text{if ill}$$
$$= 0 \qquad \text{if not ill}$$

The probabilities associated with each level of the response are

$$\Pr\{\text{ill} \mid \mathbf{X}\} = \Pr\{Y = 1 \mid \mathbf{X}\} = P(\mathbf{X})$$

and

$$\Pr\{\text{not ill} \mid \mathbf{X}\} = \Pr\{Y = 0 \mid \mathbf{X}\} = 1 - P(\mathbf{X})$$

In this section several models for binary responses are described.

Linear logistic model. A commonly used model for binary response data is the linear logistic model (9, 10):

$$\Pr(\mathbf{X}) = \frac{\exp\{\alpha + \mathbf{X}\boldsymbol{\beta}\}}{1 + \exp(\alpha + \mathbf{X}\boldsymbol{\beta}\}} \tag{2.4}$$

The parameters from the linear logistic model are most easily interpreted in terms of the odds for disease, i.e., the ratio of the probability of disease to the probability that the disease is not present. In particular, the log odds is given by

$$\log \omega(\mathbf{X}) = \log\left\{\frac{\Pr(\mathbf{X})}{1 - \Pr(\mathbf{X})}\right\}$$
$$= \alpha + \mathbf{X}\boldsymbol{\beta}$$

which is why this model is sometimes referred to as a log-linear odds model.

If one has a single binary factor under study,

$$X = 0 \qquad \text{if at level 1 (absent)}$$
$$= 1 \qquad \text{if at level 2 (present)}$$

then the odds for disease is given by $\exp\{\alpha\}$ and $\exp\{\alpha + \beta\}$ for levels 1 and 2, respectively. One risk measure is the relative odds for disease, or *odds ratio*, given by

$$\Omega(1,0) = \omega(1)/\omega(0)$$
$$= \exp\{\beta\}$$

Hence, the regression parameter from the linear logistic model, β, can be interpreted in terms of the log odds ratio for disease.

If the variable under consideration is continuous, then the shape of the $\Pr(X)$ curve for the linear logistic model is sigmoid, as shown in Figure 2–9. To estimate the odds ratio, we choose a single level of the regressor variable as the reference value, X_0, and the odds ratio becomes

$$\Omega(X_1, X_0) = \exp\{(X_1 - X_0)\beta\}$$

so that the interpretation of β is in terms of the change in the log odds ratio per unit change in X, or the slope of the line, for log $\Omega(X, X_0)$ plotted against X. In cases where there are two binary regressor variables under study, the four possible combinations of the two regressor variables can be represented by the three regressor variables defined in Table 2–1. The handling of these parameters is much the same as in the section "Models for Rates," only the measure under consideration is the odds ratio instead of the hazard ratio.

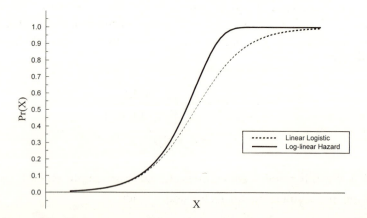

Figure 2–9 Plot of the sigmoid curves for the probability of disease under the linear logistic and the log-linear hazard models.

Complementary log-log model. It has already been noted that the probability of disease can be directly derived from the hazard function. Details of how this arises are discussed further in Appendix 1, in the section "Relationship between Models for Rates and Proportions," but the ultimate result is what is called the complementary log-log model (11) which has the form $\Pr(\mathbf{X}) = 1 - \exp\{-\exp[\alpha(\tau) + \mathbf{X}\boldsymbol{\beta}]\}$, where $\alpha(\tau)$ is the log cumulative hazard over the duration of follow-up for the risk group with $\mathbf{X} = \mathbf{0}$. A plot of the resulting sigmoid curve that describes the relationship between a single covariate, X, and the probability of disease is shown in Figure 2–9.

In Chapter 6 there is a discussion of methods for fitting this particular model to data, but two things should be pointed out at this stage. First, it is clear that by representing the outcome only after a fixed period of time, one necessarily loses information about details of the hazard function, $\lambda_0(t)$, in that one can only estimate the cumulative hazard, $\alpha(\tau)$. This limitation not only results in the loss of a potentially interesting detail but also reduces the power of a study. One way to see this is to consider what would happen if the duration of a study is so long that nearly all subjects have developed the disease by the end, leaving essentially no information for differentiating the magnitude of risk in the subgroups. However, a knowledge of the actual times to diagnosis could still be used to estimate the hazard ratio, even when all subjects have been observed to failure.

An advantage of this model over the linear logistic is that the regression parameters may be interpreted in terms of the hazard ratio because the formulation arises from the log-linear hazards model. This can be particularly useful when one wishes to compare parameters from an analysis in which the failure times are available with those in which we only know disease status after a fixed period of time. Hence, one is able to focus on substantive reasons for potential differences and need not be concerned that the choice of model is affecting the parameter estimates.

How does the linear logistic model compare with the log-linear hazard model, or the complementary log-log model? As can be seen in Figure 2–9, both models have a basic sigmoid shape and when the probability of disease is small they are virtually identical. However, for larger probabilities they are somewhat different, in that the linear logistic model is symmetric about the disease probability, $1/2$, while the log-linear hazard model exhibits a more rapid approach to the asymptote, 1.

Other models. The linear logistic model implies that the log odds is a linear function of the covariates. An alternative model analogous to the linear proportional hazards model is the linear odds model, where $\omega(X) =$

$P(\mathbf{X})/[1 - P(\mathbf{X})] = \alpha + \mathbf{X}\beta$. An example of the use of this model is the linear risk model for the effect of low doses of ionizing ratiation on cancer risk (12). While this model can be used in principle, it suffers some of the same disadvantages observed in the linear proportional hazards model, in that it can yield inadmissible values for the probabilities—probabilities that are less than zero. Hence, when fitting this particular model, we must be careful to be sure that the fitted probabilities are in the usual range for all values of $\mathbf{X}$. Other models can also be considered, but further discussion on these is held for Chapter 6, where a general approach for fitting models to the probability of disease is considered.

Summary

This chapter discusses the concept of a model for the disease process, emphasizing simple and very general models that can be used to study a variety of diseases. Quantities that are used to describe this fundamental model are the *hazard function*, $\lambda(t)$; the *survival function*, $\mathcal{F}(t)$; and, the *failure time density function*, $f(t)$. Each of these quantities can be derived from one of the others, so that they are really different expressions of the same underlying concept. Two forms are often used for the hazard: a constant hazard and a Weibull hazard. In many applications, however, it is not feasible to adequately describe the hazard by a simple mathematical function, which is one reason for the availability of non-parametric or semi-parametric methods.

Risk factors may modify a disease model in a variety of ways. The level of exposure to a putative risk factor for a person is described by one or more covariates that can be included in a regression model. These variables exhibit their effect on the disease process by modifying the rate, the risk, and the disease density function for the times to failure. An assortment of models is available, and these may be defined in terms of modifying one of these fundamental quantities. In many instances there may be no strong reason to choose among these various models, but sometimes one model may require fewer parameters, thus providing a more parsimonious summary of the data. However, when the probability of disease in a specified period of time is small, some models, including the linear logistic model and the log-linear hazards model, produce very similar results.

References

1. Armitage P, Doll R. Stochastic models for carcinogenesis. 4th Berkeley Symposium on Mathematics, Statistics and Probability 1961:19–38.

2. Hyman LH. *The Invertebrates*. New York: McGraw-Hill, 1951.
3. Nasell I. *Hybrid Models of Tropical Infections*. Berlin: Springer-Verlag, 1985.
4. Macdonald G. The dynamics of helminth infections, with special reference to schistosomiasis. *Transactions of the Royal Society of Tropical Medicine and Hygiene* 1965;59:489–506.
5. Cox DR. Regression models and life-tables (with discussion). *Journal of the Royal Statistical Society, Series B* 1972;B34:187–220.
6. Thomas DC. General relative risk models for survival time and matched case-control analysis. *Biometrics* 1981;37:673–686.
7. Rothman KJ. Synergy and antagonism in cause–effect relationships. *American Journal of Epidemiology* 1974;99:385–388.
8. Rothman KJ. Causes. *American Journal of Epidemiology* 1976;104:587–592.
9. Cox DR. *Analysis of Binary Data*. London: Methuen, 1970.
10. Hosmer DW, Lemeshow S. *Applied Logistic Regression*. New York: Wiley, 1989.
11. McCullagh P, Nelder JA. *Generalized Linear Models*. London: Chapman and Hall.
12. Edwards M. Models for estimating risk of radiation carcinogenesis. In: WR Hendee and FM Edwards (eds.) *Health Effects of Exposure to Low-level Ionizing Radiation*. Bristol: Institute of Physics Publishing, 1999.

II

NON-REGRESSION METHODS

3

Analysis of Proportions

Time is a critical factor for the development of disease; in some instances, however, time can effectively be ignored, allowing one to consider only the proportion of individuals who become ill. In this chapter, methods of analysis for proportions are described, and these methods can be relatively easy to compute; in fact, for small tables they can readily be carried out on a hand calculator. In later chapters, methods that incorporate time into the analysis are discussed; these methods can have considerably more power when detailed information on the time of disease onset is available and when a high proportion of the study population develops the disease.

The method of data analysis must always take into account the study design; a failure to do so can bias either the parameter estimates or the estimates of the precision of a parameter. In this chapter, we introduce simple methods that can be applied to the analysis of proportions; some typical study designs that give rise to data that can be analyzed in this form are discussed in the first section. We then proceed to discuss various methods for estimating the association between exposure to factors and risk of disease, where the exposure is measured either as simply "yes" or "no," or in greater detail that actually reflects the level of exposure. Finally, we begin to consider the problem of jointly analyzing putative risk factors by discussing methods for estimating the effect of one factor while controlling for another.

Studies That Yield Proportion Responses

We now consider three approaches for recruiting subjects into an epidemiological study: cross-sectional, cohort, and case-control. As we shall see, each design can give rise to a different set of proportions that can be estimated. We shall also understand some of the advantages of certain measures of association in that they can be estimated regardless of the type of study that has been employed.

Cross-sectional studies

The first design that we consider is one in which we obtain a random sample of n_{++} subjects from a population, and we record their exposure and disease status at that time. Table 3–1 shows how the results of such a study might be displayed in terms of a 2×2 table. Row and column sums are denoted by substituting a "+" for the index used in the summation, so that $n_{i+} = n_{i1} + n_{i2} = \sum_j n_{ij}$, for example. If our method of random selection has indeed been successful, then the distribution across the cells should reflect the distribution in the population as a whole, except for random variation. Hence, the observed proportion in each cell, p_{ij}, will provide a valid estimate of the proportion from the general population, π_{ij}. The observed numbers of subjects in cells of the table (n_{11} n_{12} n_{21} n_{22}), have a multinomial distribution for the n_{++} subjects with probability π_{ij} for each of the respective cells.

While cross-sectional studies have a certain intuitive appeal because they can be directly related to a population at a particular point in time, they often suffer from severe limitations that hamper the conclusions that can be drawn from the data. We can especially see this problem when we consider the type of information that is typically available on disease status from such a study. Subjects who are diseased at the time of recruitment would include those who were newly diagnosed, along with others who have remained ill for a prolonged period of time. Individuals who have died of their illness will not, of course, be available for recruitment. Hence, entry into our classification as "diseased" will be influenced not only by factors that increase risk of disease occurrence but also by those that prolong the disease or change the risk of death from the disease. As these effects are hopelessly entangled or confounded, we generally prefer a study that permits us to determine the stage of the disease process that is affected by the factors, because this will enable us to develop better strategies for controlling the disease.

Table 3–1. A typical 2×2 table from a study of a single risk factor

	Disease status (j)		
Factor (i)	Healthy	Diseased	Total
Level 1	n_{11}	n_{12}	n_{1+}
Level 2	n_{21}	n_{22}	n_{2+}
Total	n_{+1}	n_{+2}	n_{++}

Cohort studies

In a cohort study, risk groups of healthy individuals are identified and then followed to determine whether the disease occurs. Thus, we have a more natural framework for conducting a study of factors associated with the occurrence of disease in that we are actually following the natural chronology of events. One pattern of disease incidence that can be analyzed by these methods has a hazard, or incidence intensity, which is positive for a relatively short period of time. An example of such a situation would be the effect of a potential teratogen on congenital malformations. For many malformations, one can assume that the clinical symptoms would be manifested shortly after the birth of the child, and the response, or disease status, is identified by whether a congenital malformation occurs. The shape of the hazard might have the form shown in Figure 3–1, which is positive only during the pregnancy, but the available data only indicate whether the malformation is present at birth. Thus, we do not have the exact time at which the teratogen had its effect on the fetus. In this case, it would not be possible to learn about the shape of the hazard, but one could still obtain very important information about the overall probability of a congenital malformation.

A second study design where these methods can be applied is in the situation where all subjects are followed for the same length of time. One such example would be the recruitment of students who matriculate on a given day and are then followed forward in time until the end of the school

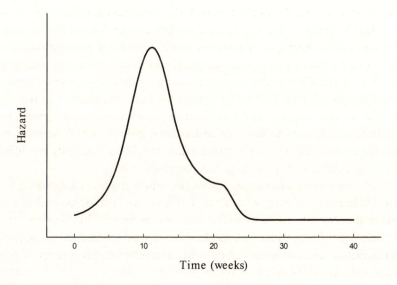

Figure 3–1 Hypothetical hazard for a teratogen that effects the fetus early in pregnancy.

year. If the response of interest is a well-defined event, such as the first occurrence of a disease, and complete follow-up information is available on all subjects, then the methods discussed in this chapter can be appropriately applied. It is not always possible or desirable to conduct a study in this way, however. Often, follow-up varies from person to person because some individuals are lost to follow-up or are recruited at different points in time. In addition, for some outcomes, like death, following subjects for a sufficiently long period of time will guarantee that the probability of failure is identical, namely 1, for all subjects, and no differences would be observed among different risk groups. A much more informative study would make use of detailed information on time until death, and the methods discussed in Chapter 4 may be used.

For the typical data display shown in Table 3–1, we regard the row totals fixed by design, so that the cell frequency has a binomial distribution for the n_{i+} individuals with probability $\pi_{j \mid i}$ for disease category j in row i. In general, we would not select n_{i+} individuals for each level of exposure in relation to the distribution in the general population but, rather, choose values that will tend to optimize the efficiency of the study design.

Case-control studies

Finally, we consider a study in which subjects with newly diagnosed disease are recruited, along with a corresponding group of controls who are free of the disease. In this instance, we compare the distribution of exposure histories among diseased cases with the corresponding distribution for the controls, which is the classic case-control design. To use the congenital malformation example, this would mean comparing the exposure distribution for a putative risk factor among the mothers of children with congenital malformations to the exposure among mothers with normal babies. In this design, we have effectively rotated the fixed elements from the row totals in the cohort study to the column totals. We are now comparing the distribution of factors in the case and control groups, but if the odds ratio is the fundamental quantity being estimated, there is usually no difference in the methods for carrying out the calculations.

This chapter considers computationally simple methods for making statistical inferences on categorical data. The methods include procedures for obtaining point estimates, as well as interval estimates. In addition, various techniques for conducting hypothesis tests are discussed. Many of these techniques can be readily carried out with an electronic spreadsheet or even a hand calculator. We describe the parameters of interest in the context of the linear logistic model, so that one can readily see their place in the more

Table 3–2. A typical 2×2 table of estimable probabilities from a cohort study of a single risk factor

	Disease status (j)		
Factor (i)	Healthy	Diseased	Total
Level 1	$\pi_{1|1}$	$\pi_{2|1}$	1
Level 2	$\pi_{1|2}$	$\pi_{2|2}$	1

general framework of models used in epidemiology. By understanding the assumptions that underlie these techniques, we can better appreciate when the methods agree with the results of more complex modeling and when they do not.

A Single Binary Risk Factor

As we have seen, the results of a study of a single factor which has only two levels can be displayed in a 2×2 table, as shown in Table 3–1. The observed frequencies in the ith row and jth column of the table are given by n_{ij}. For a cohort study, we follow individuals in different exposure groups and observe whether the disease outcome occurs, as represented by $Y = 0$ or 1, depending on whether the person is healthy or diseased. Table 3–2 shows the probabilities of the various outcomes from such a study of a single factor with just two levels of exposure, where the probability of disease, $Y = 1$, for level i of the risk factor is denoted by $\Pr\{Y = 1 \mid \text{risk group } i\} = \pi_{2|i}$ and estimated by $p_{2|i} = n_{i2}/n_{i+}$. In Chapter 2, several models for proportions were described, but in this chapter we will limit our discussion to the linear logistic model with parameters shown in Table 3–3. This suggests the odds ratio as the basic quantity of interest in determining whether a factor is associated with disease. In a cohort study, the odds for disease in

Table 3–3. Linear logistic probabilities for a factor with two levels

		Probability	
		$1 - \pi_{2|i}$	$\pi_{2|i}$
		Healthy	Diseased
Factor (i)	X_i	$(Y = 0)$	$(Y = 1)$
Level 1	0	$\dfrac{1}{1 + \exp(\alpha)}$	$\dfrac{\exp(\alpha)}{1 + \exp(\alpha)}$
Level 2	1	$\dfrac{1}{1 + \exp(\alpha + \beta)}$	$\dfrac{\exp(\alpha + \beta)}{1 + \exp(\alpha + \beta)}$

a person with level 2 of a factor, compared with a person at level 1, is represented by

$$\Omega = \frac{\pi_{2|2}/\pi_{1|2}}{\pi_{2|1}/\pi_{1|1}} = \frac{\pi_{1|1} \cdot \pi_{2|2}}{\pi_{1|2} \cdot \pi_{2|1}} = \exp\{\beta\} \qquad (3.1)$$

where β, the log odds ratio, is the regression parameter in the linear logistic model.

In a cross-sectional study, subjects are selected from a population and broken down by exposure and disease. The probability of falling into one of the four cells is shown in Table 3–4. From such data, it is also possible to estimate the proportion diseased in the two exposure groups, and the definition of conditional probability can be used to rearrange equation 3.1, so that

$$\Omega = \frac{(\pi_{11}/\pi_{1+}) \cdot (\pi_{22}/\pi_{2+})}{(\pi_{12}/\pi_{1+}) \cdot (\pi_{21}/\pi_{2+})} = \frac{\pi_{11} \cdot \pi_{22}}{\pi_{12} \cdot \pi_{21}} \qquad (3.2)$$

and π_{i+} is the proportion in exposure group i.

Finally, for a case-control study, a group of cases and a group of controls are compared for their exposure to a putative risk factor, and the estimable probabilities from such a study are shown in Table 3–5. In this instance, the random response may be regarded as the exposure information that was obtained by interviewing the cases and controls, so that disease status or the column total, n_{+j}, is fixed by the study design and the corresponding probabilities sum to 1. This allows us to determine the probability that an individual belongs to risk group i given disease status j, $\Pr\{\text{risk group } i \mid \text{disease group } j\} = \rho_{i|j}$, estimated by $r_{i|j} = n_{ij}/n_{+j}$. We can once again employ the definition of conditional probability to the cohort odds ratio as expressed in equation 3.2, then

$$\Omega = \frac{(\pi_{+2} \cdot \rho_{2|2}/\pi_{2+}) \cdot (\pi_{+1} \cdot \rho_{1|1}/\pi_{1+})}{(\pi_{+1} \cdot \rho_{2|1}/\pi_{2+}) \cdot (\pi_{+2} \cdot \rho_{1|2}/\pi_{1+})} = \frac{\rho_{1|1} \cdot \rho_{2|2}}{\rho_{2|1} \cdot \rho_{1|2}}$$

Table 3–4. A typical 2 × 2 table from a cross-sectional study of a single risk factor

Factor (i)	Disease status (j)		Total
	Healthy	Diseased	
Level 1	π_{11}	π_{12}	π_{1+}
Level 2	π_{21}	π_{22}	π_{2+}
Total	π_{+1}	π_{+2}	1

Table 3–5. A typical 2×2 table of estimable probabilities from a case-control study of a single risk factor

	Disease status (j)	
Factor (i)	Healthy	Diseased
Level 1	$p_{1\vert 1}$	$p_{1\vert 2}$
Level 2	$p_{2\vert 1}$	$p_{2\vert 2}$
Total	1	1

so that both the odds ratio for disease in a cohort study and the odds ratio for exposure in a case-control study yield the same measure of association.

The maximum likelihood estimate of $\pi_{2\vert i}$ is the observed proportion, $\hat{p}_i = n_{i2}/n_{i+}$, so we can obtain the maximum likelihood estimate of the odds ratio, by substitution:

$$\hat{\Omega} = \frac{\hat{p}_{1\vert 1} \cdot \hat{p}_{2\vert 2}}{\hat{p}_{1\vert 2} \cdot \hat{p}_{2\vert 1}} = \frac{n_{11} \cdot n_{22}}{n_{12} \cdot n_{21}} \tag{3.3}$$

where the hat indicates that this is a maximum likelihood estimator. The same expression is also used for estimating the odds ratio in a cross-sectional and a case-control study. The log odds ratio has a distribution that is more nearly normal, and because it is also the linear logistic model parameter, we can find its maximum likelihood estimate:

$$\hat{\beta} = \log \hat{\Omega}$$
$$= \log \left[\frac{n_{11} \cdot n_{22}}{n_{12} \cdot n_{21}} \right] \tag{3.4}$$

To determine the precision of the log odds ratio we compute the standard error:

$$SE(\hat{\beta}) = \sqrt{(n_{11}^{-1} + n_{12}^{-1} + n_{21}^{-1} + n_{22}^{-1})} \tag{3.5}$$

Sometimes the frequency in one of the cells is very small; in fact, it may be zero. A zero in any one of the cells would result in an undefined maximum likelihood estimator of β and its standard error. An estimator that is always defined and has been found to provide better sampling properties is obtained by adding 1/2 to all of the cell frequencies (1–3). Of course, it is most tempting to add the value only when there is a zero in a cell, but one should realize that this is just the situation where the estimator is most sensitive to the addition of an arbitrary constant. Hence, when there is a zero cell in a 2 × 2 table, a useful point estimate of the odds ratio is unavailable.

Example 3–1   To illustrate the calculations introduced thus far, consider the following data from a case-control study of congenital malformations described by Kelsey et al. (4) and displayed in Table 3–6. At this point, we are interested in the crude measure of exposure to cigarettes, not the more detailed information on the actual amount of smoking, which we will take up later. For this study, 4,337 interviews were completed, 1,369 of which were women with congenitally malformed babies, while the remaining women had normal babies.

We estimate the odds ratio by

$$\hat{\Omega} = \frac{1988 \cdot 480}{889 \cdot 980}$$

$$= 1.095292$$

and the log odds ratio is

$$\hat{\beta} = \log 1.095292$$

$$= 0.091021$$

The standard error for the estimate of the log odds ratio is

$$SE(\hat{\beta}) = \sqrt{(1/1988) + (1/889) + (1/980) + (1/480)}$$

$$= 0.068787$$

If one adds ½ to each of the frequencies, the estimates are

$$\tilde{\Omega} = \frac{1988.5 \cdot 480.5}{889.5 \cdot 980.5} = 1.095533$$

$$\tilde{\beta} = 0.091241$$

Table 3–6. Observed and expected (in parentheses) frequencies of cigarette smoking by the mother for normal babies and babies with congenital malformations (4)

Cigarette smoking (i)	Disease status (j)		Total
	Normal	Malformation	
No	1,988	889	2,877
	(1,968.8577)	(908.1423)	
Yes	980	480	1,460
	(999.1423)	(460.8577)	
Total	2,968	1,369	4,337

and

$$SE(\tilde{\beta}) = 0.068762$$

In this case the frequencies were all relatively large, so that the added constant made little difference to the numerical values of the estimates. Had one or more of the frequencies been much smaller, we might have seen a much greater effect from the added constant.

In these data, the estimate of the effect of smoking on the risk of congenital malformations is quite small; it increases the odds for a malformation by about only 10%. The magnitude of this estimate on the log scale is not much larger than the precision determined by the standard error.

Likelihood-Based Inference

To see the relationships among the various techniques for data analysis, here we describe the methods in terms of likelihood-based inference. This very powerful approach to statistical inference was invented by R. A. Fisher (5), and it can be used to justify many of the statistical methods used in epidemiology, even though it was not always used in the original derivations for some of these techniques. Nevertheless, seeing how one can arrive at these formulae from a specific epidemiologic model gives a better understanding of how the simple methods relate to the more complex multivariable modeling described in later chapters. Here we give a verbal description of the ideas behind the formulae, but in Appendix 2 these ideas are discussed with more rigorous detail.

Fundamental ideas in statistical inference include the concepts of estimation and significance testing. The likelihood gives the probability of observing the data collected in a particular study as a function of the regression parameters. Of course, these parameters are not known but are to be estimated, so that a logical choice is to obtain the most likely estimates, or the maximum likelihood estimates, which we have already seen in the previous section.

Hypothesis testing using likelihoods involves three procedures. The Wald test is perhaps the most easily understood by those with some knowledge of basic statistics, because in its simplest form it is the ratio of the parameter to its standard error, which is analogous to the z test. To apply this test, one must first fit the model to data in order to obtain the estimates of the regression parameters and their standard errors. This is usually not easy to do by hand for the models in this book, and we would ordinarily use a statistical package unless the problem is very simple. Hence, the Wald test is not used as often in this chapter as it will be in later chapters. Easier calculations are sometimes provided by the efficient score test, which was described by Rao (6). To conduct this test, we only need to fit the model implied under the null hypothesis, and this leads to some of the most widely used significance tests for contingency tables, including the Pearson chi-square. Finally, the ratio of the likelihoods for two models can be used to construct a test based on the increase in the likelihood resulting from the inclusion of additional variables in the model. Because this test generally requires the complex calculations needed for fitting two models, it suffers from the same computational difficulties as the Wald statistic. This chapter investigates several simple methods of analysis for categorical data, which often involve the use of a score statistic. In later chapters, in which some of the more general multivariate models are used, it is more common to make use of the likelihood ratio test and the Wald test.

The three tests described thus far only yield approximate p values for the hypotheses in question, and they are only useful when the sample sizes are large (more on how we define "large" later). An exact test gives a probability that does not depend on large sample theory, so it may always be used. The disadvantage of exact methods is that they very quickly become computationally difficult as the sample size increases but, thankfully, this is just the situation in which the large sample tests can be appropriately applied.

Wald test

The Wald test makes use of the estimate of the log odds ratio and its standard error. To test the null hypothesis, H_0: $\Omega = 1$, or, equivalently, H_0: $\beta = \log \Omega = 0$, we calculate

$$W = \hat{\beta}/\text{SE}(\hat{\beta}) \qquad (3.6)$$

which may be compared to a standard normal deviate. The Wald statistic is W^2, which is compared to a chi-square distribution with 1 df.

Example 3–1 (continued)   In the previous section, the maximum likelihood estimate for the log odds ratio for the association between smoking and congenital malformations was found to be $\hat{\beta} = 0.091021$ and $\text{SE}(\hat{\beta}) = 0.068787$. Hence, the Wald statistic is $W^2 = (0.091021/0.06878)^2 = 1.7509$, and when we compare it to χ_1^2 we obtain $p = .186$, which does not suggest a significant association between cigarette smoking and congenital malformations.

Score test: Pearson chi-square

The score test requires that only the parameters not restricted under the null hypothesis be estimated. In the present case, H_0: $\beta = 0$, thus, only the intercept, α, needs to be estimated. It is clear from Table 3–3 that if the null hypothesis is true, the probability of disease for both risk groups is equal, and the maximum likelihood estimate of the probability of disease is

$$\frac{\exp\{\tilde{\alpha}\}}{1 + \exp\{\tilde{\alpha}\}} = \frac{n_{+2}}{n_{++}} \tag{3.7}$$

Hence, the expected number diseased at level i of the factor under the null hypothesis is estimated by

$$\tilde{m}_{i2} = \frac{n_{i+} \cdot n_{+2}}{n_{++}} \tag{3.8}$$

and likewise

$$\tilde{m}_{i1} = n_{i+} - \frac{n_{i+} \cdot n_{+2}}{n_{++}} = \frac{n_{i+} \cdot n_{+1}}{n_{++}} \tag{3.9}$$

which are determined for all i. The statistic reduces to the Pearson chi-square

$$S^2 = \sum_{ij} \frac{(n_{ij} - \tilde{m}_{ij})^2}{\tilde{m}_{ij}} \tag{3.10}$$

which simplifies in a 2×2 table to

$$S^2 = \frac{(n_{11} \cdot n_{22} - n_{12} \cdot n_{21})^2 \cdot n_{++}}{n_{1+} \cdot n_{2+} \cdot n_{+1} \cdot n_{+2}} \tag{3.11}$$

The parameter α was not of particular interest as it is not involved in H_0, but it must be considered in the derivation of the test because it relates to the overall probability of disease. In equation 3.7, it was estimated by maximum likelihood before being incorporated into the derivation. Alternatively, we can allow for α by finding a conditional likelihood, which only depends on the parameter of interest, β. Details on the formulation of this conditional test are described in Appendix 2, and it results in a test proposed by Mantel and Haenszel (7):

$$S_c^2 = \frac{(n_{11} \cdot n_{22} - n_{12} \cdot n_{21})^2 \, (n_{++} - 1)}{n_{1+} \cdot n_{2+} \cdot n_{+1} \cdot n_{+2}} \tag{3.12}$$

The relationship between the conditional and the unconditional test is

$$S_c^2 = \left[\frac{n_{++} - 1}{n_{++}} \right] S^2$$

which shows that they are nearly equal if the total sample size, n_{++}, is large. We will see later that conditional tests can be valid in situations where unconditional tests are not, but for the simple 2×2 table there is generally little difference.

Frequencies take only integer values, but the chi-square distribution, which is used in these large sample approximations, is continuous. In an attempt to improve the accuracy of this approximation, Yates (8) suggested a continuity correction for equation 3.11:

$$S_Y^2 = \frac{(|n_{11} \cdot n_{22} - n_{12} \cdot n_{21}| - n_{++}/2)^2 \cdot n_{++}}{n_{1+} \cdot n_{2+} \cdot n_{+1} \cdot n_{+2}} \tag{3.13}$$

Whether this correction of a test that arises from the standard application of likelihood-based inference actually achieves the desired effect of improving the approximation for the p values is debatable (9–11). In any event, S_Y^2 is less than S^2, so that it always yields a larger p value. The difference between these two statistics is generally not so large as to have a very profound effect on the conclusions from an analysis. Situations in which Yates's correction does have a substantial effect on the conclusions are usually tables with small cells, so that any approximate test would not be expected to perform well. These are just the instances where we should use an exact test instead.

Example 3–1 (continued) Finding the score test for the association between cigarette smoking and congenital malformations using the data in Table 3–6 we obtain

$$S^2 = \frac{[1988 \cdot 480 - 889 \cdot 980]^2 \cdot 4337}{2968 \cdot 1369 \cdot 2877 \cdot 1460}$$

$$= 1.7514$$

which is compared to χ_1^2 ($p = .186$), and is almost identical to the results obtained using the Wald test. If one uses the conditional test instead, the result is

$$S_c^2 = \frac{[1988 \cdot 480 - 889 \cdot 980]^2 \cdot 4336}{2968 \cdot 1369 \cdot 2877 \cdot 1460}$$

$$= 1.7510$$

($p = .186$), which is once again almost identical. Finally, if we employ Yates's correction,

$$S_Y^2 = \frac{[1988 \cdot 480 - 889 \cdot 980 - 4337/2)]^2 \cdot 4337}{2968 \cdot 1369 \cdot 2877 \cdot 1460}$$

$$= 1.6611$$

($p = .197$). The results from all three of these tests are essentially the same because of the large number of subjects in the study.

Likelihood ratio test

The likelihood ratio statistic is often used as an alternative to the Pearson chi-square, especially to test the goodness of fit of a particular model. To test the null hypothesis, $H_0: \beta = 0$, this approach evaluates the goodness of fit for the null model by using the statistic

$$G^2 = 2 \sum_{ij} n_{ij} \log(n_{ij}/\tilde{m}_{ij}) \tag{3.14}$$

where $\tilde{m}_{ij}$ is defined in equations 3.8 and 3.9. This statistic would once again be compared to a chi-square distribution with 1 df.

Example 3–1 (continued)   For the data on cigarette smoking and congenital malformations shown in Table 3–6, the expected frequencies are given in parentheses below the observed frequencies. Using equation 3.14 we obtain

$$G^2 = 2 \cdot [1988 \cdot \log(1988/1968.8577) + 889 \cdot \log(889/908.1423)$$

$$+ 980 \cdot \log(980/999.1423) + 480 \cdot \log(480/460.8577)]$$

$$= 1.7453$$

($p = .186$). For this particular example, the Wald, score, and likelihood ratio statistics are nearly identical. This is to be expected because we are, after all, dealing with a large sample size. For smaller samples, particularly when the smallest expected frequency is less than 5 for the score test or the smallest observed frequency is less than 5 for the Wald test, the agreement may not be as good, and it is for these cases that we require the exact test.

Exact test

In situations where cell frequencies are too small for the appropriate use of a large sample test, an exact test can be employed instead. An exact p value for testing $H_0: \beta = 0$ can be computed by Fisher's exact test (12).

The probability of a particular realization of a 2×2 table under the null hypothesis, removing the effect of the intercept parameter α through conditioning, has a hypergeometric distribution (13). Once the margins of a table have in effect been fixed by a conditional argument, the frequency in the (1,1)-cell is sufficient for determining the remaining cells in the table. Hence, the resulting hypergeometric probability is given by

$$p(n_{11}) = \frac{n_{1+}! \cdot n_{2+}! \cdot n_{+1}! \cdot n_{+2}!}{n_{11}! \cdot n_{12}! \cdot n_{21}! \cdot n_{22}! \cdot n_{++}!} \tag{3.15}$$

For the particular table

2	5
12	3

the probability that this occurred by chance is

$$p(2) = \frac{7! \cdot 15! \cdot 14! \cdot 8!}{2! \cdot 5! \cdot 12! \cdot 3! \cdot 22!} = .029881$$

To find the appropriate tail probability of observing this table or one that is more extreme, it is necessary to also consider the more extreme tables that hold the marginal tables fixed:

1	6
13	2

and

0	7
14	1

giving probabilities

$$p(1) = \frac{7! \cdot 15! \cdot 14! \cdot 8!}{1! \cdot 6! \cdot 13! \cdot 2! \cdot 22!} = .002299$$

and

$$p(0) = \frac{7! \cdot 15! \cdot 14! \cdot 8!}{0! \cdot 7! \cdot 14! \cdot 1! \cdot 22!} = .000047$$

Hence, the probability of observing the original or a more extreme table is given by the sum

$$p = p(2) + p(1) + p(0) = .0322$$

When considering the significance of this p value, it is important to remember that the more extreme tables were considered in one direction only. In general, we are interested in either positive or negative associations—that is, two-tailed tests—so we must compare the p value from this test to $\frac{1}{2}$ the nominal significance level. For example, if we are using a 5% significance level, we would declare statistical significance if the exact p value was 2.5% or less. The preceding example just fails to reject the null hypothesis by this criterion, so that the conclusion would be that there is no strong evidence of an association.

As we have already noted, exact tests require considerably more computation than any of the other procedures given in this section. These calculations can be especially lengthy when frequencies in the table are large, but as we also noted, these are the tables for which the large sample tests work well. A rule of thumb would be to always use the exact test instead of the Pearson chi-square test when the expected frequencies given by equation 3.8 or 3.9 is less than 5 (14). We might apply a similar rule of thumb to the observed frequencies when using a Wald test. A computer program is useful in doing the calculations for even moderately sized tables, and these are now implemented in a number of standard statistical packages.

Example 3–2   Harlow and Weiss (15) report the results of a case-control study of borderline ovarian tumors and their possible association with perineal exposure to talc. Table 3–7 gives the data from this study looking at the risk for women who use deodorizing powder only, compared to women who have no perineal exposure to powder. Notice that the smallest expected value is 6.16, which is greater than 5, thus satisfying the usual rule of thumb for using the large sample Pearson chi-square test. Values for the large sample test statistics are $S^2 = 4.646$ ($p = .0311$) for the Pearson chi-square; $S_Y^2 = 3.515$ ($p = .0608$) for Yates's corrected chi-square; $W^2 = 4.193$ ($p = .0406$) for the Wald statistic; and $G^2 = 4.680$ ($p = .03052$) for the likelihood ratio statistic. There are some differences in the conclusions based on these tests, as the corrected chi-square does not achieve statistical significance at the nominal .05 level, while the other tests do. A p value of .06 should not lead

Table 3–7. Observed and expected (in parentheses) frequencies of perineal exposure to deodorizing powder in controls and cases of borderline ovarian tumors (15)

Perineal powder exposure (i)	Disease status (j)		Total
	Control	Case	
None	94	67	161
	(90.1600)	(70.8400)	
Deodorizing only	4	10	14
	(7.8400)	(6.1600)	
Total	98	77	175

to a drastically different conclusion than a value of .04 or .03, because the weight of evidence against the null hypothesis is similar in either case. However, because the sample size is only marginally adequate for a large sample test, the exact test might be more appropriate to use in this instance. The one-tailed exact test gives a *p* value of .0304, which is greater than .025, the critical value in a single tail if a .05 critical value is used. Hence, in this instance, the association does not quite achieve statistical significance.

Interval Estimates of the Odds Ratio

Significance tests are useful for demonstrating whether a factor and disease are associated. However, they do not indicate the magnitude of the association, nor do they determine the accuracy with which the effect is estimated. An alternative summary that does convey the magnitude and the precision of an estimate is the confidence interval. In this section, three methods for determining confidence intervals for the odds ratio are discussed: the logit method, Cornfield's method, and an exact method. When cell frequencies are large, there is very good agreement among the methods, but for small frequencies—tables with cell frequencies less than about 5—the exact method is preferred, with Cornfield's method giving a better approximation than the logit method (16).

Logit method

The logit method makes use of the point estimate of the log odds ratio, its standard error, and the fact that the estimator has an approximate normal distribution. To form $100(1 - \alpha)\%$ confidence intervals for the log odds ratio, we calculate $\hat{\beta} \pm z(\alpha/2) \, \text{SE}(\hat{\beta})$, where $z(\alpha/2)$ is the standard normal deviate for the $\alpha/2$ significance level.

Example 3–1 (continued)   Returning once again to the study of congenital malformations, the results from the section "A Single Binary Risk Factor" yielded an estimate of the log odds ratio, 0.091021, with a standard error, 0.068787. Thus, the 95% confidence limits for the log odds ratio is

$$(0.091021) \pm (1.96)(0.068787) = (-0.0438, 0.2258)$$

Taking antilogarithms, we obtain confidence limits for the odds ratio, (0.957, 1.253), which includes the null value. Inclusion of the null value within the confidence interval for a single parameter leads to an identical conclusion to that of the corresponding Wald test.

Cornfield's method

An alternative method for computing confidence limits is based on the Pearson chi-square statistic, using an approach suggested by Cornfield (17), which may be expressed as

$$S(\breve{m}_{11})^2 = \frac{(n_{11} - \breve{m}_{11})^2}{V(n_{11})} \tag{3.16}$$

where n_{11} and $\breve{m}_{11}$ are the observed and expected frequency in cell (1,1), and

$$V(n_{11}) = (\breve{m}_{11}^{-1} + \breve{m}_{12}^{-1} + \breve{m}_{21}^{-1} + \breve{m}_{22}^{-1})^{-1}$$

We first find a confidence interval for m_{11} by finding the values, $\breve{m}_{11}$, such that S^2 equals chi-square for the appropriate confidence level, $\chi^2(\alpha)$. In general, there are two solutions, given by

$$\frac{n_{11} - \breve{m}_{11}\,(L)}{\sqrt{V(n_{11})}} = \chi(\alpha) \tag{3.17}$$

and

$$\frac{n_{11} - \breve{m}_{11}\,(U)}{\sqrt{V(n_{11})}} = -\chi(\alpha) \tag{3.18}$$

for $100(1 - \alpha)\%$ confidence limits, where $\chi(\alpha) = z(\alpha/2)$ is the critical value for the standard normal deviate. Notice that α is the upper-tail area for a χ^2 distribution, but there are two roots, one positive and the other negative. Hence, by allocating $\alpha/2$ to each tail, we arrive at what is the equivalent of the corresponding area for each tail of the standard normal deviate. Once the values of $\breve{m}_{11}(L)$ and $\breve{m}_{11}(U)$ have been obtained, the corresponding odds ratios are given by

$$OR(\cdot) = \frac{\breve{m}_{11}(\cdot)[n_{22} + \breve{m}_{11}(\cdot) - n_{11}]}{[n_{1+} - \breve{m}_{11}(\cdot)][n_{+1} - \breve{m}_{11}(\cdot)]} \tag{3.19}$$

Finding, the solutions to equations 3.17 and 3.18 can be achieved through an iterative technique, which involves guessing a value for $m_{11}(\cdot)$ and then improving that guess until the equation is solved. This can be accomplished using a spreadsheet, by establishing a formula for a cell that yields the result of calculating equation 3.16 as a function of a second cell that contains m_{11}. We then use a solution function to find the value for m_{11} that yields the appropriate value for S^2. The advantage of Cornfield's limits is that they achieve a better approximation to exact limits (16), which are described in the next section. Another variation on this approach is to modify equations 3.17 and 3.18 so that one includes Yates's continuity correction. Pros and cons for including this correction factor are presumably similar to the pros and cons for using the factor in the computation of chi-square.

Example 3–1 (continued)   For the data on the association between cigarette smoking and congenital malformations shown in Table 3–3 the solution to equation 3.17 is $m_{11}(L) = 1959.727$. This gives a lower confidence limit of

$$OR(L) = \frac{(1959.727)(480 + 1959.727 - 1988)}{(2877 - 1959.727)(2968 - 1959.727)}$$

$$= 0.957$$

In a similar manner, the upper limit is $m_{11(U)} = 2016.665$ and

$$OR(U) = \frac{(2016.665)(480 + 2016.665 - 1988)}{(2877 - 2016.665)(2968 - 2016.665)}$$

$$= 1.253$$

For this particular example there is excellent agreement between the Cornfield and the logit limits because of the large sample size, but in general the results are not identical.

Exact method

The exact method of forming confidence limits is to the exact test, as Cornfield's method is to the Pearson chi-square test. Instead of chi-square, we employ the exact probability for the occurrence of the observed or more extreme tables as a function of the odds ratio. Gart (18) gives the equations to be solved as

$$\frac{\displaystyle\sum_{k=n_{11}}^{\min(n_{+1},n_{1+})} \binom{n_{+1}}{k}\binom{n_{+2}}{n_{1+}-k} \cdot OR(L)^k}{\displaystyle\sum_{k=\max(0,n_{1+}-n_{+2})}^{\min(n_{+1},n_{1+})} \binom{n_{+1}}{k}\binom{n_{+2}}{n_{1+}-k} OR(L)^k} = \frac{\alpha}{2} \tag{3.20}$$

and

$$\frac{\sum_{k=\max(0,n_1-n_{+2})}^{n_{11}} \binom{n_{+1}}{k}\binom{n_{+2}}{n_{1+}-k} OR(U)^k}{\sum_{k=\max(0,n_{1+}-n_{+2})}^{\min(n_{+1},n_{1+})} \binom{n_{+1}}{k}\binom{n_{+2}}{n_{1+}-k} OR(U)^k} = \frac{\alpha}{2} \tag{3.21}$$

The lower and upper limits, $OR(L)$ and $OR(U)$, are the solutions to equations 3.20 and 3.21, respectively. The two tails of the exact test of H_0: $OR = 1$ are found by substituting $OR = 1$ into the formulae on the left-hand side of equations 3.20 and 3.21.

Equations 3.20 and 3.21 are fairly complicated expressions to solve computationally, and it is really not feasible to solve them without the aid of a computer. Mehta and Patel (19) have developed efficient computational algorithms for many exact methods, and these and their generalizations have been incorporated into software packages that are commonly used in the analysis of epidemiological data.

Example 3–2 (continued)   In the previous analysis of the data in Table 3–7 on the association between use of deodorizing powder and ovarian tumors, the exact test did not achieve statistical significance. The exact confidence interval for these data is (0.954, 15.886), with a point estimate of 3.507. Because the null value, 1, is included in this confidence interval, there is a consistency of interpretation with the exact test. It is interesting to compare this value with the logit limits (1.055, 11.659) and the Cornfield limits (1.110, 11.013) both of which exclude the null. While the differences among the lower limits are rather small in magnitude, we can see that the upper limits are really quite different. Overall, the large sample limits are considerably narrower than the exact limits.

Example 3–3   It is not uncommon in smaller studies to observe zero in a particular cell of a 2 × 2 table. An example of such an instance is found in a report by Hedberg et al. (20) of an outbreak of psittacosis in a turkey processing plant. Table 3–8 shows the number of cases among workers in the "mink room" where

Table 3–8. Observed frequency of psittacosis among workers in the "mink room" compared to other areas of the processing plant (20)

Work area (i)	Disease status (j)		Total
	No psittacosis	Psittacosis	
Other areas	242	0	242
Mink room	3	2	5
Total	245	2	247

viscera and other inedible parts were processed, as compared to cases among workers who did not work in such areas. The point estimate of the odds ratio is infinite, so that there is clearly no finite upper limit to a confidence interval. However,
it is possible to find a lower confidence limit by solving equation 3.20, which gives
an exact 95% interval estimate of (10.33, ∞). Hence, we can conclude with 95%
confidence that the odds ratio for psittacosis is greater than 10, a sizeable risk indeed. When there is a zero cell, the variance for the logit limits is undefined, so the
logit limits cannot be determined unless we add a constant to each cell of the table.
The Cornfield limits, by contrast, may still be defined, and for this example the
95% interval is (32.62, ∞), which shows a much higher lower limit than that obtained by the exact method. Because of the small number of cases, 2, and the small
number of workers in the mink room, 5, we would have greater confidence in the
exact calculation for these data.

More Than Two Levels of Exposure

In our first analysis of the effect of cigarette smoking on congenital malformations, exposure was only considered at two levels: exposed and unexposed. There is clearly considerable heterogeneity in the actual exposure
level among the women who smoke cigarettes, and intuition would suggest
that taking advantage of more detailed information may be advantageous.
When exploring the association between a putative risk factor and disease,
it is important to look for a dose–response relationship, which can be used
as one piece of evidence to suggest causality. The question often facing an
investigator is how to best summarize the dose–response relationship. Usually one does not understand enough about the underlying biology to be
able to specify the mathematical form for the relationship, so that some effort must go into determining the dose–response curve. We will consider
this problem in more detail in Chapter 7, but one simple approach is to
break up the exposure into nominal categories, which allows the data to
reveal the form for the relationship. The penalty for this absence of specificity in the shape of the curve is a loss of power, as we shall see. This section demonstrates how one can use nominal categories to explore the shape
of a dose–response curve, thus validating assumptions that underlie more
specific methods.

Nominal categories

Table 3–9 gives the form for a typical $I \times 2$ contingency table showing the
frequency of I levels of exposure observed by disease status. To consider
an association in a larger table, we need to designate one level of exposure
as the reference. Sometimes the selection of a reference level makes intuitive sense, such as the comparison of the risk for various smoking cate-

Table 3–9. A typical $I \times 2$ table from a study of a single risk factor

Factor (i)	Disease status (j)		Total
	Healthy	Diseased	
Level 1	n_{11}	n_{12}	n_{1+}
Level 2	n_{21}	n_{22}	n_{2+}
$\vdots$	$\vdots$	$\vdots$	$\vdots$
Level i	n_{i1}	n_{i2}	n_{i+}
$\vdots$	$\vdots$	$\vdots$	$\vdots$
Level I	n_{I1}	n_{I2}	n_{I+}
Total	n_{+1}	n_{+2}	n_{++}

gories to nonsmokers, the clear choice as the referent group. However, there are other times when the reference level is completely arbitrary. For example, suppose we are interested in the association between geographic latitude and the risk of malignant melanoma. Should the reference level be the equator? a pole? the latitude of the investigator's residence? In these situations we can readily re-express a measure of association, like the odds ratio, using an alternative reference, but it is essential that the reference be clearly specified.

For the typical display shown in Table 3–9, let level 1 be the arbitrary reference level. Using the approach described in the section "A Single Binary Risk Factor," the odds ratio for level i compared to level 1 is

$$\hat{\Omega}_i = \frac{n_{11} \cdot n_{i2}}{n_{12} \cdot n_{i1}}$$

where $\Omega_1 = 1$ by definition. Sometime we can make a more powerful statement if we specify a mathematical equation to describe the exposure-response curve for Ω_i as a function of dose, X_i. For example, the linear logistic model implies that

$$\log \Omega_i = (X_i - X_1) \cdot \beta \tag{3.22}$$

where X_1 is the reference exposure, thus giving rise to a linear relationship between dose and the log odds ratio.

An overall indication of whether there is a relationship between exposure categories and disease can be addressed by testing the null hypothesis, $H_0: \Omega_1 = \Omega_2 = \ldots = \Omega_I = 1$—that is, all of the odds ratios are equal to 1. Under the null hypothesis, the proportion diseased is the same for all levels of exposure; applying this overall proportion to each category yields an estimate of the expected frequency in the ith row and jth column, $\tilde{m}_{ij} = n_{i+}n_{+j}/n_{++}$. The resulting score test is once again the Pearson chi-square statistic

$$S^2 = \sum_{ij} \frac{(n_{ij} - \tilde{m}_{ij})^2}{\tilde{m}_{ij}}$$

which we compare to a chi-square distribution with $(I - 1)$ df. Another alternative is the likelihood ratio statistic

$$G^2 = 2 \cdot \sum_{ij} n_{ij} \log(n_{ij}/\tilde{m}_{ij})$$

which we also compare to chi-square on $(I - 1)$ df. Of course, both of these tests are large sample tests and only valid for fairly large samples.

Example 3–1 (continued)   To illustrate the analysis of more than two exposure levels, let us go back to the data on the effect of smoking on congenital malformations, this time using the more detailed exposures shown in Table 3–10. Odds ratios using nonsmokers as the reference are shown in the fifth column. For example, $\Omega_2 = (1988 \times 182) / (889 \times 426) = 0.995$. Notice that women who smoked 31+ cigarettes had an odds ratio of 1.864—an 86% excess odds of congenital malformations. In addition, there appears to be a fairly clear trend of increasing risk with the number of cigarettes smoked. Figure 3–2 gives a graphical display of the log odds ratio by the number of cigarettes smoked. A comparison of this trend with a straight line suggests that a linear logistic model may well give a reasonable description of the dose–response relationship, although the fit is not perfect. A ques-

Table 3–10. Observed and expected (in parentheses) frequencies of the amount of cigarette smoking by the mother for normal babies and babies with congenital malformations (4)

Cigarettes per day (i)	Disease status (j)		Total	Odds ratio (Ω_i)
	Normal	Malformation		
None	1988 (1968.8577)	889 (908.1423)	2877	1.000
1–10	426 (416.0812)	182 (191.9188)	608	0.995
11–20	420 (426.3463)	203 (196.6537)	623	1.081
21–30	86 (96.4925)	55 (44.5075)	141	1.430
31+	48 (60.2223)	40 (27.7777)	88	1.864
Total	2968	1369	4337	

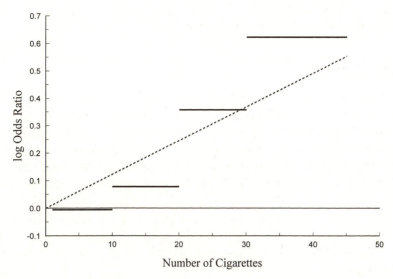

Figure 3–2 Plot of log odds ratio of congenital malformations against number of cigarettes smoked per day.

tion that we will address later is whether the departures from linear can be explained as chance variations.

The Pearson chi-square test of no association is given by

$$S^2 = \frac{(1988 - 1968.8577)^2}{1968.8577} + \frac{(889 - 908.1423)^2}{908.1423} + \cdots + \frac{(40 - 27.7777)^2}{27.7777}$$

$$= 13.1109$$

which is compared to a chi-square distribution with $5 - 1 = 4$ df ($p = .011$), leading to a rejection of the null hypothesis of no association. The corresponding likelihood ratio statistic for these data is

$$G^2 = 2 \cdot \left[1988 \cdot \log\left(\frac{1988}{1968.8557}\right) + 889 \cdot \log\left(\frac{889}{908.1423}\right) \right.$$

$$\left. + \cdots + 40 \cdot \log\left(\frac{40}{27.7777}\right) \right]$$

$$= 12.525$$

which we also compare to a chi-square distribution with 4 df ($p = .014$), resulting in the same conclusion.

The fact that more detailed information on amount of smoking leads to a statistically significant result, while the crude initial analysis gave virtually no indication that there was an effect, demonstrates the value of precise measures of exposure. This test of significance, along with the inspection of the odds ratios, strongly suggests a dose–response relationship between risk of congenital malformations and smoking. In the next section, we will consider an even more powerful test by specifying a particular form for this relationship.

Ordered categories

In general, a global hypothesis, such as the hypothesis discussed in the section "Normal Categories," that all the odds ratios are 1, is more difficult to reject than a hypothesis that is more specific. One such specific hypothesis results from the linear logistic model, which assumes that there is a linear relationship between the log odds for disease and the dose, as shown in equation 3.22. The null hypothesis that there is no association between dose and risk of disease can be expressed in terms of the regression parameter, $H_0: \beta = 0$. Hence, instead of comparing $(I - 1)$ odd ratios to their null value, this test involves just a single regression parameter and results in a more focused, and thus a more powerful, test if, in fact, the model is appropriate.

For a single binary regressor variable, the maximum likelihood estimator for β has the closed form, which we have already noted as the log odds ratio. But, in general, no simple formula exists, and we are instead required to employ an iterative technique to find the maximum likelihood estimate. Without the estimator, $\hat{\beta}$, it is not possible to conduct either a Wald test or a likelihood ratio test. However, a score test is still possible because we are only required to fit the null model that depends on the overall proportion diseased. The unconditional version of the score test (21) is

$$S^2 = \frac{n_{++}^3 \left[\sum_i X_i \left(n_{i2} - \tilde{m}_{i2}\right)\right]^2}{n_{+1} \, n_{+2} \left[n_{++} \sum_i X_i^2 n_{i+} - \left(\sum_i X_i \, n_{i+}\right)^2\right]} \tag{3.23}$$

where $m_{i2} = n_{1+} \cdot n_{+2}/n_{++}$, which is compared to a chi-square distribution with 1 df. The conditional version of the test (22) is given by

$$S_c^2 = \frac{n_{++}^2 \, (n_{++} - 1)\left[\sum_i X_i \left(n_{i2} - \tilde{m}_{i2}\right)\right]^2}{n_{+1} \, n_{+2} \left[n_{++} \sum_i X_i^2 n_{i+} - \left(\sum_i X_i \, n_{i+}\right)^2\right]} \tag{3.24}$$

which is once again related to the unconditional test by $S_c^2 = S^2(n_{++} - 1)/n_{++}$. Clearly both of these statistics agree well when the total number of observations, n_{++}, is large.

Example 3–2 (continued)   To illustrate the computations for the trend test, we consider once again the data on cigarette smoking and congenital malformations. In this case, the values for the smoking dose used in the calculations are values that

Table 3–11. Intermediate calculations for the tests for trend in equations 3.23 and 3.24 using the data on the association between cigarette smoking and congenital malformations

X_i	n_{i2}	$\tilde{m}_{i2}$	n_{i+}	$X_i \cdot n_{i2}$	$X_i \cdot \tilde{m}_{i2}$	$X_i^2 \cdot n_{i+}$	$X_i \cdot n_{i+}$
0	889	908.1423	2877	0	0.0000	0	0
5	182	191.9188	608	910	959.5940	15,200	3,040
15	203	196.6537	623	3045	2949.8055	140,175	9,345
25	55	44.5075	141	1375	1112.6875	88,125	3,525
35	40	27.7777	88	1400	972.2195	107,800	3,080
Total	1369	1369.0000	4337	6730	5994.3065	351,300	18,990

are within each of the smoking categories: 0, 5, 15, 25, and 35. Some variation of dose within each of these categories remains, but we ignore these in this approach. As intermediate steps, it is necessary to calculate $\sum_i X_i \cdot n_{i2}$; $\sum_i X_i \cdot \tilde{m}_{i2}$; $\sum_i X_i^2 \cdot n_{i+}$; and, $\sum_i X_i \cdot n_{i+}$. These are shown in Table 3–11. Substituting these values into equation 3.23 yields

$$S^2 = \frac{(4337)^3 \cdot [6730 - 5994.3065]^2}{(2968) \cdot (1369) \cdot [(4337)\cdot(351,300) - (18,990)^2]}$$

$$= 9.3439$$

which is compared to chi-square with 1 df ($p = .0022$). This test strongly suggests that there is an association between the number of cigarettes smoked and the risk of congenital malformations. Alternatively, the conditional score test yields

$$S_c^2 = \frac{(4337)^2 \cdot (4377 - 1) \cdot [6730 - 5994.3065]^2}{(2968) \cdot (1369) \cdot [(4337) \cdot (351,300) - (18,990)^2]}$$

$$= 9.3417$$

($p = .0022$), and the conclusion is identical to that of the unconditional test. These two tests are once again in close agreement because of the large number of observations in this data set, and in general there is little reason to choose between S^2 and S_c^2. Notice that the magnitude of the test statistic for trend is quite near the test for nominal categories, 9.3439 versus 13.1109, thus giving rise to a much smaller p value because it is based on fewer degrees of freedom. While this also suggests that a large proportion of the cigarette effect is accounted for by linear trend, we can address this more formally by a test of goodness of fit shown in Chapter 6.

Stratified Analysis

The preceding two sections considered the association between disease and a single factor. In most epidemiological studies, however, it is necessary to consider more than one factor at a time. For instance, it is common to focus primarily on one factor while at the same time controlling for a second, potentially confounding, factor. The concern about a potential confounder is that its distribution in the population under study could somehow bias the primary association of interest. One approach to controlling for this possibility in the data analysis is to stratify by potential confounders in order to determine whether the primary effect remains unchanged after an appropriate adjustment.

To illustrate the problem, consider the study of congenital malformations once again, but this time we will investigate the effect of tranquilizer use by the mother during the first trimester. A preliminary analysis suggests that cigarette smokers are more likely to use tranquilizers during pregnancy than are nonsmokers. We already know from our earlier analysis that women who smoke heavily during pregnancy have increased risk of giving birth to babies with congenital malformations. Hence, to provide a valid inference on the association between tranquilizer use and malformations, it is essential that we adjust for the amount of smoking by the mother.

Consider a further breakdown of the data in Table 3–9, into K strata, as shown in Table 3–12. As before, $i(= 1, \ldots, I)$ represents the exposure

Table 3–12. A typical $I \times 2 \times K$ table from a study of a single risk factor considered in a stratified analysis

| Factor (i) | Disease status (j) | | Total |
	Healthy	Diseased	
STRATUM 1			
Level 1	n_{111}	n_{121}	n_{1+1}
Level 2	n_{211}	n_{221}	n_{2+1}
$\vdots$	$\vdots$	$\vdots$	$\vdots$
Level I	n_{I11}	n_{I21}	n_{I+1}
Total	n_{+11}	n_{+21}	n_{++1}
STRATUM 2			
Level 1	n_{112}	n_{122}	n_{1+2}
Level 2	n_{212}	n_{222}	n_{2+2}
$\vdots$	$\vdots$	$\vdots$	$\vdots$
Level I	n_{I12}	n_{I22}	n_{I+2}
Total	n_{+12}	n_{+22}	n_{++2}
$\vdots$	$\vdots$	$\vdots$	$\vdots$
STRATUM K			
Level 1	n_{11k}	n_{12k}	n_{1+k}
Level 2	n_{21k}	n_{22k}	n_{2+k}
$\vdots$	$\vdots$	$\vdots$	$\vdots$
Level I	n_{I1k}	n_{I2k}	n_{I+k}
Total	n_{+1k}	n_{+2k}	n_{++k}

level for the putative risk factor, and $j(= 1,2)$ represents disease status. The additional index, $k(= 1, \ldots, K)$, gives the particular stratum under consideration, so that the frequency in a single cell of the three-dimensional table is given by n_{ijk}, with expected frequencies m_{ijk}. In a cohort study, the proportion in disease group j is represented by π_{ijk}. In this section, we discuss analytic methods that allow for stratification of data by first considering a score test for combining information on the exposure–disease association over the K strata. We will also see that this approach is best employed when there is a single odds ratio across strata, and we consider ways in which this can be more formally investigated.

Cochran and Mantel–Haenszel tests

Initially, suppose that there are just two levels of exposure, indicated by the regressor variable $X = 0,1$, which can be represented in the linear logistic equation by

$$P\{Y = 1 \mid X, k\} = \frac{\exp\{\alpha_k + X\beta\}}{1 + \exp\{\alpha_k + X\beta\}} \tag{3.25}$$

where the intercept, α_k, may vary over strata. This model implies that the odds ratio for the kth stratum is

$$\Omega_k = \frac{\Pr\{Y = 1 \mid X = 1, k\} \cdot \Pr\{Y = 0 \mid X = 0, k\}}{\Pr\{Y = 0 \mid X = 1, k\} \cdot \Pr\{Y = 1 \mid X = 0, k\}} = \exp\{\beta\}$$

which is identical for all strata. It should be emphasized that equation 3.25 allows the probability of disease to vary over the strata, even though the odds ratio remains constant.

The score test that controls for stratification by estimating the stratum parameters, α_k, gives rise to Cochran's test (14) for combining 2×2 contingency tables, as shown in Appendix 2, under "Score Statistics for Combining $I \times 2$ Tables." The expected frequency for a diseased subject at level 2 of the factor in the kth stratum, under the null hypothesis, $H_0: \beta = 0$ is

$$\tilde{m}_{22k} = \frac{n_{2+k} \cdot n_{+2k}}{n_{++k}} \tag{3.26}$$

A variance for the corresponding observed frequency, n_{22k}, is

$$V(n_{22k}) = \frac{n_{1+k} \cdot n_{2+k} \cdot n_{+1k} \cdot n_{+2k}}{n_{++k}^3} \tag{3.27}$$

Cochran's test is then computed by

$$S^2 = \frac{(\sum_k n_{22k} - \sum_k \tilde{m}_{22k})^2}{\sum_k V(n_{22k})} \tag{3.28}$$

which is compared to a chi-square distribution with 1 df.

An alternative to Cochran's unconditional test is the conditional statistic proposed by Mantel and Haenszel (7). The only real difference between the two tests is in the variance, where the conditional variance for the kth stratum is given by

$$V_c(n_{22k}) = \frac{n_{1+k} \cdot n_{2+k} \cdot n_{+1k} \cdot n_{+2k}}{n_{++k}^2 \cdot (n_{++k} - 1)} \tag{3.29}$$

with the corresponding score test

$$S_c^2 = \frac{(\sum_k n_{22k} - \sum_k \tilde{m}_{22k})^2}{\sum_k V_c(n_{22k})} \tag{3.30}$$

When the strata, n_{++k}, are large, the variances in equations 3.27 and 3.29 are in good agreement, but we shall encounter study designs in which the stratum size is small, even though the overall sample size for the study may be large. Pair-wise matching is such an extreme case in which we may regard each stratum as consisting of only two subjects, $n_{++k} = 2$, giving rise to $V_c(n_{22k}) = 2 \cdot V(n_{22k})$. In this instance, the Cochran test is twice the Mantel–Haenszel test (23). If both tests were appropriate, this would suggest more power for Cochran's statistic, but they are not. In fact, the Mantel–Haenszel statistic yields McNemar's (24) test for paired observations in this special case (see Chapter 10), and, in general, it produces a more appropriate significance test than Cochran's for small strata. There are no readily defined situations where Cochran's test is substantially superior to the Mantel–Haenszel test, so that it is generally safe to routinely make use of the latter.

Example 3–4   The data in Table 3–13 are from a case-control study described by Bracken and Holford (25) which included an analysis of the potential effect of tranquilizer use by a mother during pregnancy. This tabulation gives the distribution of tranquilizer use and the number of cigarettes for mothers with congenitally malformed babies and their controls. Intermediate calculations, shown in Table 3–14,

Table 3–13. Observed number of women using tranquilizers during pregnancy by number of cigarettes smoked for cases and controls (25)

Tranquilizer use (i)	Disease status (j)		Total	Odds ratio (Ω_i)
	Normal	Malformation		
NONSMOKERS				
No	1916	848	2764	1.442
Yes	47	30	77	
Total	1963	878	2841	
1–20 CIGARETTES				
No	826	361	1187	3.696
Yes	13	21	34	
Total	839	382	1221	
21+ CIGARETTES				
No	122	75	197	3.660
Yes	8	18	26	
Total	130	93	223	

give the observed and expected number of tranquilizer users among cases, along with the corresponding variances. Thus, Cochran's test is

$$S^2 = \frac{(69 - 45.2768)^2}{28.6865} = 19.6187$$

which we compare to chi-square with 1 df ($p = .00002$). This suggests strong evidence of an association between tranquilizer use and congenital malformations adjusting for smoking. The corresponding Mantel–Haenszel statistic is

$$S_c^2 = \frac{(69 - 45.2768)^2}{28.7231} = 19.5937$$

($p = .00002$), giving the same conclusion as the Cochran test. This good agreement results from the large stratum sizes in this example.

Table 3–14. Intermediate calculations for the Cochran and Mantel–Haenszel tests using the data in Table 3–13

Stratum[1]	n_{22k}	$\tilde{m}_{22k}$ [2]	$V(n_{22k})$ [3]	$V_c(n_{22k})$ [4]
1	30	23.7966	15.9967	16.0023
2	21	10.6372	7.1057	7.1115
3	18	9.8430	5.5841	5.6092
Total	69	45.2768	28.6865	28.7231

[1] Smoking categories.

[2] Calculations using equation 3.26.

[3] Calculations using equation 3.27.

[4] Calculations using equation 3.29.

Mantel–Haenszel estimator for the odds ratio

In addition to a significance test for combining information in K 2 $\times$ 2 tables, Mantel and Haenszel (7) proposed an estimator for the odds ratio:

$$\tilde{\Omega} = \frac{\sum_k n_{11k}\, n_{22k}/n_{++k}}{\sum_k n_{12k}\, n_{21k}/n_{++k}} = \exp(\tilde{\beta}) \qquad (3.31)$$

While this is not a maximum likelihood estimator, it does behave rather well when compared to the maximum likelihood estimator (18), and the relative ease of computation makes it a good choice for hand or spreadsheet calculations.

While the Mantel–Haenszel estimator was suggested very early in the development of statistical methods in epidemiology, its variance proved to be more difficult to derive, and there was a long lag between the proposed estimator and a good estimate of its variance (26). We will once again work with the log odd ratio, $\log(\tilde{\Omega}) = \tilde{\beta}$, which has a variance that can be estimated by

$$\mathrm{Var}(\tilde{\beta}) = \frac{\sum_k P_k \cdot R_k}{2 \cdot R_+^2} + \frac{\sum_k (P_k \cdot S_k + Q_k \cdot R_k)}{2 \cdot R_+ \cdot S_+} + \frac{\sum_k Q_k \cdot S_k}{2 \cdot S_+^2} \qquad (3.32)$$

where
$$P_k = (n_{11k} + n_{22k})/n_{++k}$$
$$Q_k = (n_{12k} + n_{21k})/n_{++k}$$
$$R_k = n_{22k} \cdot n_{11k}/n_{++k}$$
$$S_k = n_{12k} \cdot n_{21k}/n_{++k}$$

Once the variance has been calculated, the construction of confidence limits is similar to the logit method for 2 $\times$ 2 tables, $\tilde{\beta} \pm z(\alpha/2) \cdot \sqrt{\mathrm{Var}(\tilde{\beta})}$, where $z(\cdot)$ is the standard normal deviate, and the corresponding limits for the odds ratio are determined by taking antilogarithms.

Example 3–4 (continued) To estimate the overall odds ratio for the data on the association between tranquilizer use and congenital malformations shown in Table 3–13, it is necessary to first obtain the intermediate sums shown in Table 3–15. The Mantel–Haenszel estimate of the common odds ratio is $\tilde{\Omega} = 44.2862/20.5630 = 2.154$, so that the estimated log odds ratio is $\tilde{\beta} = 0.7672$. The variance estimator is

$$\mathrm{Var}(\tilde{\beta}) = \frac{29.8957}{2(44.2862)^2} + \frac{13.9649 + 14.3905}{2 \cdot (44.2862) \cdot (20.5630)} + \frac{6.5982}{2(20.5630)^2}$$
$$= 0.0309925 = (0.17605)^2$$

Table 3–15. Intermediate calculations for the variance of the Mantel–Haenszel estimate using the data in Table 3–13

Stratum k[1]	P_k^2	$Q_k = (1 - P_k)^2$	$R_k = \dfrac{n_{11k} \cdot n_{22k}}{n_{++k}}$[2]	$S_k = \dfrac{n_{12k} \cdot n_{21k}}{n_{++k}}$[3]	$P_k \cdot R_k^2$	$P_k \cdot S_k^2$	$Q_k \cdot R_k^2$	$Q_k \cdot S_k^2$
1	0.684970	0.315030	20.2323	14.0289	13.8585	9.6094	6.3738	4.4195
2	0.693694	0.306306	14.2064	3.8436	9.8549	2.6663	4.3515	1.1773
3	0.627803	0.372197	9.8475	2.6906	6.1823	1.6892	3.6652	1.0014
Total			44.2862	20.5630	29.8957	13.9649	14.3905	6.5982

[1] Smoking categories.

[2] Intermediate calculations for equations 3.31 and 3.32.

[3] Intermediate calculations for equation 3.32.

Hence, 95% confidence limits for the log odds ratio are $0.7672 \pm (1.96) \cdot (0.17605) = (0.4221, 1.1122)$, and the corresponding limits for the odds ratio are $(1.525, 3.041)$.

Testing for homogeneity of the odds ratio

A fundamental assumption we used in our rationale for the Cochran and Mantel–Haenszel statistics was that the effects are homogeneous across strata. In fact, a single estimator of effect is most easily interpreted when that effect is the same for all of the strata. When effects are not identical for all strata, the application of these statistical methods involve statistical inference for an average effect (27). This is not a simple average but a weighted average, however; the weights are related to the precision achieved for the estimate in each stratum. This weight may well be unrelated to the public health significance of that stratum, in which case the estimate of overall effect may have little value.

Before routinely applying a method for pooling information across strata, it is important to inspect the individual results to make sure they can be meaningfully pooled. A visual check can be supplemented with a test for homogeneity, because it may point out instances where chance variation can clearly be ruled out as an explanation of the observed fluctuations. If the effect of interest is the odds ratio, then the null hypothesis for homogeneity is $H_0: \Omega_1 = \Omega_2 = \cdots = \Omega_K = \Omega$—that is, all odds ratios take a common value, Ω.

One approach to this problem is to compare the individual estimates of the log odds ratios to their weighted average (28). An optimal choice of weights are the reciprocals of the variances, so that for the kth log odds ratio estimate, $\hat{\beta}_k$, we have the weight

$$w_k = 1/\mathrm{Var}(\hat{\beta}_k) = [n_{11k}^{-1} + n_{12k}^{-1} + n_{21k}^{-1} + n_{22k}^{-1}]^{-1} \qquad (3.33)$$

The weighted average of the log odds ratio is

$$\bar{\beta} = (\textstyle\sum_k w_k \hat{\beta}_k)/(\textstyle\sum_k w_k) \qquad (3.34)$$

which has estimated variance

$$\mathrm{Var}(\bar{\beta}) = [\textstyle\sum_k w_k]^{-1} \qquad (3.35)$$

An overall test for association—or a test of the null hypothesis, $H_0: \beta = 0$—is given by the corresponding Wald statistic

$$W_{\mathrm{assoc}}^2 = \bar{\beta}^2/\mathrm{Var}(\bar{\beta}) \qquad (3.36)$$

which is compared to a chi-square distribution with 1 df. The difference between individual log odds ratios and $\bar{\beta}$ gives the test of homogeneity of the log odds ratio

$$W^2_{\text{homog}} = \sum_k w_k (\beta_k - \bar{\beta})^2$$
$$= (\sum_k w_k \beta_k^2) - W^2_{\text{assoc}}$$

(3.37)

This test for homogeneity of the log odds ratio can be quite readily applied in most cases, but when one cell of a table is zero, the variance and the weights are undefined. Hence, the use of the weighted average and the corresponding test of homogeneity of effect has practical value only when the sample size is large enough to ensure no zero cells. Of course, one solution that will result in a statistic that is always defined is to add a small number like $\frac{1}{2}$ to each cell of the table before applying the test. But this would not resolve the problem entirely for many of the same reasons discussed earlier.

Example 3–4 (continued)   To illustrate the problem of evaluating homogeneity of the odds ratio, consider the tranquilizer use data once again. Table 3–13 shows the odds ratios for each of the three smoking categories. Among nonsmokers the odds ratio is only 1.4, while for the smoking group the odds ratios are 3.7 and 3.3 for light and heavy smokers, respectively. This suggests that the effect may not be homogeneous, in that the effect of tranquilizers appears to be much stronger among smokers than nonsmokers.

Table 3–16 shows the intermediate calculations needed to evaluate the individual log odds ratios. The weighted mean of the log odd ratios is $\bar{\beta} = 23.0945/30.488 = 0.7575$ with a standard error of $SE(\bar{\beta}) = (30.488)^{-1/2} = 0.1811$. These estimates, $\bar{\beta}$ and $SE(\bar{\beta})$, provide yet another estimate of the overall odds ratio, $\exp\{0.7575\} = 2.133$, and 95% confidence intervals can be constructed by find-

Table 3–16. Intermediate calculations for analyzing the log odds ratio using the data in Table 3–13

Stratum k[1]	$\hat{\beta}_k = \log(\hat{\Omega}_k)$[2]	$\text{Var}(\hat{\beta}_k)$[3]	w_k[3]	$w_k \cdot \hat{\beta}_k$[4]	$w_k \cdot \hat{\beta}_k^2$[5]
1	0.3662	0.05631	17.758	6.5025	2.3810
2	1.3073	0.12852	7.781	10.1717	13.2973
3	1.2975	0.20209	4.948	6.4204	8.3302
Total			30.448	23.0945	24.0085

[1] Smoking categories.

[2] Stratum-specific effects.

[3] Calculations using equation 3.33.

[4] Intermediate calculation for equations 3.34 and 3.35.

[5] Intermediate calculation for equation 3.37.

ing $\exp\{0.7575 \pm 1.96 \cdot (0.1811)\} = (1.496, 3.042)$. The results are very similar to estimates obtained using the Mantel–Haenszel method, which is to be expected, given the relatively large sample sizes for the strata involved.

Testing for homogeneity, we obtain $S^2_{homog} = 24.0085 - (23.0945)^2/(30.488) = 6.515$, which is compared to a chi-square distribution with $(3 - 1) = 2$ df ($p = .038$), thus implying that the null hypothesis should be rejected at the 5% significance level. This suggests that the effect of tranquilizers is not the same for all women in the study and provides support for the hypothesis that the effect is indeed stronger among smokers than nonsmokers.

Breslow and Day (29) propose an alternative test for homogeneity of the odds ratios that makes use of the Mantel–Haenszel estimator for the odds ratio, as well as the familiar Pearson chi-square statistic. Because the Mantel–Haenszel estimator is reasonably close to the maximum likelihood estimator for the combined odds ratio, it is interesting to compare the fit of a series of expected tables that forces the odds ratios to take this common value, with a table of observed frequencies. If $\tilde{\Omega}$ is the Mantel–Haenszel estimator of the odds ratio, then let $\tilde{m}_{ijk}$ be the expected frequencies for each cell of the kth table, such that

$$\frac{\tilde{m}_{11k} \cdot \tilde{m}_{22k}}{\tilde{m}_{12k} \cdot \tilde{m}_{21k}} = \tilde{\Omega}$$

subject to the condition that the row and column totals for the expected table are equal to the observed totals. In the case of $\tilde{m}_{22k}$, this can be accomplished by solving a quadratic equation $(a \cdot \tilde{m}^2_{22k}) + b \cdot \tilde{m}_{22k}) + c = 0$, where $a = (\tilde{\Omega} - 1)$, $b = -n_{++k} - (\tilde{\Omega} - 1) \cdot (n_{2+k} + n_{+2k})$, and $c = \tilde{\Omega} \cdot n_{2+k} \cdot n_{+2k}$. This quadratic equation has two roots, one of which is out of the range of legitimate solutions, leaving only one valid solution. The remaining cells can be readily found by using the row and column totals: $\tilde{m}_{12k} = n_{+2k} - \tilde{m}_{22k}$; $\tilde{m}_{21k} = n_{2+k} - \tilde{m}_{22k}$; and $\tilde{m}_{11k} = n_{11k} - n_{22k} + m_{22k}$. Once these expected frequencies are determined, homogeneity is tested using the Pearson chi-square statistic:

$$S^2 = \sum_{ijk} \frac{(n_{ijk} - \tilde{m}_{ijk})^2}{\tilde{m}_{ijk}}$$

This is then compared to a chi-square distribution with $(K - 1)$ df. Because the difference between the observed and expected frequencies is identical in absolute magnitude for each stratum, a computationally simpler version of this formula is

$$S^2 = \sum_{k} (n_{22k} - \tilde{m}_{22k})^2 \cdot (\tilde{m}_{11k}^{-1} + \tilde{m}_{12k}^{-1} + \tilde{m}_{21k}^{-1} + \tilde{m}_{22k}^{-1}) \quad (3.38)$$

Example 3–4 (continued)   Returning once again to the data addressing the tranquilizer use and congenital malformation association shown in Table 3–13, recall that we have already found the Mantel–Haenszel estimator of the odds ratio to be $\hat{\Omega} = 2.154$ in the section "Mantel–Haenszel Estimator for the Odds Ratio." This implies that for the first table, $a = 1.15368$, $b = -2841 - (1.15368) \cdot (77 + 878) = -3942.768$, and $c = (2.15368) \cdot (77) \cdot (878) = 145{,}601.94$. A solution to the quadratic equation is found by

$$\frac{-b \pm \sqrt{b^2 - 4ac}}{2a} = \frac{-(-3942.768) \pm \sqrt{(-3942.768)^2 - 4(1.15368)(145{,}601.94)}}{2(1.15368)}$$

The solution found by adding the radical, 3380.21, is greater than the number in the table, and so is clearly out of range, leaving the estimate of the expected frequency, $\tilde{m}_{221} = 37.337$. The expected frequencies for the remaining cells are shown in Table 3–17, and the contribution to the goodness-of-fit test by this first table is

$$S^2 = (30 - 37.337)^2 \left(\frac{1}{1923.337} + \frac{1}{840.663} + \frac{1}{39.663} + \frac{1}{37.337} \right)$$

$$= 2.891$$

Each of the remaining contributions are shown in Table 3–17, giving a total chi-square test of the homogeneity of the odds ratio, 6.626 with 2 df ($p = .036$). The conclusion is much the same as in the weighted analysis; that is, there is evidence of a lack of homogeneity in the odds ratios for these data.

Stratified analysis of trends

In the section "Ordered Categories" it was noted that the test for association in a simple 2×2 table could readily be generalized to the consideration of trends in an $I \times 2$ table where

$$\Pr\{Y = 1 \mid X, k\} = \frac{\exp\{\alpha_k + X\beta\}}{1 + \exp\{\alpha_k + X\beta\}}$$

Table 3–17. Intermediate calculations for computing Breslow and Day's (1987) test for homogeneity of the odds ratio using the data in Table 3–13

Stratum k[1]	a[2]	b[2]	c[2]	Expected	$(\tilde{m}_{ijk})^2$	S^2[2]
1	1.154	−3,942.768	145,601.94	1,923.337	840.663	2.891
				39.663	37.337	
2	1.154	−1,700.932	27,972.04	821.633	365.367	2.320
				17.367	16.633	
3	1.154	−360.288	5,207.61	119.193	77.807	1.415
				10.807	15.193	
Total						6.626

[1] Smoking categories.

[2] Preliminary calculations for equation 3.38.

Mantel (22) describes a test for the common trend for $K I \times 2$ tables which can once again be considered as a score test. Details on the derivation of this test statistic as it is related to the linear logistic regression model are discussed in Appendix 2, under "Score Statistics for Combining $I \times 2$ Tables," for both the unconditional and the conditional approaches. An inspection of the formulae for these tests reveals elements that are familiar from the two-way contingency table. In fact, the numerator and the denominator are both sums of similar terms used in the test for trend in a single table. The score test is

$$S^2 = \frac{[\sum_{ik} X_i (n_{i2k} - m_{i2k})]^2}{\sum_k \text{Var}_k} \tag{3.39}$$

where the variance term is calculated for each stratum. The test is actually the same as a test for linear trend in the proportions (21). For the unconditional test, the variance is given by

$$\text{Var}_{ck} = \frac{n_{+1k} \, n_{+2k}}{n_{++k}^3} \left\{ n_{i++} \cdot \sum_i X_i^2 n_{i+k} - \left(\sum_i X_i \, n_{i+k} \right)^2 \right\} \tag{3.40}$$

As before, the only difference between the conditional and the unconditional test lies in the formulation of the variance, which for the condition test is

$$\text{Var}_{ck} = \frac{n_{+1k} \, n_{+2k}}{n_{++k}^2 \, (n_{++k} - 1)} \left\{ n_{i++} \cdot \sum_i X_i^2 n_{i+k} - \left(\sum_i X_i \, n_{i+k} \right)^2 \right\} \tag{3.41}$$

Once again, these tests are very similar for large strata (when the n_{++k} are large). If all of the strata are small, which is generally the case when a matched study design is used, then these two tests can give quite different results. Because of the preference for the conditional test when one is analyzing small strata and the fact that results are essentially the same for large strata, an effective strategy is to always use the conditional variance.

Summary

This chapter has focused on computationally simple methods of analyzing contingency tables that are useful for the analysis of epidemiological data. The methods of statistical inference included significance testing, as well as point and interval estimates of a design and risk factor association that uses the odds ratio. Initially these analyses were limited to looking at just a single stratum and providing a summary of the results displayed in either a 2×2 or an $I \times 2$ table, but these were then extended to the combination of K such tables by using the approaches originally described by Cochran (14) and Mantel and Haenszel (7). All of these approaches to data analysis are particularly useful when the overall sample sizes are fairly large so that the asymptotic theory gives a good approximation to the true results.

When a table has small frequencies, the large sample theory does not give accurate results and it cannot be relied on. When the Pearson chi-square is used, small expected frequencies are critical. When using a Wald statistic or constructing logit confidence limits for the odds ratio, a small observed frequency can cause the results to be unreliable. For 2×2 tables this chapter described the use of Fisher's (12) exact test and the corresponding exact confidence intervals for tables with small frequencies. When in doubt as to the adequacy of a large sample procedure, it is generally preferable to use an appropriate exact method. Knowledge about the use and construction of exact tests is continuing to develop, including its use for investigating trends and the combination of several tables. This is beyond the scope of this book, but there are useful software implementations of current methods in StatXact (19) and LogXact (30). Because of the increased availability of improved numerical algorithms used in the calculations, these exact methods can be applied much more readily.

It should be emphasized that the score tests considered in this chapter have centered primarily on a single parameter—the odds ratio, or the slope in the linear logistic model. More general hypotheses can be investigated using this approach, which provides even further extensions to the Cochran–Mantel–Haenszel methodology.

While the methods described in this chapter are very powerful, and useful in practical situations, they are limited in what they can accomplish. For example, when one is controlling for multiple factors using a stratified analysis, it is not at all uncommon to obtain sample sizes that are so small in each stratum that there is no remaining information available to test the association of interest. In addition, there are better ways to deal with factors that are continuous, because categorizing them for tabulation necessarily results in some loss of information. In subsequent chapters, we will consider some general approaches that will provide even more powerful methods of data analysis.

Exercises

3.1. La Vecchia et al. (31) present data from a case-control study that investigated the relationship between myocardial infarction and coffee consumption among Italian women. The cases occurred between 1983 and 1987, and controls were selected from the women admitted for acute care in the same hospitals. Some results of this study are tabulated here:

Cups per day	Controls	Cases
0	85	30
≤1	434	232

a. Test the significance of the association between whether a woman drank coffee and myocardial infarction using:
  i. The score test or Pearson chi-square
  ii. Chi-square with Yates's correction
  iii. The Wald test
  iv. The likelihood ratio statistic
b. Find a point estimate for the odds ratio, the log odds ratio, and the standard error of the log odds ratio.
c. Calculate 95% confidence limits for the odds ratio using:
  i. The logit method
  ii. The Cornfield method

3.2. A more detailed breakdown of the data in exercise 3.1 is given in the following table:

Cups per day	Controls	Cases
0	85	30
1	124	43
2	132	61
3	95	46
≤4	83	82

a. Estimate the odds ratio for each level of coffee consumption using 0 cups per day as the reference level.
b. Draw a graph showing the relationship between the log odds ratio for myocardial infarction and the number of cups of coffee consumed per day.
c. Test for the significance of the trend in the log odds ratio with the number of cups of coffee consumed.

3.3. In a study of the association between obesity and risk of ovarian cancer, Farrow et al. (32) report the following results from their case-control study for the subgroup of premenopausal women with endometrioid ovarian cancer:

Quetelet index	Controls	Cases
<22.3	173	2
≥22.3	82	8

a. Test the null hypothesis that there is no association between obesity, as measured by Quetelet's index, and ovarian cancer.
b. Estimate the odds ratio for these data.
c. Give a 95% confidence interval for the estimate of the odds ratio.

3.4. Rosenberg et al. (33) used a case-control study to investigate the relationship between epithelial ovarian cancer and the use of combination oral contraceptives. The data are stratified by age and summarized in the following table:

Age	Combination oral contraceptive	Control	Case
18–29	Nonuser	12	5
	User	37	6
30–39	Nonuser	39	13
	User	49	10
40–49	Nonuser	128	40
	User	80	13
50–59	Nonuser	173	45
	User	21	4

a. Compute a score statistic for the association between use of combination oral ontraceptives and risk of ovarian cancer adjusting for the effect of age using:
  i. Cochran's test
  ii. The Mantel–Haenszel statistic
b. Compute the Mantel–Haenszel estimate of the odds ratio.
c. Find a 95% confidence interval for the Mantel–Haenszel estimate of the odds ratio.
d. Estimate the odds ratio for the association between use of oral contraceptives and risk of ovarian cancer separately for each age group, and comment on the adequacy of the analysis in parts a–c.
e. Give a test of homogeneity of the odds ratio for the oral contraceptive use and ovarian cancer association.

References

1. Anscombe FJ. On estimating binomial response relations. *Biometrika* 1956;43: 461–464.

2. Gart JJ. Alternative analysis of contingency tables. *Journal of the Royal Statistical Society, Series B* 1966:164–179.

3. Gart JJ, Zweifel JR. On the bias of various estimators of the logit and its variance, with application to quantal bioassay. *Biometrika* 1967;54:181–187.

4. Kelsey JL, Dwyer T, Holford TR, Bracken MB. Maternal smoking and congenital malformations: an epidemiological study. *Journal of Epidemiology and Community Health* 1978;32:102–107.

5. Fisher RA. On the mathematical foundations of theoretical statistics. *Philosophical Transactions, Series A* 1921;222:309.

6. Rao CR. *Linear Statistical Inference and Its Applications.* New York: Wiley, 1973.

7. Mantel N, Haenszel W. Statistical aspects of the analysis of data from retrospective studies of disease. *Journal of the National Cancer Institute* 1959;22:719–748.

8. Yates F. Contingency tables involving small numbers and the χ^2 test. *Journal of the Royal Statistical Society Supplement* 1934;1:217–235.

9. Conover WJ. Uses and abuses of the continuity correction. *Biometrics* 1968;24:1028.

10. Grizzle JE. Continuity correction in the χ^2 test for 2×2 tables. *American Statistician* 1967;21:28–32.

11. Mantel N, Greenhouse SW. What is the continuity correction? *American Statistician* 1968;22:27–30.

12. Fisher RA. The logic of inductive inference (with discussion). *Journal of the Royal Statistical Society* 1935;98:39–54.

13. Cox DR. *Analysis of Binary Data.* London: Methuen, 1970.

14. Cochran WG. Some methods for strengthening the common χ^2 tests. *Biometrics* 1954;10:417–451.

15. Harlow BL, Weiss NS. A case-control study of borderline ovarian tumors: the influence of perineum exposure to talc. *American Journal of Epidemiology* 1989;130:390–394.

16. Gart JJ, Thomas DG. Numerical results on approximate confidence limits for the odds ratio. *Journal of the Royal Statistical Society, Series B* 1972:441–447.

17. Cornfield J. A statistical problem arising from retrospective studies, 1956.

18. Gart JJ. The comparison of proportions: a review of significance tests, confidence intervals and adjustments for stratification. *Review of the International Statistical Institute* 1971;39:148–169.

19. Mehta C, Patel N. 1996. *StatXact 3 for Windows.* Cambridge, MA: CYTEL Software, 1996.

20. Hedberg K, White KE, Forfang JC, Korlath JA, Friendshuh AJ, Hedberg CW, MacDonald KL, Osterholm MT. An outbreak of psittacosis in Minnesota turkey industry workers: implications for modes of transmission and control. *American Journal of Epidemiology* 1989;130:569–577.

21. Armitage P. Test for linear trend in proportions and frequencies. *Biometrics* 1955;11:375–386.

22. Mantel N. Chi-square tests with one degree of freedom: Extensions of the Mantel–Haenszel procedure. *Journal of the American Statistical Association* 1963;58:690–700.

23. Pike MC, Casagrande J, Smith PG. Statistical analysis of individually matched case-control studies in epidemiology: Factor under study a discrete variable

taking multiple values. *British Journal of Social and Preventive Medicine* 1975; 29:196–201.

24. McNemar Q. Note on the sampling error of the difference between correlated proportions on percentages. *Psychometrika* 1947;12:153–157.

25. Bracken MB, Holford TR. Exposure to prescribed drugs in pregnancy and association with congenital malformations. *Obstetrics and Gynecology* 1981;58: 336–344.

26. Robins J, Breslow N, Greenland S. Estimators of the Mantel–Haenszel variance consistent in both sparse data and large-strata limiting models. *Biometrics* 1986;42:311–323.

27. Greenland S, Neutra R. Control of confounding in the assessment of medical technology. *International Journal of Epidemiology* 1980;9:361–367.

28. Fleiss JL. *Statistical Methods for Rates and Proportions*. New York: Wiley, 1981.

29. Breslow NE, Day NE. *Statistical Methods in Cancer Research*. Lyon: International Agency for Research on Cancer, 1987.

30. Mehta C, Patel N. *LogXact for Windows*. Cambridge, MA: CYTEL Software, 1996.

31. La Vecchia C, Gentile A, Negri E, Parazzini F, Franceschi S. Coffee consumption and myocardial infarction in women. *American Journal of Epidemiology* 1989;130:481–485.

32. Farrow DC, Weiss NS, Lyon JL, Daling JR. Association of obesity and ovarian cancer in a case-control study. *American Journal of Epidemiology* 1989; 129:1300–1304.

33. Rosenberg L, Shapiro, S., Slone, D., et al. Epithelial ovarian cancer and combination oral contraceptives. *Journal of the American Medical Association* 1982; 247:3210–3212.

4

Analysis of Rates

Atkins et al. (1) report the results of a 10-year cohort study of 210 women with breast cancer who were treated at Guy's Hospital, London. Of particular interest was the type of treatment received by these patients: 116 radical mastectomy, 23 simple mastectomy, 71 not treated. By the end of the study, all but 12 of the patients had died, and even among those there was considerable variability in the length of time they had been followed. In this example we have the type of data that is very common in epidemiologic studies in which the response of interest is the time till the outcome, in this case death, occurs. Clearly, if the investigators had been able to follow each of these patients long enough, there would ultimately have been no survivors, so there would be no useful information left in an analysis of the proportion of survivors.

In the preceding chapter, we justified the analysis of proportions for studies in which all subjects were effectively followed for the same length of time. This nonvariability is rather uncommon, however, as we generally must recruit subjects over a period of time in order to build up a sample population that is large enough to yield meaningful results. In the breast cancer example, women were enrolled at the time the diagnosis was made, so when the study stopped, inevitably some had been followed for longer periods than others. Hence, at the time of analysis, some subjects have complete information about the time to the outcome, and others have been *withdrawn-alive* from the study. Because the length of time a subject is followed is directly related to the likelihood that the outcome will be observed, we would be remiss if we conducted an analysis that ignored this critical feature of the data.

Another factor that often affects the length of time an individual is under observation is whether they are *lost to follow-up*, perhaps because an individual moved out of the area in which the study is being conducted. In one way, individuals who are lost to follow-up appear to be similar to those who have truncated observations because the study ended. However, because those lost to follow-up may represent a self-selected group, we need to understand the reasons individuals are lost to the study. For example, if patients no longer return to a clinic because the treatment is not curing their illness, then this could mean that the outcome of interest is about to occur but we are not able to observe it. As we shall see, it is common to assume that the reason a subject produces only partial information is unrelated to the outcome, but subjects who are lost to follow-up may potentially violate that assumption, thus opening the door to bias and invalid statistical inferences.

A fundamentally different way in which rates are generated by epidemiologists is through the data provided by vital registries, which are often used for descriptive epidemiology. In this case, the rate is produced by taking the ratio of number of cases to mid-year population. Instead of analyzing times, we are now considering counts of events, which on the surface may appear to be fundamentally very different entities. But as we shall see, these two types of data result in estimates and inference formulae that are identical, so we shall consider these two types of data together in this discussion.

In this chapter we limit our discussion to fairly simple methods for comparing groups and summarizing data. Hence, the chapter provides a description of methods for rates that are analogous to the methods for proportions discussed in Chapter 3. Regression methods that allow us to simultaneously consider many factors in the analysis are left to Chapter 8.

Rates as an Outcome

Let us now consider methods for estimating rates, as well as some simple tests for comparing subgroups and testing for trend. We first consider these methods in the context of data on time until an event occurs, then discuss the rationale for using these techniques in the context of vital rates and standardized ratios. The formulae are identical, so we only need to be aware of the variations in interpretation of the results.

Censored observations with constant hazard

In a typical cohort study, subjects in a specified population are recruited for a period of time and then are followed to determine whether a failure occurs—that is, whether the disease is diagnosed or death occurs. Figure 4–1 shows a chronological representation of such a study, which begins on a particular date when recruitment begins, followed by a date when no ad-

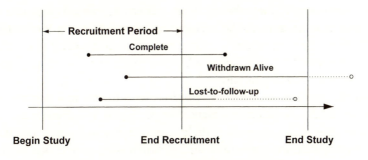

CHRONOLOGICAL REPRESENTATION

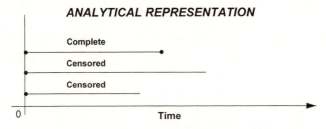

ANALYTICAL REPRESENTATION

Figure 4–1 Chronological and analytical representation of typical observations that arise in a cohort study.

ditional subjects are entered. The follow-up continues until the study ends, when no further information is obtained and the results are analyzed. Also shown in Figure 4–1 are some typical examples of the types of subjects we might encounter. First, we see a complete observation of an individual who was observed until the failure occurred, so that we accurately know the length of time until the event. Often, the study will end before some subjects have failed, resulting in an individual being withdrawn alive from the study. Hence, we only have partial information on these individuals, because we know that if the failure occurred, it was sometime after the end of the study. Finally, we have individuals lost to follow-up, for whom follow-up ends for reasons other than the end of the study.

We have already alluded to the bias that can arise when subjects are lost to follow-up, so it is important in conducting a study to minimize the number in this category. One rule of thumb is that this number should be kept under 10%. When the outcome is death, one can almost always obtain this minimal information on essentially all subjects, so that one can at least analyze survival without serious bias due to loss to follow-up. However, if the outcome requires a subtle diagnostic procedure, then we could have a serious problem if our study was unable to maintain fairly complete follow-up on all subjects. The interpretation of results of a study often requires careful thought, especially when specific causes of failure are of interest. For example, a survival study of cancer patients may consider a patient who is in an automobile accident as essentially being lost to follow-up; alternatively, if somehow a treatment was putting patients at increased risk of fatal accidents, then we would miss this result if we simply ignored this possibility in our analysis.

For the analysis, we generally consider time from entry into the study, as shown in the analytical representation in Figure 4–1. Hence, the origin for each individual depends on their date of entry into the study. We not only need to determine the time during which each subject was under active follow-up, but we also need to determine their status at the end of follow-up. For the ith subject, let t_i represent the time under observation and δ_i the status at the end of follow-up, where $\delta_i = 1$ for a complete observation and $\delta_i = 0$ for a censored observation, so that the available information on the outcome is the pair (t_i, δ_i).

If the hazard is a constant over time, $\lambda(t) \equiv \lambda$, then we have an exponential distribution of the times until failure, and the maximum likelihood estimate of the hazard is given by the failure rate:

$$\hat{\lambda} = \frac{\text{Number of failures}}{\text{Total person-years experience}}$$

$$= \frac{\sum_i \delta_i}{\sum_i t_i} = \frac{n}{D} \tag{4.1}$$

where n represents the total number of failures and D, represents the total person-years of follow-up observed in the study. It is interesting to note that if all subjects are observed until failure—if n is the sample size—then the failure rate is the reciprocal of the sample mean. This mirrors the fact that the mean of the exponential distribution that arises from the assumption of a constant hazard is $1/\lambda$.

The variance of the failure rate is given by

$$\text{Var}(\hat{\lambda}) = \frac{\lambda^2}{n} \tag{4.2}$$

but for most purposes we will make our inferences on the log rate, because its distribution is more nearly normal for modest samples sizes, and

$$\text{Var}(\log \hat{\lambda}) = \frac{1}{n} \tag{4.3}$$

In setting confidence limits about an estimated failure rate, we will generally employ equation 4.3 to set the interval about the logarithm before summarizing the final results by taking the antilog.

Example 4–1 The Paris Prospective Study investigated the occurrence of myocardial infarction (MI) among male workers in the Paris city government (2). A total of 104 experienced an MI during a total of 47,179 person-years of follow-up, yielding the estimated rate

$$\hat{\lambda} = \frac{104}{47,179} = 22.0 \times 10^{-4}$$

which we read as 22 per 10,000 person-years. We can give an interval estimate for the rate by making use of the standard error of the log rate,

$$SE(\log \hat{\lambda}) = \sqrt{\frac{1}{104}} = 0.09806$$

so that a 95% confidence interval is given by

$$\hat{\lambda} \cdot \exp\{\pm z_{0.05/2} \cdot SE(\log \hat{\lambda})\} = 22.0 \times 10^{-4} \cdot \exp\{\pm 1.96 \times 0.09806\}$$
$$= (18.2, 26.7) \times 10^{-4}$$

Population rates

Summary rates provide a useful description of the overall experience of a population with respect to disease or mortality, and this may be estimated by

$$\hat{\lambda} = \frac{\text{Number of failures}}{\text{Mid-year population}}$$

$$= \frac{n}{D} \tag{4.4}$$

The numerator is a count of the number of outcome events that are observed, but the denominator is viewed as a fixed constant that is known without error. If we think of our population as undergoing dynamic changes in which people are constantly moving in and out, then the mid-year population may be thought of as an approximation to the total person-years' experience, so in that sense it is similar to the denominator considered in equation 4.1. However, in the situation we are now describing, the denominator is a fixed quantity while our earlier rationale made it a sum of random times, and in that sense it is fundamentally different. In the present context, the random aspect of equation 4.4 arises in the numerator, n. Brillinger (3) discussed a variety of stochastic models for the number of events in a population and showed that under fairly general conditions we can regard the distribution of n as Poisson with mean λD. Despite this somewhat different process for the mechanism giving rise to the data, the maximum likelihood estimate of λ is identical to what we saw in equation 4.1, and the variance formulae shown in equations 4.2 and 4.3 still apply.

Standardized ratios

Standardized mortality, or standardized morbidity, ratios (SMRs) compare the experience of a specified population with the experience of a standard population. For example, in a study of the mortality experience of workers in a Montana smelter, we might compare their mortality to that of the United States or to the entire state of Montana. We can begin by assuming that these workers are just like those in the general population when they started, so that if they are worse off then we can obtain a measure of the effect of their work environment.

A serious limitation of this approach is that the infirm would not be likely to obtain or even to seek such employment, so that typically workers in an occupation such as this start out healthier than the population as a whole. This "healthy worker effect" results in a bias in favor of workers, so that in general we would tend to underestimate any deleterious effect of a particular type of employment on the health of the workers.

The expected mortality experience of the ith worker depends on when they began employment, and we can trace that experience with a Lexis diagram, shown in Figure 4–2. Time must be considered from two perspectives, in that as a worker ages, chronological time is also passing, so that they would be expected to experience the same effects of changes in health care as the general population. If a worker's job did not affect risk of disease, then his expected mortality rate at age t would be the same as that of the general population, $\lambda_i^*(t)$. If the job did change risk by a proportional constant (4), however, the actual rate for the individual would be $\lambda_i(t) = \psi \cdot \lambda_i^*(t)$. The contribution of the ith individual, who was first employed at age t_{0i} and last observed at age t_{1i}, to the expected number of failures is given by the area under the appropriate standard rate curve, $\Lambda_i = \int_{t_{0i}}^{t_{1i}} \lambda_i^*(u)\, du$, and the total expected number of events is $E = \sum_i \Lambda_i$. Calculation of the expected number of failures is generally based on rates, which are typically tabulated on a rectangular grid in which age and calendar year are divided into 5- or 10-year categories, as shown in Figure 4–2. Notice

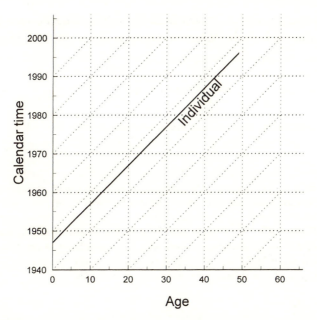

Figure 4-2 Lexis diagram representing the follow-up experience for an individual born in 1947.

that the diagonal line that traces the time course for an individual traverses different parts of the grid for varying lengths of time, so that we need to carefully determine the length of time that a particular rate applies to an individual. Let us represent the cutpoints in the observed time line by the set of points $\{\tau_{i0} = t_{0i}, \tau_{i1}, \tau_{i2}, \ldots, \tau_{i\mathcal{J}} = t_{1i})$, where $\lambda_{j,i}^{*}$ is the corresponding mortality or morbidity rate for the time interval $(\tau_{i,j-1}, \tau_{i,j}]$ which yields $E = \sum_{j=1}^{\mathcal{J}} (\tau_{j,i} - \tau_{j-1,i}) \cdot \lambda_{j}^{*}$. The maximum likelihood estimate of the relative magnitude of the hazard in the group of interest is

$$\hat{\psi} = \frac{n}{\sum_{i} E_{i}} \qquad (4.5)$$

where n is the observed number of failures and $\hat{\psi}$ is the estimated SMR (4). Notice that the form for the estimator is essentially the same as the one we saw in equation 4.1, only now the denominator cumulates the expected values, E_{i}, rather than the observed follow-up times. Otherwise, inference on the parameter remains essentially the same as before, and

$$\mathrm{Var}(\log \hat{\psi}) = \frac{1}{n}$$

A score test of H_0: $\psi = 1$ takes the familiar form of the Pearson chi-square statistic, which relates the observed and expected number of failures:

$$S^2 = \frac{(n - \Sigma_i E_i)^2}{\Sigma_i E_i} \qquad (4.6)$$

which is compared to a chi-square distribution with 1 df (4).

Example 4–2   Breslow et al. (5) describe the experience of 8,014 workers at a Montana smelter who had been employed for at least a year. Follow-up for each individual began at the end of the first year of employment or 1938, whichever was later, and recruitment continued through the end of 1956. By the end of follow-up in 1963, a total of 1,877 had died, 5,397 were withdrawn alive, and 773 had been lost to follow-up. Among workers who had been born in the United States, 75 had died, while 36.15 were expected to die, based on the mortality experience of the U.S. population. Hence, our estimate of the SMR is

$$\hat{\psi} = \frac{75}{36.15} = 2.07 \qquad (4.7)$$

The standard error of the log rate is $\sqrt{(1/75)}$, so that a 95% confidence interval for our estimate is

$$2.07 \cdot \exp\{\pm(1.96) \cdot \sqrt{1/75}\} = 2.07 \cdot \exp\{\pm 0.2263\} = (1.65, 2.60)$$

Finally, if we wish to conduct a score test of whether there is a significant excess mortality among these smelter works, we have

$$S^2 = \frac{(75 - 36.15)^2}{36.15} = 41.75$$

which is clearly significant when compared to chi-square with 1 df ($p < .0001$). Therefore, we have strong evidence to show that the mortality experience of these men is higher than that of the general population.

Comparing Nominal Groups

We now consider methods for comparing rates among different groups that are computationally relatively easy to conduct, and they are analogous to the methods we gave for proportions in Chapter 3. All three methods for constructing significance tests apply, and the formulae used in conducting the tests take a form that is similar to those seen earlier.

First, let us consider the comparison of just two groups, with hazards λ_1 and λ_2. Data have been summarized so that there are n_1 and n_2 failures with denominators D_1 and D_2, respectively, for each group. The measure of association we use in this discussion is the hazard ratio

$$\psi = \frac{\lambda_2}{\lambda_1}$$

so that the relationship between the hazards may be expressed as $\lambda_2 = \psi \cdot \lambda_1$. An alternative way of representing these two rates is to use a log-linear model

$$\lambda(X) = \exp\{\alpha + X\beta\} \tag{4.8}$$

in which the two groups are represented by a binary regressor variable, where $X = 0$ for group 1 and $X = 1$ for group 2. Hence, $\lambda_1 = \exp\{\alpha\}, \lambda_2 = \exp\{\alpha + \beta\}$ and the hazard ratio becomes

$$\psi = \frac{\exp\{\alpha + \beta\}}{\exp\{\alpha\}} = \exp\{\beta\}$$

We can see that the regression parameter, β, is equivalent to the log hazard ratio.

The maximum likelihood estimate for the hazard ratio is

$$\hat{\psi} = \frac{n_2 \cdot D_1}{n_1 \cdot D_2} \tag{4.9}$$

As in the case of the odds ratio, we shall work with the log hazard ratio in constructing significance tests and confidence intervals, because the distribution is less skewed, and

$$\mathrm{Var}(\log \hat{\psi}) = \mathrm{Var}(\hat{\beta}) = \frac{1}{n_1} + \frac{1}{n_2} \tag{4.10}$$

Thus, the Wald test of H_0: $\psi = 1$ or $\beta = 0$ is given by

$$W^2 = \frac{\hat{\beta}^2}{\mathrm{Var}(\hat{\beta})} \tag{4.11}$$

which is compared to a chi-square distribution with 1 df.

For an alternative test of the null hypothesis, H_0: $\psi = 1$ or $\beta = 0$, we can compute the expected number of failures in each category by allocat-

ing the total failures in direct proportion to the relative size of the denominators for the rates:

$$m_i = n_+ \cdot \left(\frac{D_i}{D_+} \right) \tag{4.12}$$

In this way we can obtain a likelihood ratio test by employing

$$G^2 = 2 \cdot \sum_i n_i \cdot \log\left(\frac{n_i}{m_i} \right) \tag{4.13}$$

which is compared to a chi-square distribution with 1 df. Similarly, we can
construct a score test from the familiar formula

$$S^2 = \sum_i \frac{(n_i - m_i)^2}{m_i} \tag{4.14}$$

which is also compared to a chi-square distribution with 1 df.

The score and likelihood ratio tests can immediately be generalized to
compare $I > 2$ groups, in order to test $H_0: \lambda_1 = \lambda_2 = \ldots = \lambda_I$. We can also
represent this hypothesis in terms of the hazard ratio, if we arbitrarily use
the first group as the reference, so that $H_0: \psi_2 = \ldots = \psi_I = 1$. In this case,
we can still use equation 4.12 to calculate the expected number of failures
in each groups, and then apply either equation 4.13 or 4.14, depending on
whether we wish to use the likelihood ratio or the score statistic. Either statistic is compared to a chi-square distribution with $I - 1$ df.

Example 4–1 (continued)   Continuing our consideration of the Paris Prospective
Study (2), a summary of some of the results are given in Table 4–1. In this study,
7,000 male employees of the Paris city government were followed, and the results
in this analysis are for those ages 43–53. The response of interest was the occurrence of a myocardial infarction (MI), and we are particularly interested in exploring the effect of leukocyte count, which is divided into three categories (<5,500;
5,500–6,799; ≥6,800). We are secondarily interested in the effect of cigarette smoking, because it has already been well established that smoking is associated with an
increased risk of heart disease. Hence, at some point we will be interested in controlling for this factor in our analysis. A somewhat peculiar five-level categorization
is reported here (never smoked, ex-smokers, noninhalers, partial or former inhalers,
and inhalers). However, in this first cut of the analysis for these data, we shall ignore this variable in order to look at the unadjusted effect, leaving the adjustment
for later.

If there truly is a steady trend in the risk of MI with leukocyte count, as suggested by the estimates of the failure rates, then the greatest difference would be

Table 4-1. Summary of results from the Paris Prospective Study, showing the number of myocardial infarctions, person-years follow-up, and the incidence rate by smoking status and leukocyte count (2)

	Leukocyte count/mm³ No./person-years (rate × 1000)		
Smoking status	<5,500	5,500–6,799	≥6,800
Never smoked	2/4,056 (0.5)	4/2,892 (1.4)	2/1,728 (1.2)
Ex-smoker	2/4,172 (0.5)	3/3,467 (0.9)	1/2,173 (0.5)
Noninhaler	7/4,616 (1.5)	6/3,835 (1.5)	6/3,102 (1.9)
Partial or former inhaler	2/888 (2.3)	5/1,101 (4.5)	2/1,674 (1.2)
Inhaler	6/2,456 (2.4)	10/3,740 (2.7)	46/7,269 (6.3)
Total	19/16,188 (1.2)	28/15,035 (1.9)	57/15,956 (3.6)

found between the lowest and the highest categories, so that we might first conduct a significance test comparing these two groups. Our estimate of the hazard ratio is

$$\hat{\psi} = \frac{57 \cdot 16,188}{19 \cdot 15,956} = 3.044$$

and the standard error of its logarithm is

$$SE(\log \hat{\psi}) = \sqrt{\frac{1}{19} + \frac{1}{57}} = 0.2649$$

We can construct a Wald test of the null hypothesis of no association between lymphocyte count and the rate of MIs, $H_0: \log(\psi) = \beta = 0$, by finding

$$W^2 = \left(\frac{\log(3.044)}{0.2649}\right)^2 = 4.2017^2 = 17.65$$

which is compared to a chi-square distribution (1 df, $p < .0001$). Alternatively, we can calculate a likelihood ratio statistics, making use of estimates of the expected frequencies in this two-category comparison:

$$\hat{m}_1 = \frac{(19 + 57) \cdot 16,188}{16,188 + 15,956} = 38.274, \qquad \hat{m}_2 = \frac{(19 + 57) \cdot 15,956}{16,188 + 15,956} = 37.726$$

yielding

$$G^2 = 2 \cdot \left[19 \cdot \log\left(\frac{19}{38.274}\right) + 57 \cdot \log\left(\frac{57}{37.726}\right) \right] = 20.44$$

Likewise, the corresponding score test becomes

$$S^2 = \left[\frac{(19 - 38.274)^2}{38.274} + \frac{(57 - 37.726)^2}{37.726} \right] = 19.55$$

both of which are compared to a chi-square distribution with 1 df, and both are highly significant if we were to employ the usual criteria for statistical significance.

Instead of only comparing the extreme categories, we can also conduct an overall test, comparing the MI rates across the three lymphocyte categories, thus testing H_0: $\lambda_1 = \lambda_2 = \lambda_3$, or, equivalently, H_0: $\log(\psi_2) = \log(\psi_3) = 0$. The relevant expected frequencies are shown in Table 4–2, and the likelihood ratio test becomes

$$G^2 = 2 \cdot \left[19 \cdot \log\left(\frac{19}{35.684}\right) + 28 \cdot \log\left(\frac{28}{33.143}\right) + 57 \cdot \log\left(\frac{57}{35.173}\right) \right] = 21.64$$

which we now compare to chi-square with 2 df ($p < .0001$), because there are two unique parameters under consideration in the null hypothesis. It is interesting to note that the magnitude of the statistic has changed little from what we obtained by just comparing the extreme categories, suggesting that our first analysis actually captured most of the trend for these data. The corresponding score statistic is

$$S^2 = \left[\frac{(19 - 35.684)^2}{35.684} + \frac{(28 - 33.143)^2}{33.143} + \frac{(57 - 35.173)^2}{35.173} \right] = 22.14$$

which is very similar to the value obtained for the likelihood ratio statistic, and our interpretation of the results is essentially the same.

Table 4–2. Worksheet for intermediate calculations for the trend test, using data from Table 4–1

$x_j{}^1$	$n_j{}^2$	$D_j{}^3$	$m_j{}^4$	$x_j n_j$	$x_j m_j{}^5$	$x_j D_j{}^5$	$x_j{}^2 D_j{}^5$
1	19	16,188	35.6844	19.0000	35.6844	16,188	16,188
2	28	15,035	33.1427	56.0000	66.2854	30,070	60,140
3	57	15,956	35.1729	171.0000	105.5188	47,868	143,604
Total	104	47,179	104.0000	246.0000	207.4886	94,126	219,932

[1] Exposure level.

[2] Observed number of failures.

[3] Total person-years of follow-up.

[4] Expected number of failures.

[5] Intermediate calculations for equation 4.15.

The methods we have described in this section can also be applied to the problem of comparing SMRs. Recall that the SMR already is an estimate of the ratio of two hazard functions, the hazard that applies to the study population and the hazard for the standard population, and we already gave a test for this quantity in equation 4.6. We now wish to test the equality of two SMRs—that is, $H_0: \psi_1 = \psi_2$, or $H_0: \psi_2/\psi_1 = 1$. The problem now has the same form as the one we used for rates, so we can test this null hypothesis using the same approach, as we shall see in the following example.

Example 4–2 (continued) If we continue our analysis of mortality among the Montana smelter workers (5), we might next wish to compare the experience of foreign-born workers with those born in the United States. The SMR among foreign-born workers is

$$\hat{\psi}_2 = \frac{67}{13.78} = 4.86$$

while equation 4.7 estimates $\hat{\psi}_1$. Hence, we estimate that the foreign-born workers have

$$\frac{\hat{\psi}_2}{\hat{\psi}_1} = \frac{67/13.78}{75/36.15} = 2.34$$

times the risk as similar U.S.-born workers at this smelter. Under the null hypothesis, $H_0: \psi_1 = \psi_2$, the expected number of deaths would be allocated in proportion to the number expected, based on the mortality experience for the standard population:

$$\hat{m}_1 = \frac{142 \cdot 36.15}{36.15 + 13.78} = 102.810 \qquad \hat{m}_2 = \frac{142 \cdot 13.78}{36.15 + 13.78} = 39.190$$

Thus, we can calculate the score test,

$$S^2 = \left[\frac{(75 - 102.810)^2}{102.810} + \frac{(67 - 39.190)^2}{39.190} \right] = 27.26$$

which we compare to a chi-square distribution with 1 df ($p < .0001$). This strongly suggests that the foreign-born workers are at an even higher mortality risk than are their U.S.-born counterparts. However, we need to conduct further analyses to see whether we can find reasons that might explain this difference. For example, the foreign-born workers may have been given jobs that exposed them to higher levels of toxic chemicals that were generated during the smelting processes.

Score Test for Trend

In the previous section we considered the comparison of groups that were represented by nominal categories, and no structure was imposed on the relationships among them. In cases where the categories give an ordinal measure of exposure, however, we can generally achieve greater power for a test of significance of an association if we are able to characterize the form for the relationship. Let us at first suppose that we can characterize the association between the rate for group j and the exposure measure, X_j, by a log-linear model in which

$$\lambda(X_j) = \exp\{\alpha + X_j \cdot \beta\}$$

Thus, we are proposing a linear relationship between the logarithm of the rate and exposure. The null hypothesis of no association, H_0: $\beta = 0$, can be tested by using the score statistic:

$$S^2 = \frac{(\sum_j x_j \cdot n_j - \sum_j x_j \cdot m_j)^2}{(n_+/D_+^2) \cdot [D_+ \cdot \sum_j x_j^2 D_j - (\sum_j x_j D_j)^2]} \tag{4.15}$$

which is compared to a chi-square distribution with 1 df (6).

Example 4–1 (continued)   Continuing our discussion of the data from the Paris Prospective Study (2), let us consider a test for trend across the three categories of leukocyte counts. Let the categories be represented by $x = 1, 2, 3$, shown in the first column of Table 4–2. Columns 2 and 3 give the numerator and denominator for the respective rates. The expected number of MIs for $X = 1$ is

$$m_1 = \frac{104 \cdot 16,188}{47,179} = 35.6844$$

and the other expected frequencies are calculated in a similar fashion. The remainder of the table contains a worksheet showing the intermediate calculations necessary for obtaining the relevant score statistic. Substituting into equation 4.15, we obtain

$$S^2 = \frac{(246 - 207.4886)^2}{(104/(47,179)^2) \cdot [(47,179)(219,932) - (94,126)^2]}$$

$$= 20.93$$

which we compare to chi-square with 1 df ($p < .0001$). Notice that this is only slightly smaller than the test with 2 df, which we obtained when we treated leukocyte as nominal categories. In this case, the trend is so great that both tests are highly significant, but in situations where the results are not so clear cut, an appropriate trend test can yield considerably more power, especially when there are many categories that provide greater leverage at the extreme exposures.

Stratification

We now consider the problem of comparing rates between two groups, controlling for one or more covariates by stratification, thus extending the Cochran (7) and Mantel–Haenszel (8) tests for proportions to the analysis of rates. The rate for the ith ($i = 1,2$) group in the jth ($j = 1, \ldots, \mathcal{J}$) stratum is given by λ_{ij}, which we assume takes the form

$$\lambda_{1j} = \exp\{\alpha_j\} \tag{4.16}$$

$$\lambda_{2j} = \exp\{\alpha_j + \beta\}$$

Notice that under this form for the model, the stratum-specific hazard ratios are constant over the strata

$$\psi_j = \frac{\lambda_{2j}}{\lambda_{1j}} = \exp\{\beta\}$$

in much the same way that we assumed the odds ratio was identical for all strata when we developed the Cochran and Mantel–Haenszel statistics. We can express the null hypothesis that the groups have identical rates by considering, $H_0: \beta = 0$.

A score test that the common hazard ratio across strata is one is given by

$$S^2 = \frac{[\sum_j (n_{2j} - n_{+j} P_{2j})]^2}{\sum_j n_{+j} P_{2j}[1 - P_{2j}]} \tag{4.17}$$

where $P_{ij} = D_{ij}/D_{+j}$, the proportion of the denominator total for the jth stratum that is observed in group i. With this modification to the calculation of the proportions, it is interesting that the form for the test statistic is otherwise identical to the statistic given by Cochran (7) for proportions.

Example 4–1 (continued) We have already seen a very strong association between the risk of MI and leukocyte count in the data from the Paris Prospective Study (2). However, it is also important to notice in Table 4–1 that there is a considerable imbalance in the distribution of follow-up experience among the leukocyte categories by smoking status. For example, we see that among those who never

Table 4–3. Worksheet for intermediate calculations for the test combining information across strata, using data from Table 4–1

Strata[1]	$n_{1j}{}^2$	$D_{1j}{}^2$	$n_{2j}{}^2$	$D_{2j}{}^2$	$m_{2j} = n_{+j} - \pi_{2j}$ [3]	Var_j [3]
1	2	4,056	2	1,728	1.1950	0.8380
2	2	4,172	1	2,183	1.0305	0.6765
3	7	4,616	6	3,102	5.2249	3.1249
4	2	888	2	1,674	2.6136	0.9059
5	6	2,456	46	7,269	38.8677	9.8158
Total			57		48.9317	15.3612

[1] Smoking status categories.

[2] Required elements from Table 4–1.

[3] Intermediate calculations for equation 4.17.

smoked, the total person-years of follow-up is greatest for the low leukocyte category, and for the inhalers the most follow-up is seen in the highest category. It is well known that cigarette smoking is associated with risk of MI; in fact, we can see evidence for that association in Table 4–1. Hence, we might ask whether the effect of leukocyte count is still seen after adjustment for the cigarette smoking categories.

The relevant stratum-specific data in Table 4–1 are extracted into Table 4–3, which forms the basis for a worksheet for making the relevant intermediate calculations for the score test by combining information across strata. From these values we can calculate the expected number of MIs in group 2 for the first stratum by

$$m_{21} = \frac{(2 + 2) \cdot 1,728}{(4,056 + 1,728)} = 1.1950$$

and the corresponding variance for the observed number of cases is

$$Var_1 = \frac{(2 + 2) \cdot 4,056 \cdot 1,728}{(4,056 + 1,728)^2} = 0.8380$$

If we make similar calculations for the other strata, we can obtain the necessary totals for the test that combines information over the strata by substitution into equation 4.17:

$$S^2 = \frac{[57 - 48.9317]^2}{15.3612} = 4.24$$

which is compared to chi-square with 1 df ($p = .0395$). Hence, we see that the association remains statistically significant, although the strength of the evidence has diminished considerably from the unadjusted analysis.

The information on cigarette smoking has explained some, but not all, of the observed association between MI and leukocyte count. This particular form for collecting exposure to cigarettes is unusual, and we might wonder whether data on the number of cigarettes smoked would be even more strongly associated with the outcome, thus explaining even more of the effect of leukocyte count. We might also carefully consider the implications of this analysis. Cigarette smoking could independently affect both leukocyte count and the physiological factors that lead to an MI. Alternatively, leukocyte count could be indicative of an intermediate step in the mechanism by which cigarette smoking leads to an increased risk of MI. Either way, we would expect a similar result from making these calculations on the available data, and further work is needed to better understand the process that gave rise to them.

Summary Rates

Summary rates offer a common way of summarizing a set of rates among groups that have been stratified on some well-known risk factor that is not of particular interest for the immediate study objectives. Age, for example, is such a variable because it is generally associated with disease risk and thus should not be ignored. Suppose we are interested in comparing incidence rates among different geographic regions; it would be important to be sure that our summary statistic adjusts for any differences in the age distributions that might occur among regions. It is common to relate such a summary to a hypothetical population that represents a standard basis for comparison.

For purposes of this discussion, let us assume that the log-linear model for a rate is true, so that we can represent equation 4.16 in terms of a multiplicative model,

$$\lambda_{ij} = \psi_i \cdot \theta_j \tag{4.18}$$

where $I(=1, \ldots, I)$ represents the groups to be compared, $j(=1, \ldots, \mathcal{J})$ the strata to be controlled, and $\sum_i \log(\psi_i) = 0$. In addition, let D_{ij} represent the relevant population size or person-years experience for the (i,j) group. Following the argument by Freeman and Holford (9), the simplest summary is the *crude rate*, which is the ratio of the total number of cases divided by the total of the denominators, and is thus not adjusted for strata. The expected value for the crude rate is

$$\bar{\lambda}_{Ci} = \frac{m_{i+}}{D_{i+}} = \frac{\sum_j D_{ij} \cdot \psi_i \cdot \theta_j}{\sum_j D_{ij}} = \psi_i \cdot \bar{\theta}_{i\cdot} \tag{4.19}$$

where $\bar{\theta}_{i\cdot}$ is a weighted average of the stratum effects. If we wish to compare two regions by taking the ratio of crude rates, we obtain

$$\frac{\bar{\lambda}_{Ci}}{\bar{\lambda}_{Ci^*}} = \left(\frac{\psi_i}{\psi_{i^*}}\right) \cdot \left(\frac{\bar{\theta}_{i\cdot}}{\bar{\theta}_{i^*\cdot}}\right)$$

which does not only reflect the ratio of the group parameters, ψ_i/ψ_i^*, but also the weighted means of the stratum effects. Hence, this summary is biased by a factor that reflects differences in the age distribution among the groups, and thus it is not a useful summary statistic.

The crude rate can be seen as a weighted average of the stratum-specific rates, and the bias results from the fact that we are using a different set of weights for each comparison group. One solution is to use an identical set of weights, derived to reflect the distribution in a standard population. If we are making comparisons among different regions of the United States, we might use the population in a particular year, say 1970. Alternatively, international comparisons often make use of an international standard population, which is designed to more nearly reflect the age distribution of the world. If we let D_{Sj} represent the standard population size for the jth stratum, then we can use as a summary statistic

$$\bar{\lambda}_{Di} = \frac{\sum_j D_{Si} \cdot \psi_i \cdot \theta_j}{\sum_j D_{Sj}} = \psi_i \cdot \bar{\theta}_S. \tag{4.20}$$

which is the *direct adjusted rate*. The variance of an estimated direct adjusted rate is

$$\text{Var}(\bar{\lambda}_{Di}) = \left(\frac{1}{D_{S+}}\right)^2 \cdot \sum_j \frac{(D_{Si}\lambda_{ij})^2}{n_{ij}}$$

We generally use the log rate in setting confidence intervals and conducting Wald tests, and its variance is

$$\text{Var}(\log\bar{\lambda}_{Di}) = \left(\frac{1}{\bar{\lambda}_{Di}}\right)^2 \cdot \text{Var}(\bar{\lambda}_{Di})$$

If we wish to compare two groups, then we may take the ratio of two direct adjusted rates,

$$\frac{\bar{\lambda}_{Di}}{\bar{\lambda}_{Di^*}} = \frac{\psi_i}{\psi_i^*}$$

By using a common standard, the direct adjusted rate has avoided the bias that we found in the crude rate, so this clearly offers a better summary of the results (9).

In calculating the direct adjusted rates, we employed a common standard population distribution to the rates for the different groups, but suppose we instead used a standard set of rates in making the adjustment. If

λ_{Sj} is the standard rate for the jth stratum, the *indirect adjusted rate* is the ratio of the observed cases in the ith group to the expected number based on the standard set of rates:

$$\bar{\lambda}_{Ii} = \frac{n_{i+}}{\sum_j D_{ij} \cdot \lambda_{Sj}} = \frac{\sum_j D_{ij} \cdot \lambda_{ij}}{\sum_j D_{ij} \cdot \lambda_{Sj}} \tag{4.21}$$

If we assume that the number of cases in the jth stratum has a Poisson distribution, then the total overall strata is also Poisson, and by making the additional assumption that the standard rates are given without error, we can obtain the variance:

$$\text{Var}(\bar{\lambda}_{Ii}) = \frac{n_{i+}}{\left(\sum_j D_{ij}\lambda_{Sj}\right)^2}$$

The variance of its logarithm is

$$\text{Var}(\log \bar{\lambda}_{Ii}) = \frac{1}{n_{i+}}$$

To give the magnitude for this summary, it is sometimes multiplied by the crude rate for the standard population; otherwise, the summary is primarily used as relative measure of the difference between the ith group and the standard. In that sense, we can see a clear relationship with the SMR given in equation 4.5. To eliminate bias when comparing ratios of indirect adjusted rates, it is necessary for the standard rates to belong to the same multiplicative model as the groups to be compared (9); thus, $\lambda_{Sj} = \psi_S \cdot \theta_j$. Hence, the indirect summary rate becomes

$$\bar{\lambda}_{Ii} = \frac{\sum_j D_{ij} \cdot \psi_i \cdot \theta_j}{\sum_j D_{ij} \cdot \psi_S \cdot \theta_j} = \frac{\psi_i}{\psi_S} \tag{4.22}$$

and we can see that ratios of these statistics directly measure ratios of the group effects, ψ_i/ψ_i^*.

Direct adjusted rates are often preferred by practitioners because they are more easily understood, reflecting as they do the hypothetical experience of populations that have identical distributions over the strata. In addition, the indirect adjustment requires an additional assumption that the standard rates belong to the same multiplicative class. However, the indirect adjustment method does offer other strengths that give it a practical advantage in some circumstances. Notice, for example, that the numerator in equation 4.22 is the observed number of cases for the ith group, which is the only disease-related data necessary for calculating this summary rate of a population. Sometimes, stratum-specific numerators are unavailable for a population, making it impossible to calculate the individual rates, but all that is required for calculating the indirect adjusted rate is the total number of cases, which can be especially helpful when systems for collecting vital statistics are not highly developed. More important, the indirect adjusted rate is related to the maximum likelihood estimate of the group effect (10), which brings to the group comparisons better optimality properties in terms of generally smaller variances. This can be especially important when one is dealing with relatively small populations or rare diseases in which there are few cases of the outcome of interest.

Example 4–3 Mantel and Stark (11) present the data displayed in Table 4–4 on rates of Down syndrome per birth in Michigan from 1950 to 1964. Of particular interest is the effect of birth order on the risk, and as we can see in Table 4–4, the

Table 4–4. Number of Down syndrome births, number of live births, and rate of Down syndrome in Michigan from 1950 to 1964, by maternal age and and birth order (11)

| Maternal age | Birth order | | | | | |
	1	2	3	4	5+	Total
NO. OF DOWN SYNDROME BIRTHS						
<20	107	25	3	1	0	136
20–24	141	150	71	26	8	396
25–29	60	110	114	64	63	411
30–34	40	84	103	89	112	428
35–39	39	82	108	137	262	628
40+	25	39	75	96	295	530
Total	412	490	474	413	740	2,529
NO. OF LIVE BIRTHS						
<20	230,061	72,202	15,050	2,293	327	319,933
20–24	329,449	326,701	175,702	68,800	30,666	931,318
25–29	114,920	208,667	207,081	132,424	123,419	786,511
30–34	39,487	83,228	117,300	98,301	149,919	488,235
35–39	14,208	28,466	45,026	46,075	104,088	237,863
40+	3,052	5,375	8,660	9,834	34,392	61,313
Total	731,177	724,639	568,819	357,727	442,811	2,825,173
RATE OF DOWN SYNDROME BIRTHS 10,000 BIRTHS						
<20	4.65	3.46	1.99	4.36	0.00	4.25
20–24	4.28	4.59	4.04	3.78	2.61	4.25
25–29	5.22	5.27	5.51	4.83	5.10	5.23
30–34	10.13	10.09	8.78	9.05	7.47	8.77
35–39	27.45	28.81	23.99	29.73	25.17	26.40
40+	81.91	72.56	86.61	97.62	85.78	86.44
Total	5.63	6.76	8.33	11.55	16.71	8.95

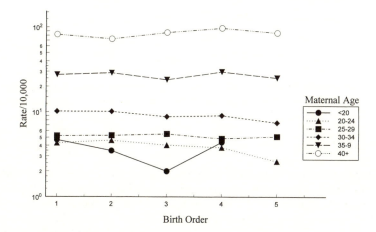

Figure 4–3 Rate of Down syndrome per 10,000 live births in Michigan from 1950 to 1964, by birth order and maternal age.

overall or crude rates of Down syndrome steadily increase with birth order. However, it is also well known that maternal age affects the risk of Down syndrome, and we can also see from these data that older women are more likely to have had previous births, as we would expect. Thus, we need to make an adjustment for age when presenting a summary of the results. In a later chapter, we shall describe a more formal test of whether the rates behave in a way that we might expect based on a log-linear model, but for now let us consider a graphical approach to the question by plotting the age-specific rates against birth order using a log scale for the vertical axis, as shown in Figure 4–3. We would expect the lines to be parallel under this model, and the departures from that assumption do not appear to be seriously violated in these data, except perhaps for the youngest ages. Notice that the estimated rate of 0 for birth order 5+ in the youngest age group does not appear because its logarithm is undefined. Small numbers of cases also result in less precision for the log rate, so that we would expect greater variation in the higher birth orders in the younger maternal ages because of the small number of cases, so that the departure from parallelism may be due, at least in part, to random variation.

To compute the direct adjusted rate for birth order 1, we shall use the total number of births by age, giving

$$\lambda_{D1} = [(319{,}933)(4.65) + (931{,}318)(4.28) + \cdots + (61{,}313)(81.91)]/(2{,}825{,}173)$$

$$= 9.23$$

and its variance is

$$\text{Var}(\lambda_{D1}) = \frac{\left[\dfrac{(319{,}933)^2(4.65)^2}{107} + \dfrac{(931{,}318)^2(4.28)^2}{141} + \cdots + \dfrac{(61{,}313)^2(81.91)^2}{25}\right]}{(2{,}825{,}173)^2}$$

$$= 0.3919$$

We can calculate the standard error for the log rate by

$$SE[\log(\lambda_{D1})] = \frac{\sqrt{0.3919}}{9.23} = 0.068$$

Using similar calculations for the other groups, we can obtain the estimates and the corresponding standard errors for the other birth order, and these are shown in Table 4–5. Also shown are the differences in log rates, which we call the effect in relation to birth order 1, along with the corresponding standard errors and a Wald test. None are significant except for birth order 5+ in which we see a lower rate than in birth order 1.

To illustrate the calculation of the indirect adjusted rate, we use as the standard rates the overall age-specific rates from these data. In general, this marginal rate will violate the requirement that the standard rate belongs to the same class of multiplicative models as the individual rates that have been combined in its formation. This will result in some bias in the estimated effect, but the bias is usually small. The indirect adjusted rate for birth order 1 is

$$\lambda_{I1} = \frac{412}{[(230,061)(4.25) + (329,449)(4.25) + \cdots + (3,052)(86.44)]/10,000}$$

$$= 1.039$$

and the standard error of its logarithm is

$$SE(\log\lambda_{I1}) = \sqrt{1/412} = 0.049$$

Similar calculations can be made on the other birth orders, and these are displayed in Table 4–5. Notice that the standard error for the effects are generally slightly

Table 4–5. Direct and indirect adjusted rates of Down syndrome by birth order for the data in Table 4–4

	Birth order				
Summary statistic	1	2	3	4	5+
DIRECT ADJUSTED					
Rate	9.23	9.12	8.51	9.27	7.55
log(Rate)	2.223	2.210	2.141	2.227	2.022
(SD)	0.068	0.051	0.048	0.073	0.054
Effect ($\log[\bar{\lambda}_{Di}/\bar{\lambda}_{D1}]$)	0	−0.012	−0.082	0.004	−0.201
(SD)	—	0.085	0.083	0.099	0.087
Wald test	—	−0.146	−0.979	0.045	−2.308
p-value	—	0.884	0.327	0.964	0.021
INDIRECT ADJUSTED					
Rate	1.039	1.035	0.976	1.053	0.947
log(Rate)	0.039	0.035	−0.025	0.052	−0.054
(SD)	0.049	0.045	0.046	0.049	0.037
Effect ($\log[\bar{\lambda}_{Ii}/\bar{\lambda}_{I1}]$)	0	−0.004	−0.063	0.013	−0.093
(SD)	—	0.067	0.067	0.070	0.061
Wald test	—	−0.055	−0.939	0.187	−1.508
p-value	—	0.956	0.348	0.851	0.132

smaller for the indirect adjusted method, which we might expect because it is more closely related to the maximum likelihood estimator for the effect, and hence more nearly optimal.

While we saw a positive association between birth order and the rate of Down syndrome in the crude rates, that disappeared when we adjusted for maternal age. In fact, there was a suggestion of a lower rate for birth order 5+ when compared to birth order 1. Hence, we have fairly strong evidence that the trend for the crude rates is due to confounding with the much stronger effect of maternal age. In a later chapter, we will be able to more formally investigate the simultaneous effect of birth order and maternal age. Even though the standard error is smaller for the indirect adjusted rate, the comparison of birth order 5+ with birth order 1 achieves statistical significance for the direct adjusted rate, while the indirect does not. This reflects the relatively small point estimate of the direct adjusted summary rates that resulted from a greater weight being placed on the rates in the younger ages. The model for the effect of maternal age and birth order on the rates of Down syndrome is rather critical here, so it could be useful to explore this in greater detail when we consider more formal regression methods.

Summary

Rates can arise from a variety of stochastic mechanisms, including the occurrence of events in time and space. If the outcome is time to the occurrence of a failure, then a constant hazard or an exponential distribution of the failure times is required if we are to obtain a reasonable summary of a set of data using failure rates. Alternatively, rates may arise from counts of the number of events occurring in a defined geographic region, which are assumed to have a Poisson distribution with a mean that is proportional to the midyear population. Either mechanism gives rise to identical formulae for estimating the rates and conducting fundamental significance tests.

In this chapter we have seen methods for testing hypotheses comparing two or more rates, testing for trend, and combining rates over different strata. These methods are directly analogous to methods for analyzing proportions that we saw in Chapter 3; in fact, in several instances, we could observe certain similarities between the formulae for the methods. The methods were more similar to the unconditional methods of inference because we employed unconditional approaches when we established the rationale for the methods. We might expect similar limitation to those we saw in our study of proportions, and we should be especially careful about employing these formulae in situations where the number of events is small. This can be especially easy to overlook when combining large numbers of strata, each of which contains tiny numbers of events, thus resembling the situation that gives rise to a matched design for proportions.

Finally, we discussed the direct and indirect methods for calculating summary rates. We saw that either method could be used to give a reasonable summary of a common multiplicative effect, although the indirect method required an additional assumption that the standard rates also conform to the same underlying multiplicative model. The method of direct adjustment is often preferred by practitioners because it is more readily interpreted, but the indirect method appears to offer greater precision and power when it is appropriate to use. We shall see in our discussion of model fitting that with this approach we can capture a summary that is directly interpretable while preserving the optimal properties of our summary rates.

Exercises

4.1. Laird and Olivier (12) present data from a study of survival following heart valve replacement and the results are tabulated here:

| | | Type of heart valve | |
Age	Item	Aortic	Mitral
<55	Deaths	4	1
	Total months exposed	1,259	2,082
55+	Deaths	7	9
	Total months exposed	1,417	1,647

   a. Test whether there is a significant difference in survival by type of valve, adjusting for age.
   b. Calculate the age-specific death rates and the age-specific relative risks found in this study.
   c. Give the assumptions on which your test in (a) is based. In each instance, either show how you would determine that the assumption was appropriate or describe a further analysis that you might do with more time or more complete data.

4.2. The data in the following table are from a study of patients with advanced breast cancer treated at Guy's Hospital, London (1). There are three factors of interest: type of operation (adrenalectomy or hypophysectomy); type of mastectomy (none, simple, or radical); and age (−40, 41–45, 46–50, or 51–55). Shown in the table are the number of deaths and the person-days of follow-up (in parentheses).

Type of	Age			
mastectomy	−40	41–45	46–50	51–55
ADRENELECTOMY				
None	3	7	8	19
	(522)	(1,355)	(790)	(9,421)
Simple	4	4	1	1
	(3,071)	(796)	(273)	(752)
Radical	12	17	15	18
	(4,756)	(7,529)	(6,033)	(10,328)
HYPOPHYSECTOMY				
None	4	8	7	13
	(2,392)	(4,804)	(3,551)	(4,068)
Simple	6	3	1	2
	(2,616)	(1,905)	(1,172)	(862)
Radical	6	18	8	13
	(6,352)	(7,105)	(6,960)	(8,509)

   a. Estimate the unadjusted rate ratio for adrenalectomy compared to hypophysectomy, and then provide a 95% confidence limit for this estimate.

   b. Compute a score test comparing the relative risk for adrenalectomy with hypophysectomy, controlling for age and type of mastectomy.

4.3. This example makes use of data from a clinical trial for hypernephroma. A listing of the variables are shown below, and a copy of the data is stored on the web site in a dataset named TRIAL.DAT. Each item is coded as follows:

ITEM	DESCRIPTION
1	Patient number
2	Sex (1, male; 2, female)
3	Age in years
4	Nephrectomy (0, no; 1, yes)
5	Treatment (1, combined chemotherapy and immunotherapy; 2, others)
6	Response to therapy (0, no response; 1, complete response; 2, partial response; 3, stable; 4, increasing disease; 9, unknown)
7	Survival time
8	Status (0, alive; 1, dead)
9	Lung metastasis (0, no; 1, yes)
10	Bone metastasis (0, no; 1, yes)

    a. Estimate the mortality rates for each treatment group.
    b. Give an estimate of the rate ratio, along with a 90% confidence interval.
    c. Estimate the mortality rates broken down by treatment, gender, and nephrectomy.
    d. Estimate the rate ratio for treatment, controlling for gender and nephrectomy. Did the adjustment for gender and nephrectomy change the estimated effect of treatment? Why?

4.4. Doria et al. (13) conducted a study to evaluate the risk of a second cancer among Hodgkin's disease patients after cancer treatment. Tabulated below are the observed number of second primary cancers broken down by type of treatment. Also shown are the expected number of cancers, based on incidence rates from the Connecticut Tumor Registry.

Treatment	No. of cancers	
	Observed	Expected
Radiation	6	4.386
Combined Modality Therapy	19	4.635
All patients	25	9.021

    a. Find the standardized mortality ratio (SMR), and test whether there is evidence for an increased risk of a second cancer:
       i. In all patients
      ii. Within each treatment group
    b. Give a test of whether the SMR is the same for each treatment group, and discuss its implications.
    c. Describe a model under which the SMRs calculated in (a) and (b) give a reasonable summary of these data.

References

1. Atkins H, Bulbrook RD, Falconer MA, Hayward JL, MacLean KS, Schurr PH. Ten years' experience of sterioid assays in the management of breast cancer: a review. *Lancet* 1968;2:1255–1260.
2. Zalokar JB, Richard JL, Claude JR. Leukocyte count, smoking, and myocardial infarction. *New England Journal of Medicine* 1981;304:465–468.
3. Brillinger DT. The natural variability of vital rates and associated statistics. *Biometrics* 1986;42:693–734.
4. Breslow N. Some statistical models useful in the study of occupational mortality. In: A. Whittamore (ed.) *Environmental Health: Quantitative Methods*, pp. 88–103. Philadelphia: SIAM, 1977.
5. Breslow NE, Lubin JH, Marek P, Langholz B. Multiplicative models and cohort analysis. *Journal of the American Statistical Association* 1983;78:1–12.
6. Armitage P. Test for linear trend in proportions and frequencies. *Biometrics* 1955;11:375–386.

7. Cochran WG. Some methods for strengthening the common χ^2 tests. *Biometrics* 1954;10:417–451.
8. Mantel N, Haenszel W. Statistical aspects of the analysis of data from retrospective studies of disease. *Journal of the National Cancer Institute* 1959;22: 719–748.
9. Freeman DH, Holford TR. Summary rates. *Biometrics* 1980;36:195–205.
10. Breslow NE, Day NE. Indirect standardization and multiplicative models for rates, with reference to the age adjustment of cancer incidence and relative frequency data. *Journal of Chronic Diseases* 1975;28:289–303.
11. Mantel N, Stark CR. Computation of indirect-adjusted rates in the presence of confounding. *Biometrics* 1968;24:997–1005.
12. Laird N, Olivier D. Covariance analysis of censored survival data using loglinear analysis techniques. *Journal of the American Statistical Association* 1981;76: 231–240.
13. Doria R, Holford TR, Farber LR, Prosnitz LR, Cooper DL. Second solid malignancies after combined modality therapy for Hodgkin's disease. *Journal of Clinical Oncology* 1995;13:2016–2022.

5

Analysis of Time to Failure

We have so far considered the analysis of cohort data in which subjects were all followed for the same length of time or else the hazard was assumed to be a constant over time. These are clearly not realistic assumptions in general, so it is important that we have the ability to relax such restrictive assumptions. In this chapter we consider methods that are directed toward making inferences on the survival distribution, which can be more easily handled using methods that do not require severe parametric assumptions. As we shall see, these can provide us with tools for checking the validity of the assumptions used in dealing with highly parametric methods, and they also provide their own non-parametric methods of inference.

Estimating Survival Curves

We first consider the problem of estimating the survival function in a manner that does not simply involve taking a function of parameters in a particular distribution. Some of the original ideas for this statistical problem go back to the work of John Graunt, who in 1662 published his "Observations upon Bills of Mortality" which sought to understand the distribution for the length of human life (1). The actuarial method is closely related to approaches used in demography, and while it is not optimal in the same way as the other methods we discuss, it does work reasonably well, especially when dealing with large data files, such as those provided by vital statistics registries. The piecewise constant method is a direct extension of the idea of constant hazards, in that the hazard is assumed to be a constant during a particular interval of time but may vary from interval to interval. Finally, we consider the product limit method that is completely nonparametric, as well as a maximum likelihood estimate of the survival function.

Actuarial estimate

In this method for estimating the survival function, the period of follow-up is divided into intervals using cutpoints, as shown in Figure 5–1. Let x_i ($i = 0, \ldots I$) be the ith cutpoint, where $x_0 = 0$. A total of l_i individuals may enter an interval alive and be under active follow-up at that point in time. Of these, d_i will die before the next interval, thus resulting in a complete observation. Alternatively, the time of recruitment and the end of the study may result in an individual being withdrawn alive before the end of the interval, which occurs to w_i subjects. The final type of observation that can arise occurs when a subject is lost to follow-up at a point that lies within an interval, which happens to u_i subjects. These last two outcomes are incomplete or censored observations, and in a sense they are essentially only a partial observation of what occurred to a subject during an interval. As noted in Chapter 4, observations that are lost to follow-up are of greater concern because of the possible bias that can result when the reason for the loss is related to the outcome. The method, however, assumes that they are unrelated, so for purposes of these calculations it is only necessary to consider the total number of censored individuals, $W_i = w_i + u_i$. Because dying or being censored exhausts the possible survival events that can occur to a subject during an interval, the number entering the next interval is given by $l_{i+1} = l_i - d_i - W_i$.

A fundamental quantity that we estimate for an interval is the probability of dying for an individual who enters the interval alive, q_i. The obvious estimate when all observations are complete, $W_i = 0$, is the proportion who die, $\hat{q}_i = d_i/l_i$. As the censored observations only represent partial observations, it has been suggested on somewhat heuristic grounds that they should only be counted as $\frac{1}{2}$ of a complete observation (2). This gives rise to a hypothetical quantity referred to as the "effective number at risk," in which we reduce the number entering an interval alive by $\frac{1}{2}$ for each individual who is censored in the interval, $l_i' = l_i - \frac{1}{2} \cdot W_i$. Thus, the estimate of the proportion dying becomes, $\hat{q}_i = d_i/l_i'$.

The final step in the actuarial calculation requires that we use the probability of surviving an interval, given that a subject entered the interval

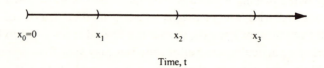

Time, t

Figure 5–1 Division of follow-up time into intervals for actuarial estimate.

alive, $p_i = 1 - q_i$, which is estimated by $\hat{p}_i = 1 - \hat{q}_i$. Survival to x_i requires survival of each preceding interval, so that

$$\mathscr{F}_i = \Pr\{\text{Alive at } x_1 \mid \text{Alive at } x_0\} \times \Pr\{\text{Alive at } x_2 \mid \text{Alive at } x_1\} \times \cdots$$

$$\times \Pr\{\text{Alive at } x_i \mid \text{Alive at } x_{i-1}\}$$

$$= p_0 \, p_1 \cdots p_{i-1}$$

$$= \prod_{j=0}^{i-1} p_j$$

and the estimate is found by substituting the estimator for p_i. An approximate variance estimate is provided by Greenwood's formula (3)

$$\text{Var}(\hat{\mathscr{F}}_i) = \mathscr{F}_i^2 \sum_{j=0}^{i-1} \left(\frac{1}{l'_j - d_j} - \frac{1}{l'_j} \right)$$

This can be used to construct confidence intervals or significance tests at specified times by applying the normal approximation when the total number of observations is reasonably large and the estimates are not too close to the 0/1 boundary.

The somewhat ad hoc basis in which we arrived at the quantity l'_i and the fact that it was not derived using a rigorous development should give us pause. A study of the properties of the actuarial estimate by Breslow and Crowley (4) revealed that in practice the estimator behaved reasonably well, provided that one was careful in selecting a sufficient number of interval cutpoints. Bias in this estimator can be reduced by choosing more interval cutpoints, and they indicate that the bias is usually negligible if one chooses at least 10 to 15 intervals.

Example 5–1 Table 5–1 gives remission times from a study of two treatments for leukemia patients (5). Subjects were randomly assigned to two groups: the first was a placebo-treated control group, and the second were given the drug 6-mercap-

Table 5–1. Remission times (weeks) for 21 control and 21 6-MP treated leukemia patients (5)

Treatment	Remission time (weeks) by subject
Control	1, 1, 2, 2, 3, 4, 4, 5, 5, 8, 8, 8, 8, 11, 11, 12, 12, 15, 17, 22, 23
6-MP	6*, 6, 6, 6, 7, 9*, 10*, 10, 11*, 13, 16, 17*, 19*, 20*, 22, 23, 25*, 32*, 32*, 34*, 35*

* Censored observation (subject in remission at time of last follow-up).

topurine (6-MP). An asterisk is used to indicate that a subject was still in remission at the time of last follow-up—that is, a censored observation. Hence, we see that all of the controls are complete observations, but 12 in the 6-MP group are incomplete or censored observations.

To illustrate the calculations for the actuarial life table, let us consider subjects in the 6-MP group. The first step is to divide the follow-up time into intervals, in order to tabulate the data by whether the observed length of follow-up ended with a failure. We shall use 3-week intervals, which results in a total of nine intervals, which is close to the Breslow–Crowley rule of thumb. Table 5–2 gives the number of failures in each interval, d_i, along with the number censored, W_i. There are a total of 21 observations in this group, all of which enter the first interval, $l_1 = 21$. By subtracting the number of failures or losses that occur in each interval, we obtain the number who enter alive into the next interval, thus $l_3 = 21 - 3 - 1 = 17$, and the remaining elements of the column labeled l_i are similarly obtained.

Once the raw tabulations have been obtained, we can determine the effective number at risk, $l_2' = 21 - \frac{1}{2}(1) = 20.5$. We can now obtain our estimate of the conditional probability of surviving the second interval, given that a subject entered the interval alive:

$$\hat{p}_2 = 1 - \frac{3}{20.5} = 0.8537$$

The survival curve starts at 1, or $\hat{\mathcal{F}}_0 = 1$, and successive estimates can be obtained by the recursive use of $\hat{\mathcal{F}}_i = \hat{p}_i \cdot \hat{\mathcal{F}}_{i-1}$. Hence, $\hat{\mathcal{F}}_3 = (0.8537) \cdot (0.9394) = 0.8019$,

Table 5–2. Calculations for the actuarial lifetable using the data from 6-MP-treated patients in Table 5–1

Interval	d_i[1]	W_i[2]	l_i[3]	l_i'[4]	$\hat{p}_i$[5]	$\hat{\mathcal{F}}_i$[6]	SD($\hat{\mathcal{F}}_i$)
(0,3][7]	0	0	21	21.0	1.0000	1.0000	0.0000
(3,6]	3	1	21	20.5	0.8537	0.8537	0.0781
(6,9]	1	1	17	16.5	0.9394	0.8019	0.0888
(9,12]	1	2	15	14.0	0.9286	0.7446	0.0993
(12,15]	1	0	12	12.0	0.9167	0.6826	0.1087
(15,18]	1	1	11	10.5	0.9048	0.6176	0.1161
(18,21]	0	2	9	8.0	1.0000	0.6176	0.1161
(21,24]	2	0	7	7.0	0.7143	0.4411	0.1342
(24,27]	0	1	5	4.5	1.0000	0.4411	0.1342

[1] Number of remissions.

[2] Number censored.

[3] Number under follow-up at beginning of interval.

[4] Effective number at risk.

[5] Estimated condition survival probability.

[6] Survival probability.

[7] Open-closed interval, for example 3 included in this interval but not in the line below.

and the remaining elements in this column are obtained in a similar way. Finally, we can obtain an estimated variance for our estimate:

$$\text{Var}(\hat{\mathscr{F}}_3) = (0.8019)^2 \cdot \left[\left(\frac{1}{21.0 - 0} - \frac{1}{21.0} \right) \right.$$

$$\left. + \left(\frac{1}{20.5 - 3} - \frac{1}{20.5} \right) + \left(\frac{1}{16.5 - 1} - \frac{1}{16.5} \right) \right]$$

$$= 0.007892 = (0.0888)^2$$

Piecewise exponential estimate

One way of introducing flexibility in the hazard function is to divide the period of follow-up into intervals and let it take the form of a step-function with jumps at the interval cutpoints. Because the hazard is constant during the interval, the conditional density function for survival times within an interval follows an exponential distribution. Thus, the model is synonymously known as the *piecewise exponential model*. Figure 5–2 shows such a hazard function, and we can immediately see that an implausible feature is the steps themselves. While we tend to contemplate our changing mortality risk at particular birthdays, we also realize that the underlying biology is much more likely to be a smooth function, rather than one with discrete jumps. At best we can regard the step-function as an approximation to a smooth underlying hazard function. As we can also see

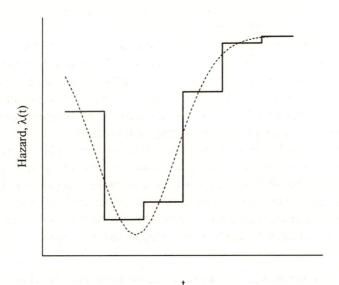

Figure 5–2 Piecewise constant approximation to a smooth hazard function.

in Figure 5–2, this approximation can be improved by taking many small intervals, and we can continue this process so that the step function becomes arbitrarily close to the underlying smooth function.

We represent the piecewise constant hazard by

$$\lambda(t) = \lambda_i \qquad \text{for } x_i < t \leq x_{i+1} \tag{5.1}$$

and we wish to find maximum likelihood estimates of the hazards associated with each interval. This is a failure rate for the interval, so we can essentially make use of the estimator we used in Chapter 4. As in the previous section, we let d_i represent the number of deaths in the ith interval. Total follow-up time during an interval can be obtained by tabulating each individual's contribution during an interval, which for the jth subject is

$t_{ij} = x_{i+1} - x_i$ if individual is under active follow-up at the end of the interval

      $= t_j - x_i$ if individual dies or is censored during the interval

and the total follow-up time for the interval is $T_i = \sum_j t_{ij}$. Thus, the maximum likelihood estimate for the hazard is $\hat{\lambda}_i = d_i/T_i$.

The log of the survival function, also known as the *cumulative hazard function*, is just a function of the step parameters, so the invariance property of maximum likelihood estimates yields the estimator

$$\hat{\Lambda}(t) = \sum_{\{i:\, x_{i+1} < t\}} (x_{i+1} - x_i) \cdot \hat{\lambda}_i + (t - x_{\text{last}})\hat{\lambda}_{\text{last}}$$

where "last" indicates the lower interval cutpoint for the interval in which t falls. This function is monotone increasing and a broken line, beginning at zero for $t = 0$. The survival function can be found by taking the antilog of the negative of this function, $\hat{\mathscr{F}}(t) = \exp\{-\hat{\Lambda}(t)\}$, which is monotone decreasing, starting at 1 for $t = 0$, but the shape is a scalloped function in which there is exponential decay during each interval.

A variety of different estimators have been derived under a similar underlying model, when the actual times within an interval are not available (6). However, the differences among these estimators in practical applications, especially when proper care is taken in selecting the intervals, is usually trivial, so practitioners have never seen a reason to adopt any of the alternatives, which are slightly more complicated to compute.

Example 5–1 (continued) To compare this estimator with that obtained using the actuarial approach, let us use the same data and the same choice of intervals. As before, we first tabulate the number of failures in each group, as shown in

Table 5–3. Calculations for piecewise constant lifetable using the data from 6-MP-treated patients in Table 5–1

Interval	d_i [1]	T_i [2]	$\hat{\lambda}$ [3]	$\hat{\Lambda}_i$ [4]	$\hat{\mathcal{F}}_i$ [5]
(0,3]	0	63	0.0000	0.0000	1.0000
(3,6]	3	63	0.0476	0.1429	0.8669
(6,9]	1	49	0.0204	0.2041	0.8154
(9,12]	1	40	0.0250	0.2791	0.7565
(12,15]	1	34	0.0294	0.3673	0.6926
(15,18]	1	30	0.0333	0.4673	0.6267
(18,21]	0	24	0.0000	0.4673	0.6267
(21,24]	2	18	0.1111	0.8007	0.4490
(24,27]	0	13	0.0000	0.8007	0.4490

[1] Number of failures.

[2] Total follow-up time.

[3] Estimated hazard.

[4] Estimated cumulative hazard.

[5] Estimated survival curve.

Table 5–3. To illustrate the calculation of the total follow-up time, let us consider the third interval. From Table 5–1 we see that 4 subjects either failed or were censored before this interval began at week 6, so they contribute 0 to the total. At the other end, 15 subjects were observed for more than 9 weeks, so each of these will contribute 3 weeks to the total. Adding the contributions for the two subjects who either failed or were censored during the interval yields $T_3 = (7 - 6) + (9 - 6) + (15) \cdot (3) = 49$. This, along with the number of failures, yields an estimate of the hazard function during the interval, $\hat{\lambda}_3 = 1/49 = 0.0204$. From the hazard, we can directly determine the cumulative hazard, which is the area under the hazard, function. Hence, if we wish to estimate the cumulative hazard at 10 weeks, we calculate

$$\hat{\Lambda}(10) = (3)(0.0000) + (3)(0.0476) + (3)(0.0204) + (1)(0.0250) = 0.2290$$

and the corresponding estimate of the survival function at 10 weeks is $\hat{\mathcal{F}}(10) = \exp\{-0.2290\} = 0.7953$. Table 5–3 gives the cumulative hazard, along with the estimated survival function at the interval cutpoints.

Product limit estimate

In both the actuarial and the piecewise exponential estimates we recognized that in real applications these were at best approximate methods due to the finite intervals selected. In each case, the approximation could be improved by taking a greater number of small intervals, so we now consider the problem of going to the limit—that is, letting the number of intervals go to infinity while the size of the intervals goes to zero. Figure 5–3 shows the observations on a time line in which the x's indicate times of failure and the circles show times at which individuals are censored. The

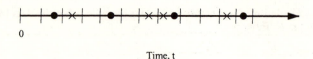

Time, t

Figure 5–3 Time line with failures (×) and censored (●) observations.

figure shows one step in the imagined process of taking a finer and finer grid on the time line—a process that will ultimately split the two observation that currently share an interval into separate intervals.

When there are ties for failure and censoring times, we adopt the rule that the censoring occurs after the death. Such ties only arise when time is measured crudely; otherwise, the probability of a tie would be zero. In practice, it is unlikely that an individual failed immediately after they were censored from the study, in that they are likely to have survived for at least a short period of time. Thus, we effectively move censored observations slightly to the right on our time line when they are tied with complete observations. The result of this is that all of the tiny intervals either have deaths or they do not, and deaths and censored observations do not occur in the same interval. As before, we let d_i represent the number of deaths in the ith interval and l_i the number alive and under active follow-up at the beginning of the interval.

Most intervals do not include failure times, and they would yield an estimate of the probability of death, $\hat{q}_i = 0$, and a conditional survival probability, $\hat{p}_i = 1$. Hence, the estimated survival function remains unchanged for each of these intervals. For the remaining intervals that contain deaths, we do not at the same time have to contend with censored observations because they have been excluded in the limiting process or they have been moved to the succeeding interval if they are tied with a death time. During these intervals, the estimated survival function does change, and the obvious estimate of the conditional probability of failure is $\hat{q}_i = d_i/l_i$ and $\hat{p}_i = (l_i - d_i)/l_i$. Hence, the estimated survival function at time t only requires that we calculate the changes that occur at the observed failure times before t. We refer to this as the set of failure times less than t, which can be represented by $\{i: T_i < t\}$, and the estimator is given by

$$\hat{\mathcal{F}}(t) = \prod_{\{i: T_i < t\}} \frac{l_i - d_i}{l_i} \tag{5.2}$$

with variance

$$\mathrm{Var}[\hat{\mathcal{F}}(t)] = \mathcal{F}(t)^2 \cdot \sum_{\{i: T_i < t\}} \frac{d_i}{l_i \cdot (l_i - d_i)} \tag{5.3}$$

The *product limit*, or Kaplan–Meier estimator (7), is the most commonly used estimator of the survival function in cohort studies. It has clear advantages over those discussed in the previous sections because it does not require an approximation that results from an assumption about the division of follow-up time into intervals. As there is little or no loss in efficiency resulting from the completely nonparametric nature of the estimator, we essentially cannot go wrong in always using it in practice (7). The actuarial estimator is primarily used to summarize vital statistics information with respect to the survival function, and these population summaries can be based on fairly large samples. In these cases, the summary of data by intervals reduces the amount of information to be tabulated. This estimate will agree well with the product limit estimate, provided one takes a sufficiently large number of intervals (4).

Example 5–1 (continued)   Once again, we shall illustrate these calculations using the data on patients treated with 6-MP shown in Table 5–1. As we have seen, we only need to make that calculation at the observed failure times, which are displayed in the first column of Table 5–4. At each of these times we determine the number of failures, d_i, as well as the number censored before the next failure time, W_i. Recall that in the case of ties between failure and censoring times, we proposed the rule that the censored observation occurred after the failure. Hence, three failures occurred at 6 weeks, but the one observation that was censored at 6 weeks was counted among those at risk, then removed before the next failure time at 7 weeks. Calculation of number at risk of failure at each time is obtained by starting with all 21 subjects at time 0, and then subtracting the number of failures and cen-

Table 5–4. Calculations for the product limit lifetable using the data from 6-MP-treated patients in Table 5–1

Time (weeks)	d_i[1]	W_i[2]	l_i[3]	$\hat{p}_i$[4]	$\hat{\mathscr{F}}_i$[5]	SD($\hat{\mathscr{F}}_i$)
0	0	0	21	1.0000	1.0000	0.0000
6	3	1	21	0.8571	0.8571	0.0764
7	1	1	17	0.9412	0.8067	0.0869
10	1	2	15	0.9333	0.7529	0.0963
13	1	0	12	0.9167	0.6902	0.1068
16	1	3	11	0.9091	0.6275	0.1141
22	1	0	7	0.8571	0.5378	0.1282
23	1	5	6	0.8333	0.4482	0.1346

[1] Number of failures.

[2] Number censored.

[3] Number at risk of failure.

[4] Estimated conditional survival probability.

[5] Estimated survival.

sorings that occur before the next failure time. For example, the number at risk at the seventh week is $l_3 = 21 - 3 - 1 = 17$.

Once we have obtained the raw summary information, we can proceed to estimate the conditional probability of surviving at each failure time; thus for the seventh week, we have $\hat{p}_3 = (17 - 1)/17 = 0.9412$. Starting with the survival function defined to be 1 at time 0, we multiply each estimate by the corresponding conditional survival probability to obtain the next estimate of the survival function. For example, at the thirteenth week we have

$$\hat{\mathcal{F}}_5 = (1.000)(0.8571)(0.9412)(0.9333)$$
$$= (0.8067)(0.9333) = 0.7529$$

Table 5–4 gives the estimated survival function at each failure time. The estimated curve changes just at the failure time, thus retaining the value from the previous estimate until the instant before that time. Hence, the estimate of the curve is a step function, with jumps occurring at the failure times. The variance of this estimator is estimated by

$$\text{Var}(\hat{\mathcal{F}}_5) = (0.7529)^2 \cdot \left(\frac{3}{21 \cdot (21 - 3)} + \frac{1}{17 \cdot (17 - 1)} + \frac{1}{15 \cdot (15 - 1)} \right)$$
$$= 0.009282 = (0.0963)^2$$

Figure 5–4 plots all three of our estimated survival functions on a single graph. It is interesting to see that, in fact, there is very good agreement among the estimators, as would be expected when a fairly large number of intervals are used.

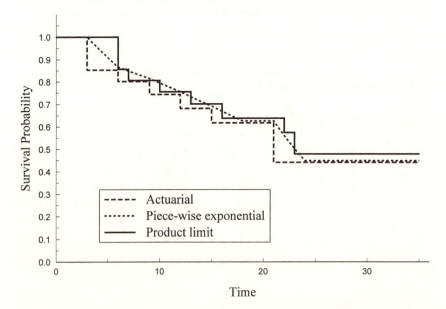

Figure 5–4 Plot of the survival curve estimates for the 6-MP data in Table 8–1.

Graphical Displays

The survival function is a useful summary of failure-time data in its own right, but it can also provide invaluable insights into the adequacy of a parametric model for the underlying disease process. We shall now consider some graphical methods that can be used to explore the underlying assumptions for some particular forms for the hazard function.

Diagnostic for constant hazard

We have already noted that for the constant hazard model, $\lambda(t) \equiv \lambda$, the survival function takes the form $\mathcal{F}(t) = \exp\{-\lambda \cdot t\}$ and its logarithm becomes $\log \mathcal{F}(t) = -\lambda \cdot t$. Hence, as graph of the log survival function on t would be expected to result in a line starting at the origin with slope $-\lambda$.

In practice, we can plot the log of the estimated survival function against time, using the estimators described in "Estimating Survival Curves" in this chapter. It takes some practice to interpret these graphs, because even if the times arise from an exponential distribution, there will be random departures from linear trend. Hence, we must use some judgment when trying to decide whether the departures are systematic or whether they are only due to random variation. Figure 5–5 shows plots of the product limit estimates for 12 samples of size 10 that were drawn from an exponential distribution with $\lambda = 1$. This is clearly a very small sample size, but from it we can see typical random fluctuations for such estimated survival functions. The graph illustrates the fact that the estimates at individual points are correlated, in that curves tend to be low (high) at an early stage tend to also be low (high) as time progresses. In addition, we can see much more variation as the time axis moves to the right. If the sample size increases to 25, Figure 5–6, then we see much more stability in our estimate of the survival curve. When using these curves as a diagnostic tool, we must be careful about concluding curvature based on just a few individuals with high times. The curves in the graphs in row 1 column 4 and row 3 column 3 (Fig. 5–6) occurred at random, but on close inspection we can see that the visual impression of curvature is a result of one or two points at the end. If we ignore these points, then the remainder is actually quite close to the theoretically true broken line.

In practice, the data we are likely to see will have censored observations, which will tend to make the observations in the upper tail even less stable. To see this, let us suppose that the censoring occurs uniformly about the median, which is 0.693 for an exponential distribution with $\lambda = 1$. Hence, for each subject we draw a survival time, t, from an exponential distribution with $\lambda = 1$, as well as a censoring time, c, from a uniform dis-

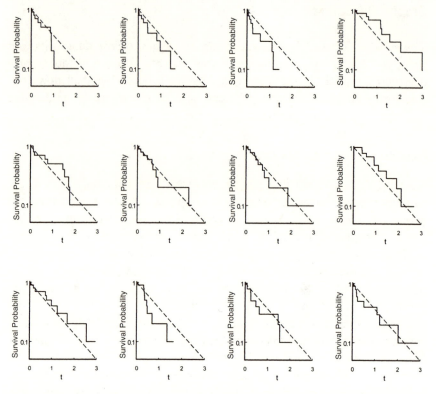

Figure 5–5 Plot of the estimated survival function (log scale) against time for samples of size 10 from an exponential distribution with $\lambda = 1$.

tribution on the interval [0.193,1.193]. The observation is complete if $t \leq c$, and censored at c if $t > c$. The probability that an observation is censored under this scenario is 49.9%. In Figure 5–7 we see plots of 12 samples of size 20, for which we expect that 10 will be censored. Of course, the actual number censored will be a random number about the expected number censored. We can see this instability in the tail of the estimated curve, especially when there is the occasional subject observed for a long period before being censored, as in the graph shown in row 2 column 2. As expected, an increase in the sample size from 20 to 50 results in more stable estimators for the survival curve, as shown in Figure 5–8. However, we still see the phenomenon in which the right end of the curve has less stability due to the censoring, which has left fewer observations for estimating this part of the curve.

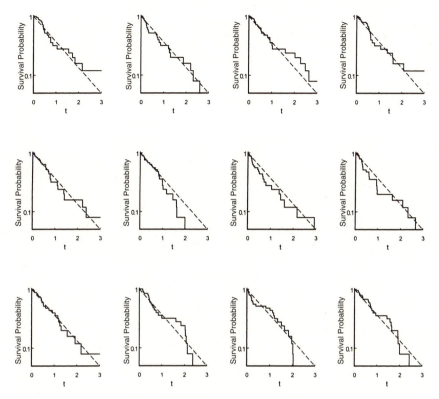

Figure 5–6 Plot of the estimated survival function (log scale) against time for samples of size 25 from an exponential distribution with $\lambda = 1$.

Example 5–1 (continued) One type of analysis we might consider for the data in Table 5–1 would employ failure rates, which are best used when the hazard is constant, as we saw in Chapter 4. Figure 5–9 plots the log survival against time for each group. We can see that both steps that estimate the survival curves are relatively close to a straight line, suggesting that the constant hazard assumption is not seriously violated for these data.

Diagnostic for Weibull hazard

For the Weibull distribution, the hazard takes the form $\lambda(t) = \lambda \cdot \gamma \cdot t^{\gamma-1}$ and the survival function is $\mathscr{F}(t) = \exp\{-\lambda \cdot t^{\gamma}\}$. If we employ the log-log transformation, we have $\log\{-\log[\mathscr{F}(t)]\} = \log \lambda + \gamma \cdot \log t$, which is linear in $\log t$, with slope γ, and intercept $\log \lambda$. Notice that the constant hazard or exponential distribution is just a special case when $\gamma = 1$, so if this is

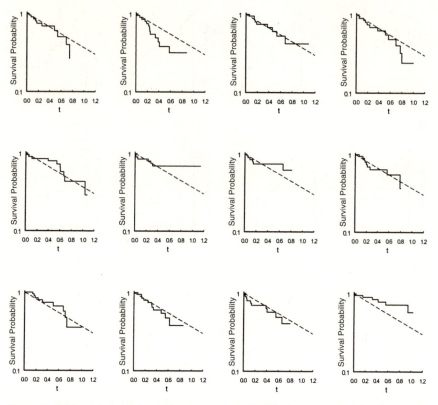

Figure 5–7 Plot of the estimated survival function (log scale) against time for samples of size 20 from an exponential distribution with $\lambda = 1$ with 50% censoring.

the correct distribution for a set of data, we would expect to see a straight line with slope 1.

Examples of the results obtained when 25 observations are drawn at random from a Weibull distribution are shown in Figure 5–10. In this case we chose $\lambda = 1$ and $\gamma = \frac{1}{2}$. The graph shows $\log\{-\log[\hat{\mathscr{F}}(t)]\}$ plotted against $\log(t)$, which is expected to be a straight line with slope $\frac{1}{2}$, as shown by the dashed line. Notice that in this case we not only have greater instability at the right end of the curve, but on the left as well. To see the effect of censoring, we once again draw samples of failure times, t, from the same Weibull distribution, but we also draw a uniform censoring time, c, from an interval about the median of our Weibull, or the interval of width 0.5 around 0.480 or $[0.230, 0.730]$. Censoring accentuates further the variability about the ends of the distribution, as we can see in the plots shown in Figure 5–11.

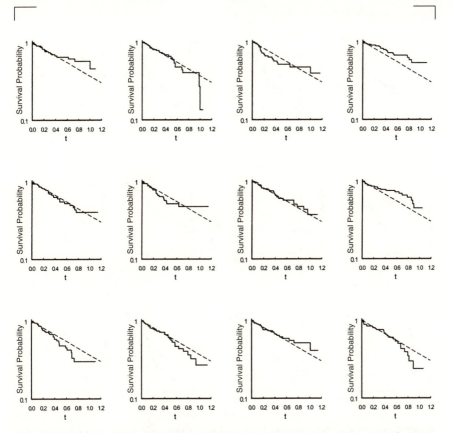

Figure 5–8 Plot of the estimated survival function (log scale) against time for samples of size 50 from an exponential distribution with $\lambda = 1$ with 50% censoring.

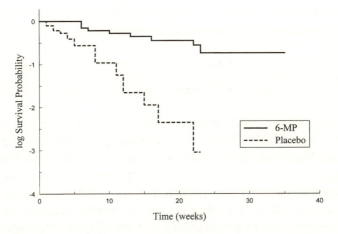

Figure 5–9 Plot of the log survival probability against time for the data in Table 5–1.

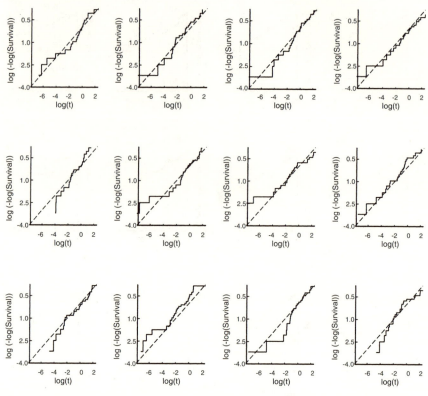

Figure 5–10 Plot of the estimate log-log survival function against time for samples of size 25 from a Weibull distribution with $\lambda = 1$ and $\gamma = \frac{1}{2}$.

Diagnostic for proportional hazards

If the hazards for two groups are proportional, then we have already seen that they are related by a constant of proportionality

$$\lambda_1(t) = \lambda_0(t)$$

$$\lambda_2(t) = \lambda_0(t) \cdot \exp\{\beta\} = \lambda_1(t) \cdot \exp\{\beta\}$$

The corresponding survival functions are related to each other by the expression $\mathscr{F}_2(t) = \mathscr{F}_1(t)^{\exp\{\beta\}}$. By once again employing the log-log transformation on these two survival functions, we obtain $\log\{-\log[\mathscr{F}_2(t)]\} = \log\{-\log[\mathscr{F}_1(t)]\} + \beta$. Hence, we can see that the two transformed functions are parallel to each other, in that they are shifted vertically by the log hazard ratio, β. Figure 5–12 displays log-log survival functions that arose from the assumption of proportionality. At first glance it may appear that these lines are not parallel, but on closer examination we can see that, in

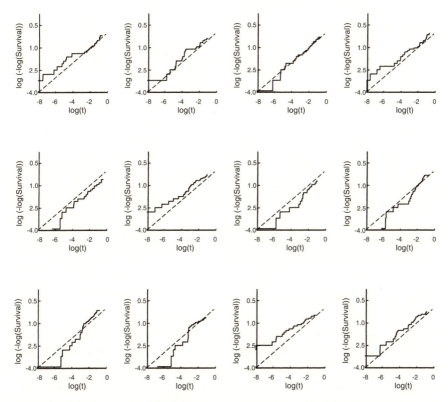

Figure 5–11 Plot of the estimated log-log survival function against time for samples of size 50 from a Weibull distribution with $\lambda = 1$ and $\gamma = \frac{1}{2}$ with 50% censoring.

fact, the vertical distance between the two curves is indeed constant, thus the lines are parallel by our definition. Parallelism is easier to see for straight lines, rather than curves, because our eyes tend to process the minimum distance between the curves rather than the vertical distance. We can often reduce this perceptual difficulty by transforming the horizontal axis so that the log-log survival curves are more nearly linear, as in Figure 5–13 which is the same as Figure 5–12 except for taking the log of time.

Example 5–1 (continued)   Continuing our exploration of the data in Table 5–1, we plot the log-log transformation of the estimated survival curves against log time in Figure 5–14. We see that the steps that estimate the survival curves indeed tend to be parallel; thus, an analysis based on the proportional hazards assumption would appear to be appropriate. Actually, the proportional hazards assumption is less restrictive than our earlier assumption of constant hazards, so it is not surprising that we would conclude that proportionality was appropriate given that we had already concluded that the hazards appeared to be constant for these data.

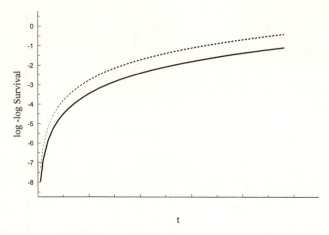

Figure 5–12 Plot of the log-log survival curve on t for two groups related by the proportional hazards model.

Tests for Comparing Hazards

In this section, we consider some significance tests for comparing hazard functions through their relationship with survival curves. These methods can be thought of as offering extensions to the score test methodology we described in Chapter 4 for comparing failure rates, which applied to the cases where the hazards were constant. The extensions considered here are directed toward an optimal test for comparing proportional hazards for the case when the hazard behaves as a step function. We then extend this to

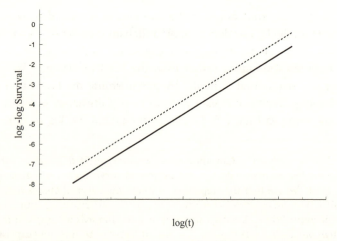

Figure 5–13 Plot of log-log survival curve on $\log(t)$ for two groups related by the proportional hazards model.

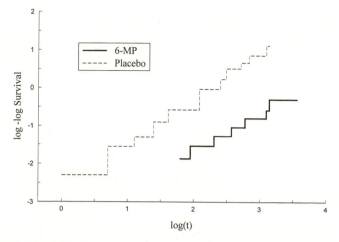

Figure 5–14 Plot of the log-log survival probability against log time for the data in Table 5–1.

the product limit case, following the same progression used in our discussion of survival curve estimation.

Piecewise constant hazards

In Chapter 4, we considered methods of analyzing a hazard function that was constant over time. We shall now allow the hazard to vary with time by dividing the period of follow-up into intervals, and then allow the hazard to change from interval to interval—that is, a piecewise constant hazard for group i in interval j:

$$\lambda_i(t) = \lambda_{ij} \qquad \text{for } \tau_j < t \le \tau_{j+1}$$

The proportional hazards model implies that the hazard for each group is given by the product of one term involving time (λ_{0j}) and a second term (θ_i) that is specific to the group:

$$\lambda_i(t) = \lambda_{0j} \cdot \theta_i = \exp\{\alpha_j + \beta_i\} \qquad \text{for } \tau_j < t \le \tau_{j+1}$$

where $\beta_1 = 0$. The null hypothesis of equal risk among the groups is given by $H_0: \beta_1 = \beta_2 = \ldots = \beta_I$. Expressed in this way, we can see that the model and the null hypothesis takes the same form as the model we used to obtain an overall test for rates for stratified data. The major difference now is that the strata are formed by observing what occurs in each interval, rather than comprise a group formed by one or more additional factors.

Because the same individual may be observed in more than one interval, we no longer have independence between intervals, in the same way that we may treat the observations for different individuals as independent. Nevertheless, the formula turns out to be identical to that which we saw in equation 4.17:

$$S^2 = \frac{[\sum_j(n_{2j} - n_{+j}P_{2j})]^2}{\sum_j n_{+j}P_{2j}[1 - P_{2j}]}$$

$$= \frac{[\sum_j n_{2j} - \sum_j E(n_{2j})]^2}{\sum_j \mathrm{Var}(n_{2j})}$$

(5.4)

which is compared to a chi-square distribution with 1 df, where $P_{2j} = T_{2j}/T_{+j}$ and T_{ij} is the total follow-up time for group i during interval j. Thus, P_{ij} is the proportion of follow-up time in interval j that occurs in group i.

Example 5–2 The Hypertension Detection and Follow-up Program (8) was a randomized trial designed to investigate the efficacy of a systematic antihypertensive treatment program called "stepped care." Patients who qualified were randomly assigned either to the group who received this form of medical care or to a control group in which they were referred to community medical therapy without systematic follow-up, called "referred care." Results after 5 years of follow-up are shown in Table 5–5, which we recognize as the raw summary data required for finding the actuarial survival curve estimates. To compare the survival experience for the two groups, we need to know the total follow-up time for each interval. If we assume that the times of death and lost to follow-up occur uniformly during the interval, then we would expect these individuals to contribute ½ year each to the total, while the remainder would contribute a full year to the total. We can represent this algebraically by $T_{ij} = l_{ij} - \frac{1}{2}(d_{ij} + W_{ij})$. Hence, for stepped care during

Table 5–5. Five-year results from the Hypertension Detection and Follow-up Program Cooperative Group (8)

Years	Stepped care			Referred care		
	l_{j1}[1]	d_{j1}[2]	W_{j1}[3]	l_{j2}[1]	d_{j2}[2]	W_{j2}[3]
(0,1]	5485	51	1	5455	67	3
(1,2]	5433	54	1	5385	77	2
(2,3]	5378	67	7	5306	73	5
(3,4]	5304	86	6	5228	111	12
(4,5]	5212	91	8	5104	91	16

[1] Number alive at beginning of interval by treatment.

[2] Number of deaths in interval by treatment.

[3] Number censored in interval by treatment.

Table 5–6. Intermediate score test calculations for the data in Table 5–5

Years	T_{j1} [1]	T_{j2} [1]	P_{j2} [2]	d_{j2} [3]	$E[d_{j2}]$ [4]	$Var(d_{j2})$ [5]
(0,1]	5459.0	5420.0	0.4982	67	58.788	29.500
(1,2]	5405.5	5345.5	0.4972	77	65.134	32.749
(2,3]	5341.0	5267.0	0.4965	73	69.512	34.998
(3,4]	5258.0	5166.5	0.4956	111	97.635	49.246
(4,5]	5162.5	5050.5	0.4945	91	90.002	45.495
Total:				419	381.072	191.988

[1] Approximate total follow-up by treatment.

[2] Proportion of follow-up observed in group 2.

[3] Observed deaths in group 2.

[4] Expected deaths in group 2.

[5] Variance of observed deaths in group 2.

the first interval we have $T_{11} = 5485 - \frac{1}{2}(51 + 1) = 5459$ years of follow-up. The remaining estimates are calculated in a similar manner and are displayed in Table 5–6.

Continuing our calculations for the first interval, the proportion of the total follow-up that occurs in the referred care group during the first interval is $p_{21} = 5459.0/(5459.0 + 5420.0) = 0.4982$, so under the null hypothesis the expected number of deaths in this group during the first interval is $E[d_{21}] = 0.4982 (51 + 67) = 58.788$. The corresponding variance is $Var(d_{21}) = (51 + 67) \cdot 0.4982 \cdot (1 - 0.4982) = 29.500$

We then carry out these calculations for the remainder of the table, shown in Table 5–6, thus yielding the total expected number of deaths, 381.072, along with the total variance, 191.988. From these values, we obtain the score test of the null hypothesis that the survival experience is the same for the two groups: $S^2 = (419 - 381.072)^2/191.988 = 7.49$, which is compared to a chi-square distribution with 1 df ($p = .0062$), thus providing strong evidence for a difference in the survival experience between the two groups. Notice that 419 deaths were observed in the referred care group, which is greater than the 381.072 expected under the null hypothesis of no difference. Hence, we can see that the stepped care group experienced a better prognosis.

Log-rank test

In our discussion of survival curve estimates, we relaxed the assumptions imposed by a step function by letting the interval widths become vanishingly small. If we invoke a similar approach when constructing a score test for a proportional hazards model, the intervals with no failures, $n_{+j} = 0$, contribute nothing to either the numerator or the denominator of the score statistic in equation 5.4. So, we only need to pay attention to intervals that include times that deaths occur. The total follow-up time for group i in the jth small interval of width Δ is approximately $l_{ij}\Delta$, which yields $P_{2j} = l_{2j}/l_{+j}$.

Thus, the statistic, which is compared to a chi-square distribution with 1 df, takes the now familiar form,

$$S^2 = \frac{[\sum_j n_{2j} - \sum_j E(n_{2j})]^2}{\sum_j \text{Var}(n_{2j})} \tag{5.5}$$

where our estimate of the expected number of failures in group 2 at failure time j is

$$E[n_{2j}] = \frac{n_{+j} \cdot l_{2j}}{l_{+j}}$$

and the variance is

$$\text{Var}(n_{2j}) = \frac{n_{+j} \cdot l_{1j} \cdot l_{2j}}{l_{+j}^2}$$

Notice that this variance is essentially the same as the variance used in calculating Cochran's statistic for comparing proportions across strata (9). Kalbfleisch and Prentice (10) present an alternative development of the test statistic, which gives rise to a variance that is analogous to the variance from a conditional argument, or:

$$\text{Var}^*(n_{2j}) = \frac{n_{+j} \cdot l_{1j} \cdot l_{2j} \cdot (l_{+j} - n_{+j})}{l_{+j}^2 \cdot (l_{+j} - 1)}$$

This test was first proposed by Mantel (11) as an extension to the Mantel-Haenszel test for comparing stratified proportions (12). Notice that when time is measured to a level of precision that avoids ties, or $n_{+j} = 1$ for each failure time, then the two variances are identical. The difference only occurs when ties exist, and in these instances the second formula yields a smaller variance, thus giving rise to a larger chi-square test statistic. Even here, the overall difference tends to be small when the sample size is reasonably large, so there is not a clear advantage of one expression over the other in practical situations.

Example 5–1 (continued)   Returning once again to the leukemia data displayed in Table 5–1, let us now determine whether the observed differences in the survival curves are statistically significant using the log-rank test. Each contribution to the statistic is identified with an observed failure time, and the requisite summary information is displayed in Table 5–7. Notice that we must identify the failure times for both treatment groups in order to determine the number of deaths expected

Table 5–7. Intermediate calculations for the log-rank test using the data in Table 5–1

Time (weeks)	Placebo d_{j1}[1]	l_{j1}[2]	6 MP d_{j2}[1]	l_{j2}[2]	$E[d_{j2}]$[3]	$Var(d_{j2})$[4]	$Var^*(d_{j2})$[5]
1	2	21	0	21	1.0000	0.5000	0.4878
2	2	19	0	21	1.0500	0.4988	0.4860
3	1	17	0	21	0.5526	0.2472	0.2472
4	2	16	0	21	1.1351	0.4909	0.4772
5	2	14	0	21	1.2000	0.4800	0.4659
6	0	12	3	21	1.9091	0.6942	0.6508
7	0	12	1	17	0.5862	0.2426	0.2426
8	4	12	0	16	2.2857	0.9796	0.8707
10	0	8	1	15	0.6522	0.2268	0.2268
11	2	8	0	13	1.2381	0.4717	0.4481
12	2	6	0	12	1.3333	0.4444	0.4183
13	0	4	1	12	0.7500	0.1875	0.1875
15	1	4	0	11	0.7333	0.1956	0.1956
16	0	3	1	11	0.7857	0.1684	0.1684
17	1	3	0	10	0.7692	0.1775	0.1775
22	1	2	1	7	1.5556	0.3457	0.3025
23	1	1	1	6	1.7143	0.2449	0.2041
Totals	21		9		19.2505	6.5957	6.2570

[1] Number of failures by treatment.

[2] Number at risk by treatment.

[3] Expected number of failures in group 2.

[4] Variance for number of failures in group 2.

[5] Kalbfleisch-Prentice variance for number of failures in group 2.

among those who are under active follow-up at that time. The first failure time was tied for two subjects, and the expected number for the 6-MP group is

$$E[d_{j2}] = \frac{(2)(21)}{21 + 21} = 1.000$$

with the corresponding variance,

$$Var(d_{12}) = \frac{(2)(21)(21)}{(21 + 21)^2} = 0.500$$

Calculations for the remaining failure times are shown in Table 5–7, along with the total expected number of deaths and the total variance. Thus, we obtain the log-rank statistic

$$S^2 = \frac{(9 - 19.2505)^2}{6.5957} = 15.93$$

which is compared to a chi-square distribution with 1 df ($p < .0001$), thus providing very strong evidence that those treated with 6-MP had longer remission times.

The alternative expression for the variance yields

$$\text{Var}(d_{21}) = \frac{(2)(21)(21)(42 - 2)}{(42)^2 \cdot (42 - 1)} = 0.4878$$

for the first failure time. Thus, the resulting score statistic becomes

$$S^2 = \frac{(9 - 19.2505)^2}{6.2570} = 16.79$$

which is slightly larger than the earlier value, and still statistically significant ($p < .0001$).

Stratified log-rank test

We have now seen that an appropriate treatment of follow-up time in the proportional hazards model results in a score test that is essentially identical to the tests that arose from a consideration of a common hazard ratio across strata. So let us now take these ideas one step further and consider a stratified proportional hazards model, which can be represented by $\lambda_{ik}(t) = \lambda_{0k}(t) \cdot \theta_i = \exp\{\alpha_k(t) + \beta_i\}$, where $\beta_1 = 0$. The underlying assumption here is that the hazards are proportional within each stratum, or $\lambda_{2k}(t)/\lambda_{1k}(t) = \theta_2$, a constant that does not depend on either time or the stratum (10). The fact that the time component of the model is allowed to be a different arbitrary function of time for each stratum, $\lambda_{0k}(t)$, makes this a very flexible assumption indeed, in that there is not an additional restriction on the functional form for the stratum effects.

For the piecewise constant hazard version of this test, the underlying model for the hazard is given by

$$\lambda_{ik}(t) = \lambda_{0jk} \cdot \theta_i = \exp\{\alpha_{jk} + \beta_i\} \qquad \text{for } \tau_j < t \le \tau_{j+1}$$

The summary statistics used in conducting the test are the number of failures in group i, interval j, and stratum k, d_{ijk}, and the corresponding total follow-up time is T_{ijk}. We now combine, across strata and time intervals, the observed and expected number of failures in group 2, along with their variances, yielding

$$S^2 = \frac{[\sum_{jk}(n_{2jk} - n_{+jk}P_{2jk})]^2}{\sum_{jk}n_{+jk}P_{2jk}[1 - P_{2jk}]}$$

$$= \frac{[\sum_{jk}n_{2jk} - \sum_{jk}E(n_{2jk})]^2}{\sum_{jk}\text{Var}(n_{2jk})}$$

(5.6)

where $P_{ijk} = T_{ijk}/T_{+jk}$. The statistic is once again compared to a chi-square distribution with 1 df.

Similarly, we can extend the log-rank test to the case of a stratified proportional hazards model (10) by calculating the expected number of failures in the comparison group and the corresponding variances within strata, and then combining these to obtain the relevant numerator and denominator:

$$ S^2 = \frac{[\sum_{jk} n_{2jk} - \sum_{jk} E(n_{2jk})]^2}{\sum_{jk} \text{Var}(n_{2jk})} \tag{5.7} $$

As usual, this statistic is compared to a chi-square distribution with 1 df.

Types of Incomplete Data

We have described one type of incomplete data that arises because the study ends or because individuals are lost to follow-up. However, other situations can also arise to provide only partial information on failure times, and in this section we briefly consider some of these.

Right censoring

Classical or *Type I censoring* results from the end of a study for a particular individual, so that the maximum length of time that an individual may be followed is the time since recruitment, as illustrated by subject B in Figure 5–15. If the time to failure for the ith individual is a random variable, t_i, and the length of time from entry to the study until the end is also a random variable, c_i, then with respect to the survival time, it is only possible for us to observe the smaller of the two, $\min(t_i, c_i)$, along with an indicator of whether the observation was complete, $\delta_i = 1$, or censored, $\delta_i = 0$. It is often reasonable for us to assume that the distribution of survival and censoring times are independent of each other, as we have done in our treatment of loss to follow-up. However, we have also noted the fact that this may not always be reasonable, in which case all methods we have discussed in this chapter would produce biased quantities.

If we try to relax the assumption of independence between the censoring and failure times, it turns out that we have an identifiability problem (13), which is to say the two distributions are inextricably linked and they cannot be disentangled. The only way in which we can make any progress in developing a method of analysis when we do not have independence between the censoring and failure times is when specific and often unverifiable assumptions apply for the relationship between failure and censoring

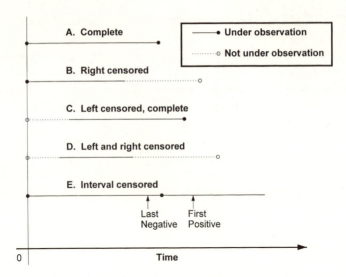

Figure 5–15 Alternative types of censoring for failure time and data.

times (14). Some approaches to dealing with the problem when something is known about the form of the dependence is discussed by Lagakos (15), but these can occur in the context of a highly parameterized model, rather than the completely flexible functions we have considered in this chapter.

In laboratory studies, a certain level of precision in the summary statistic is often desired, and rather than waiting a set length of time until the end, the study is stopped after a specified number of failures have been observed. Hence, the number of failures in such an experiment is fixed, but the total lengths of follow-up are not. This is called *Type II censoring*.

Left censoring

In left censoring, we know that the time to failure is greater than some specified value, $T_i > C_i$. Let us consider a study of the distribution of time from infection with HIV until the development of AIDS. Some of the first approaches to this problem made use of blood samples collected in conjunction with hepatitis B vaccine trials that were conducted in homosexual men. In one such trial, an initial screening blood sample was obtained, and once the trial got under way 2 years later, samples were collected quarterly and stored in a freezer. Once a blood test for HIV was developed, it became possible to construct the infection history of these individuals. The incubation period was measured by the time from the first HIV-positive blood sample until a diagnosis of AIDS. However, consider those individuals who were negative at the time the initial screening sample was collected, but positive for the sample taken 2 years later: thus, we know that $T_i < 2$. We refer to this as left censoring, and individual C in Figure 5–15 provides an illustration of such a case.

Interval censoring

If we continue our discussion of the AIDS example in the preceding section, notice that we have measured time only rather crudely, in that time from seroconversion until failure is determined only to the nearest quarter. It would be more accurate to specify the interval in which the time from seroconversion until failure might fall. This interval would be determined from the last date for a negative blood test until the first date of a positive test, or, $r_i < t_i < c_i$. Turnbull (16, 17) discusses the problem of estimating a survival curve in the situation in which the data may be left, right, or interval censored.

Summary

In this chapter we have considered nonparametric methods for summarizing the occurrence of failures over time. The survival curve is the most commonly used summary, and we discussed actuarial, piecewise constant, and product limit estimators. We saw that the degree to which the estimator was nonparametric depended on the size of the intervals to be chosen for the follow-up time, and as the product limit estimator was essentially based on infinitesimally small intervals, it is the only truly nonparametric estimator of the three. Actuarial estimators are primarily used in epidemiological research to summarize population-based statistics, which are derived from large databases. When this estimator is used, it is best to select at least 10 intervals in order to reduce potential bias. However, for typical cohort studies, the product limit estimator is most suitable.

Another use for estimates of survival curves is to validate assumptions about the distribution of times to failure that may underlie a parametric analysis. For this type of analysis we considered plots of the log and the log-log of the survival curve, which provided us with a diagnostic tool for evaluating the validity of assumed exponential, or Weibull, distributions. In addition, the parallelism of two or more log-log survival curve plots allows us to visually check the proportional hazards assumption that underlies many of the commonly used methods of analysis. We shall use these diagnostic methods further when we consider some of the regression methods in later chapters. While such diagnostic plots can be an invaluable way to explore assumptions, they do require a certain amount of judgment when applying them because of their underlying random variability. However, as we shall also see, these can suggest focused models that yield more objective criteria for distinguishing between random and systematic departures from what is expected.

Finally, we considered tests for comparing two survival curves that are best used when the proportional hazards assumption applies. The log-rank test is perhaps the most commonly used test for a typical cohort study, but there are alternatives—such as the generalized Wilcoxon test—that routinely appear as part of the output for many statistical packages. The log-rank and Wilcoxon tests are best used under different underlying models for the relationship between the groups. Hence, while both of these are nonparametric tests in that no distribution assumptions are made, there is an underlying structure for the relationship between groups. This semi-parametric aspect of the methods becomes even more pronounced in the regression models considered in Chapter 9.

Exercises

5.1. The data in the following table are from a study of survival from cancer of the cervix (18), broken down by stage and treatment.

| | Stage I | | | | | | Stage II | | | | | |
| | Treatment A | | | Treatment B | | | Treatment A | | | Treatment B | | |
Year	l_i^*	W_i^*	d_i^*	l_i	W_i	d_i	l_i	W_i	d_i	l_i	W_i	d_i
0	81	5	2	29	0	3	205	2	21	29	1	3
1	74	5	6	26	2	1	182	10	25	25	1	2
2	63	3	4	23	4	3	147	6	28	22	3	3
3	56	6	3	16	2	0	113	7	14	16	0	3
4	47	3	0	14	4	0	92	11	5	13	2	2
5	44	7	2	10	3	0	76	4	5	9	2	1
6	35	4	3	7	2	0	67	6	5	6	0	0
7	28	5	0	5	0	0	56	10	2	6	0	1
8	23	3	0	5	1	0	44	12	2	5	1	0
9	20	8	1	4	0	0	30	5	3	4	1	1

* l_i = Number alive at beginning of interval; W_i = Number censored; d_i = Number of deaths in interval.

    a. Estimate the survival curve and the corresponding 90% confidence interval for treatments A and B.

    b. Test the null hypothesis that the survival curves are equal.

    c. Estimate the survival curves for stages I and II.

    d. Prepare a graph that demonstrates the appropriateness of the proportional hazards model in representing the effect of stage on survival.

    e. Test the null hypothesis that the survival curves are equal, adjusting for stage by conducting a stratified analysis.

5.2. Tabulated here are data from a clinical trial that compared the survival experience of severely ill patients, who were treated with a new drug, with a randomly selected control group, who were treated with a placebo.

Treatment	Days to death from time enrolled in study
Drug	$10^*, 22^*, 46^*, 57, 60^*, 69, 69, 73, 74, 82, 101^*, 110, 113^*,$ 141, 144, 155, 158, 164, 170, 178, 196, 200, 243, 273, 306
Placebo	$9^*, 33, 34, 42^*, 45, 50, 52, 55, 57, 59, 71, 73, 75, 82,$ 84, 87, 97^*, 99, 99, 107, 109, 109, 110, 128, 132

* Censored times.

    a. Construct an actuarial survival curve for the subjects who were treated with the drug.

    b. Construct a survival curve using the piecewise exponential estimate for the subjects who were treated with the drug.

    c. Construct a product limit estimate of the survival curve for the subjects who were treated with the drug.

    d. Use a graphical approach to determine whether the constant hazard assumption is reasonable for the analysis of these data.

    e. Use a graphical approach to determine whether the Weibull model provides an appropriate description of the distribution of times to death.

    f. Use a graphical approach to determine whether the proportional hazards model is appropriate for these data.

    g. Test whether the survival experience is the same for these two groups.

5.3. Using the data from the clinical trial on hypernephroma first described in exercise 4.3, compare the survival experience for patients who did and did not receive nephrectomy by:

    a. Estimating the survival curve for each group

    b. Comparing the survival experience for the two groups using the log-rank test

    c. Using a graphical approach, to answer the following:

       i. Which group has the better prognosis?

      ii. Does the constant hazards assumption appear to be appropriate for these data?

     iii. Does the proportional hazards assumption appear to be appropriate for these data?

References

1. Stigler SM. *The History of Statistics: The Measurement of Uncertainty before 1900.* Cambridge, MA: Belknap Press, 1986.
2. Cutler SJ, Ederer F. Maximum utilization of the life table method in analyzing survival. *Journal of Chronic Diseases* 1958;8:699–713.
3. Greenwood M. A report on the natural duration of cancer. *Reports on Public Health and Medical Subjects* 1926;33:1–26.
4. Breslow N, Crowley J. A large sample study of the life table and product limit estimates under random censorship. *Annals of Statistics* 1974;2:437–453.
5. Gehan EA. A generalized Wilcoxon test for comparing arbitrarily singly-censored samples. *Biometrika* 1965;52:203–223.
6. Chiang CL. *The Life Table and Its Applications.* Malabar, FL: Krieger Publishing, 1984.
7. Kaplan EL, Meier P. Nonparametric estimation from incomplete observations. *Journal of the American Statistical Association* 1958;53:457–481.
8. Hypertension Detection and Follow-up Program. The effect of treatment of mortality in "mild" hypertension. *New England Journal of Medicine* 1981;307: 979–980.
9. Cochran WG. Some methods for strengthening the common χ^2 tests. *Biometrics* 1954;10:417–451.
10. Kalbfleisch JD, Prentice RL. *The Statistical Analysis of Failure Time Data.* New York: Wiley, 1980.
11. Mantel N. Chi-square tests with one degree of freedom: extensions of the Mantel–Haenszel procedure. *Journal of the American Statistical Association* 1963; 58:690–700.
12. Mantel N, Haenszel W. Statistical aspects of the analysis of data from retrospective studies of disease. *Journal of the National Cancer Institute* 1959;22: 719–748.
13. Tsiatis A. A nonidentifiability aspect of the problem of competing risks. *Proceedings of the National Academy of Science USA* 1975;72:20–22.
14. Lagakos SW, Williams JS. Models for censored survival analysis: a cone class of variable-sum models. *Biometrika* 1978;65:181–189.
15. Lagakos SW. General right censoring and its impact on the analysis of survival data. *Biometrics* 1979;35:139–156.
16. Turnbull BW. Nonparametric estimation of a survival function with doubly censored data. *Journal of the American Statistical Association* 1974;69:169–173.
17. Turnbull BW. The empirical distribution function with arbitrarily grouped, censored and truncated data. *Journal of the Royal Statistical Society, Series B* 1976; 38:290–295.
18. Hills M. *Statistics for Comparative Studies.* London: Chapman and Hall, 1974.

REGRESSION METHODS

6

Regression Models for Proportions

Significance testing is a fundamental part of many epidemiologic investigations, but its usefulness is limited to addressing the question of whether the null hypothesis is true. If one rejects the null hypothesis, other questions we might pose are the following:

How large is the effect?

Is the effect the same for different subgroups of the population?

Can we account for the effect by confounding with another known risk factor?

What is the best way to provide a quantitative description of our data?

This now involves the estimation and model-fitting side of statistical inference, which can be even more important than the question of whether the null hypothesis is true. With a very large study, it is possible to reject the null hypothesis, even though the effect may be very small and of little importance to public health. Very small effects are also more likely to be subject to subtle biases, which can result in the apparent effect being entirely attributable to an artifact.

The second error that can be made with significance testing results from a test that fails to reject the null hypothesis, which is often loosely referred to as accepting the null hypothesis. A small study, even one that is carefully designed to avoid bias, may contain so much random error that it is only possible to detect extremely large effects. Such a study could miss a risk, even though it had real importance to public health. Hence, we must be careful not to overinterpret a statement that the null hypothesis has been accepted, because this does not imply that the null hypothesis has been shown to be true. The null hypothesis can never be proven, as it is always possible that there may be a minuscule effect that a sufficiently large and powerful study could detect. An alternative that is sometimes used is to present an interval estimate of the parameter(s) of interest, as we shall see.

In Chapter 3, we described the Mantel and Haenszel (1) estimate of the odds ratio for K 2×2 tables. The limitation of this approach is that we often do not have sufficient data to simultaneously consider many strata. Suppose, for instance, that we need to adjust for eight potential confounding variables in a particular analysis. Each of these would be reported as having at least two levels, which means that there is a minimum of $2^8 = 256$ strata, or, 256 2×2 tables with an overall total of $4 \times 256 = 1,024$ cells. If the study was even moderately large, with 1,000 subjects, say, there would still only be an average of about 1 subject per cell of the table, and it is not uncommon to see epidemiological studies that are smaller than this. If we look closely at the formulae for this method we can see that those subtables with zero in either a row or a column have no effect on the resulting statistics, so this effectively removes them from playing a role in the inference. The problem is exacerbated still further when we have variables that have more than two levels. Another issue is the fact that the Mantel–Haenszel method only deals with categorical variables, so we can only deal with factors that are measured on a continuum by arbitrarily splitting up the levels into groups. Hence, we really need a more general framework for our analysis—one that allows for a structure that can handle more variables, as well as providing a more effective means of dealing with exposures that are measured on a continuum.

In this chapter we will discuss the application of regression methods for epidemiological data that arise from studies in which time of observation is fixed, so that the underlying outcome is a proportion. The most commonly used model in this situation is the linear logistic model, although this may not always give the best description of a set of data. Hence, it is also useful to have available other models, and we will discuss a general approach that is extremely flexible in allowing an analyst to consider alternative descriptions for their data. When developing a quantitative summary of a relationship between the probability of disease and putative risk factors, important questions arise as to which equation best describes the relationship and which measure of exposure should be included. This chapter primarily addresses the question of the model, beginning with the linear logistic model and then considering various alternatives. In Chapter 7 we will discuss issues related to choice of regressor variables and the interpretation of the corresponding regression parameters.

Generalized Linear Model for Proportions

As in Chapter 3, we continue our discussion of methods that deal with the analysis of proportions. For cohort data, these are assumed to arise from instances in which time can effectively be ignored, so that we are only interested in whether the disease of interest occurs. Examples we considered included studies of subjects who were all followed for the same length of time, such as diseases where the hazard is positive for a relatively short period of time, like outbreaks of food poisoning or congenital malformations that can be observed at birth. The response, Y, in these studies is binary, taking the value 1 if the disease is observed and is 0 otherwise. The probability of disease, $\pi(\mathbf{x})$, depends on a row vector of regressor variables, $\mathbf{x} = (x_1, x_2, \ldots, x_p)$. In this section, the fitting of such models is described, so that we can obtain the maximum likelihood estimates of parameters, significance tests adjusting for other factors in the model, and evidence of goodness of fit.

An essential feature of model fitting is the specification of the equation that determines how the regressor variables influence the probability of disease. For a single factor that just has two levels, this specification is not crucial because essentially all equations will give a good description of the data, and the only real decision is the measure of effect to be reported. However, as pointed out in Chapter 2, when there are more than two levels of exposure, or if there is more than one factor to be considered at the same time, the choice of equation can have a profound effect on the results.

A common feature of all the models we shall consider is that the response, Y, can be expressed as $Y = \mu(\mathbf{x}) + \epsilon$, which is the sum of two components: a systematic component or mean, $\mu(\mathbf{x})$, that depends on the regressor variables; and a random part or error, ϵ, that has a specified distribution. In ordinary regression, the error distribution is assumed to have a normal distribution with 0 mean and unspecified variance σ^2. The mean depends on the regressor variables through a linear predictor:

$$\eta = \alpha + x_1\beta_1 + x_2\beta_2 + \cdots + x_p\beta_p = \alpha + \mathbf{x}\boldsymbol{\beta}$$

In fact, for ordinary regression, $\mu = \eta$. The three essential ingredients of this model are these:

1. A linear predictor, η, describes the dependence of the outcome on the regressor variables included in the model.
2. The link function identifies the relationship between the mean, μ, and the linear predictor, η.
3. The error distribution characterizes the unexplained random variation.

The allowable error distributions belong to a broad exponential family that includes the binomial, as well as the Poisson and other probability distributions that apply to data from the types of studies that are commonly used by epidemiologists. Models that have these three ingredients are called *generalized linear models*, and they include all of the models we shall consider (2).

Let us now see how a binary response can be specified in terms of a generalized linear model. Recall that the probability of the different levels of the response are given by $\Pr\{Y = 1\} = \pi(\mathbf{x})$ and $\Pr\{Y = 0\} = 1 - \pi(\mathbf{x})$. If the data are grouped, so that n individuals are observed with the regressors, $\mathbf{x}$, the response, Y, would represent the total number of responders with a mean given by $\mu(\mathbf{x}) = n\,\pi(\mathbf{x})$. We shall see later that grouping has some advantages in assessing goodness of fit for a model, but in any event, we can still recover our original formulation by setting $n = 1$. Hence, we can express the observed response as $Y = \mu(\mathbf{x}) + \epsilon$, where the distribution of error, ϵ, is determined by the binomial distribution for the observed number of cases of disease, Y. The probability of disease, $\pi(\mathbf{x})$, depends on the regressor variables through the linear predictor, η, and, likewise, the mean depends on the same linear predictor because of its relationship with the probability of disease. In general, the mean is not equal to the linear predictor as in ordinary regression but depends on the *link function*, which defines the relationship between the mean and the linear predictor, $\eta = g(\mu)$. In the abstract, these relationships seem to be somewhat obscure, but, in fact, the relationship becomes fairly clear when we consider some specific examples.

Linear logistic model

The form for the linear logistic model which was used extensively in Chapter 3 is expressed as

$$
\begin{aligned}
\pi\{\mathbf{x}\} &= \frac{\exp\{\alpha + \mathbf{x}\boldsymbol{\beta}\}}{1 + \exp\{\alpha + \mathbf{x}\boldsymbol{\beta}\}} \\[2mm]
&= \frac{\exp\{\eta\}}{1 + \exp\{\eta\}}
\end{aligned}
\tag{6.1}
$$

Solving this expression for η yields the logit link function,

$$
\eta = \log\left(\frac{\pi}{1-\pi}\right) = \log\left(\frac{\mu}{n-\mu}\right) = g(\mu)
\tag{6.2}
$$

where n is the number of subjects in the corresponding observation.

One reason for the popularity of the linear logistic model is the ready interpretability of the model parameters, which results from the fairly simple interpretation of a change in the linear predictor. Suppose that $\mathbf{x_0}$ represents a reference level of the regressor variables, and one wishes to estimate the odds ratio for disease in a group with variables $\mathbf{x_1}$. The corresponding linear predictors for the two groups are η_0 and η_1, respectively, and the difference may be written as

$$\eta_1 - \eta_0 = (\mathbf{x_1} - \mathbf{x_0})\boldsymbol{\beta} \tag{6.3}$$

Using equations 6.1 and 6.2, we can see that this difference in linear predictors can be expressed as

$$\eta_1 - \eta_0 = \log\left(\frac{[1 - \pi(\mathbf{x_0})]\,\pi(\mathbf{x_1})}{\pi(\mathbf{x_0})\,[1 - \pi(\mathbf{x_1})]} \right) \tag{6.4}$$

which is the log odds ratio for disease. If only a single variable changes between the comparison and the reference groups, x_p, and all other variables remain the same, then equation 6.3 simplifies, and equation 6.4 may be written as

$$\eta_1 - \eta_0 = 0{\cdot}\boldsymbol{\beta_1} + 0{\cdot}\boldsymbol{\beta_2} + \cdots + (x_{p1} - x_{p0}) \cdot \beta_p + 0{\cdot}\boldsymbol{\beta}_{p+1} + \cdots$$

$$= (x_{p1} - x_{p0}) \cdot \beta_p$$

Hence, a one-unit change in the pth regressor variable, or $(x_{p1} - x_{p0}) = 1$, results in a β_p change in the log odds and an $\exp\{\beta_p\}$ multiplicative change in the odds.

Log-linear hazard model

The Cox proportional hazards model is often used for the analysis of failure time data, and in this context it is discussed in Chapter 9. As we saw in Chapter 2, the log-linear hazard model described by Cox (3) is given by

$$\lambda(t,\mathbf{x}) = \lambda_0(t)\,\exp\{\mathbf{x}\boldsymbol{\beta}\} \tag{6.5}$$

where t represents the time under observation. If all subjects are followed for the same interval of time, $(0,\tau]$, then we know that the probability a person has acquired the disease sometime during the interval is

$$\Pr(\tau;\mathbf{x}) = 1 - \exp\{-\exp[\alpha(\tau) + \mathbf{x}\boldsymbol{\beta}]\}$$

$$= 1 - \exp\{-\exp[\eta]\} = \pi$$

where $\alpha(\tau) = \log\left[\int_0^\tau \lambda_0(u)\,du \right]$.

Like the linear logistic model, this particular equation forces the range of possible values for the probability of disease to remain within the valid range, $(0,1)$. Solving for η, one can obtain the link function,

$$\eta = \log[-\log(1 - \pi)] = \log\left[-\log\left(1 - \frac{\mu}{n}\right)\right] = g(\mu)$$

which is called the *complementary log-log link* (2).

To interpret the model parameters, one can use an approach similar to that shown here earlier for the linear logistic model. The hazard ratio for a group with regressor variables $\mathbf{x_1}$ compared to the reference group with covariates $\mathbf{x_0}$ may be found from equation 6.5:

$$\frac{\lambda(t,\mathbf{x_1})}{\lambda(t,\mathbf{x_0})} = \frac{\lambda_0(t) \cdot \exp\{\mathbf{x_1}\boldsymbol{\beta}\}}{\lambda_0(t) \cdot \exp\{\mathbf{x_0}\boldsymbol{\beta}\}}$$

$$= \exp\{\eta_1 - \eta_0\}$$

Thus, the difference in the linear predictors is the log hazard ratio. Hence, if one variable, x_p, changes by one unit and all others remain constant, then the log hazard ratio changes by β_p or the hazard ratio is multiplied by $\exp\{\beta_p\}$.

One might well ask whether this model is preferred over the more popular linear logistic model. In fact, neither model has a compelling biological rationale, although there are desirable statistical properties for the linear logistic model that make it somewhat more convenient to deal with some theoretical aspects of model fitting. However, there are instances where some observations have detailed information on the length of time to the development of disease, and others only note whether the disease occurred during a specified interval of time. In the first instance, one might well use the proportional hazards model. Hence, it is most appropriate for comparison purposes to make use of the complementary log-log link for the proportions, which is essentially the same model. If one used the linear logistic model instead, it would be difficult to know whether any differences found between the two groups were in fact due to the fundamental differences in the models.

Probit model

Another multivariate model for proportions arises from using the inverse of the standard normal probability distribution as the link function, or $\eta = \Phi^{-1}(\pi) = \Phi^{-1}(\mu/n)$, where $\Phi(\cdot)$ is the standard normal distribution function. The probit model arose from work on biological assay (4–6), where one was interested in a clearly defined response of an animal to a given dose of drug. Let Z represent the tolerance of a subject to various assaults with respect to the response. We could think of z as representing a single exposure, or it could in fact arise from a linear combination of various factors, i.e., $z = c_1x_1 + c_2x_2 + \cdots + c_px_p$. If one focuses on a particular exposure level, z, then the response will be observed in an individual if the tolerance, $Z \leq z$, and it will not if $Z > z$. The proportion of individuals who respond to dose z is $\Pr\{Z \leq z\}$, and if one assumes that Z has a normal distribution with mean θ and variance σ^2, then

$$\Pr(Z \leq z) = \Phi\left(\frac{z - \theta}{\sigma}\right)$$

An advantage of the probit model is the existence of a fairly clear rationale in terms of the tolerance distribution. However, we cannot be certain that this distribution should be normal, and, unlike with the use of this distribution in multiple regression, there is no guarantee that the approximation will improve by increasing the sample size. Probably the most important reasons for not using this model in epidemiologic studies is that the parameters are not easily interpreted in terms of a risk measure. In addition, the difference in shape between the logit and the probit models is extremely small over the range of probabilities most commonly observed— that is, between .1 and .9—so, on the basis of providing a good description for a set of data, there is little reason for not choosing the linear logistic model, which is easier to handle for theoretical reasons.

Fitting Binary Response Models

Fitting the models described in the previous section is computationally tedious if it is attempted by hand. Hence, model fitting is generally accomplished by using a computer package, which provides summary statistics that may be used for statistical inference, as well as indicating the adequacy with which the data fit the model. In Appendix 5, there is a discussion of some of the issues that must be considered when fitting generalized linear models for binary responses. These details are not necessary if one is interested in fitting the most common binary response model, the linear logistic model, because software is available for just that purpose.

Fitting the linear logistic model

The logit link is typically the default when the binomial distribution is specified for the response because this is a so-called canonical link function for this distribution. Hence, we are usually not required to further specify any of the functions required to obtain maximum likelihood estimates. Let us now consider some examples of fitting this model to data.

Example 6–1   In Chapter 3 we conducted a significance test for trend using the data from a case-control study of the association between cigarette smoking and risk of giving birth to a baby with a congenital malformation, as shown in Table 3–10. We now attempt to fit a linear logistic model to these data, using a centered value to represent the smoking exposure for each category—$x = 0, 5, 15, 25,$ and 35 cigarettes per day. Figure 6–1 shows the log likelihood surface for the linear logistic model using these data, and its shape is typical of most of the problems we shall discuss in that it has a single maximum. The values of the parameters at the highest point in the likelihood surface are the *maximum likelihood estimates*, $(\hat{\alpha}, \hat{\beta})$. In addition, the overall shape resembles that of the log likelihood of a normally distributed response in which the equal likelihood contours displayed on the (α, β) plane are nearly elliptical, with vertical slices of the surface falling off as a quadratic function.

Figure 6–2 shows typical output that results from using software to fit this model (PROC GENMOD in SAS) (7). The estimated intercept gives the value for $\hat{\alpha}$, and the estimated regression coefficient for the regressor variable is $\hat{\beta}$, which estimates that the log odds changes by 0.0123 per cigarette (95% CI $= 0.0123 \pm (1.96)(0.0040) = 0.0045, 0.0201$). Hence, the estimated change in odds for a congenital malformation if a mother smokes 20 cigarettes more than her current level is $\exp\{(0.0123)(20)\} = 1.279$ (95% CI $= (1.279) \exp\{\pm(1.96)(0.0040)(20)\} = 1.093, 1.496$).

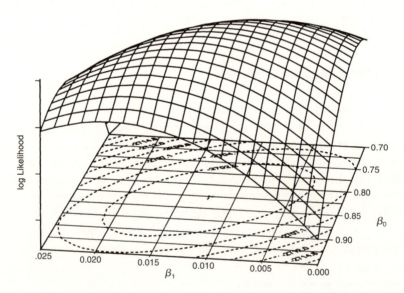

Figure 6–1 Log likelihood surface for the linear logistic model using the data on congenital malformations in Table 3–10.

```
Criteria For Assessing Goodness Of Fit

Criterion                DF        Value        Value/DF

Scaled Deviance           3        3.3830        1.1277
Pearson Chi-Square        3        3.3808        1.1269
Log Likelihood            .      -2699.7725         .


Analysis Of Parameter Estimates

Parameter    DF    Estimate    Std Err    ChiSquare    Pr>Chi

INTERCEPT     1     -0.8293     0.0377     484.5003     0.0001
X             1      0.0123     0.0040       9.2952     0.0023

Likelihood Ratio Based Confidence Intervals For Parameters

Two-Sided Confidence Coefficient: 0.9500
Parameter        Confidence Limits      Parameter Values
                                         PRM1          PRM2

PRM1         Lower       -0.9035      -0.9035      0.0162
PRM1         Upper       -0.7558      -0.7558      0.008387
PRM2         Lower        0.004355    -0.7931      0.004355
PRM2         Upper        0.0202      -0.8664      0.0202


MAL      NUM     Pred     Xbeta      Std    Resraw    Reschi    Resdev

889     2877    0.3038   -0.8293   0.0377   15.0005   0.6081    0.6071
182      608    0.3170   -0.7678   0.0327  -10.7108  -0.9336   -0.9384
203      623    0.3442   -0.6447   0.0531  -11.4257  -0.9635   -0.9677
 55      141    0.3725   -0.5216   0.0885    2.4818   0.4323    0.4310
 40       88    0.4017   -0.3986   0.1269    4.6541   1.0120    1.0058
```

Figure 6–2 Output generated by PROC GENMOD (SAS) showing results from fitting data on congenital malformations in Table 3–10.

The maximum log-likelihood is given as −2699.7725, so that the contour at −2702.2 is 2.4 lower than the maximum. Hence, the region circumscribed by the contour at −2702.2 yields the values for α and β that result in a likelihood ratio statistic that takes the value 2(2.4) = 4.8 or less. The p value from the corresponding chi-square distribution with 2 df is .09, so that the two-parameter region has a confidence level of $100(1 - .09) = 91\%$. Because we are only interested in the parameter associated with cigarette smoking, we can similarly construct a confidence interval for this parameter by only considering the profile likelihood. This curve traces the silhouette that would be formed by a parallel beam of light shining onto the β by log-likelihood plane in Figure 6–1. We can find this by fitting a linear logistic model in which we estimate α for specified values of the offset, βx_i. This curve

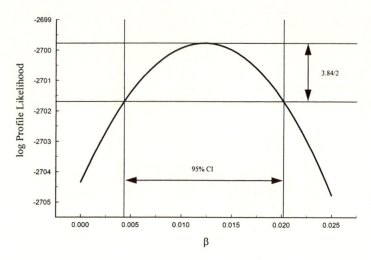

Figure 6–3 Profile likelihood for the slope using the data on congenital malformations in Table 3–10.

is shown in Figure 6–3, and the values of β that decrease the log likelihood by $\frac{1}{2}$ of the 5% critical value for a chi-square distribution with 1 df (3.84/2 = 1.92) or less comprise the 95% confidence interval (CI). These were also calculated by the software and displayed in Figure 6–2, showing the likelihood ratio interval to be (0.0043, 0.0202), which is similar to the Wald intervals, $\hat{\beta} \pm z_{\alpha/2}SE(\hat{\beta})$, we have already calculated.

When we use tabulated or grouped data, the overall adequacy of this model in describing the exposure-disease association can be assessed by either the scaled deviance ($G^2 = 3.3830$, df = 3) or the Pearson chi-square ($\chi^2 = 3.3808$, df = 3), both of which do not suggest strong evidence for lack of fit. In addition, we consider the residuals in order to determine whether any one level of exposure exhibits poor fit, or whether patterns exist. As we see in Figure 6–2, both the chi and the deviance residuals are similar because of the relatively large sample size. None of these residuals is suspiciously large; the greatest magnitude is approximately 1, which is the expected value of any standardized residual for a model that fits the data. There is some suggestion of a pattern among the residuals, in that they are negative for $I = 2,3$ and positive for the others, with the largest values at the extremes. However, we also need to keep in mind that there are only five data points, so this is not particularly surprising, and we can conclude that this model appears to be adequate for describing the relationship between exposure and disease. This formal analysis of the adequacy of fit can only be accomplished when we are working with tabulated data. Had we, instead, put in the data for each subject individually, the regression parameters would have been unchanged, but the goodness-of-fit statistics would not have been meaningful.

Fitting alternatives to the logistic model

We now consider some alternatives to the linear logistic model that are sometimes considered when they are thought to give a better representation of data. We first consider a model in which the odds for disease is linear, rather than log linear, and then extend this to the more general power family of models for the odds that allows us to address the question of whether one model offers a significantly better fit to the data.

Linear odds model. We now assume a linear relationship with the untransformed odds, so that

$$\frac{\pi(\mathbf{x})}{1 - \pi(\mathbf{x})} = \alpha + \mathbf{x}\boldsymbol{\beta} = \frac{\mu}{n - \mu} = \eta \qquad (6.6)$$

which is the linear odds link function. Because the odds is the ratio of two probabilities, it cannot be negative—that is, values of $\mathbf{x}$ such that $\mathbf{x}\boldsymbol{\beta} < -\alpha$ are inadmissable. This anomaly did not exist for either the linear logistic, the log-linear hazard, or the probit models described earlier, but one needs to keep this possibility in mind when fitting data to this model. Numerical algorithms used in fitting these models require intermediate estimates of the parameters, along with the corresponding disease probabilities. A negative fitted odds for a subject will yield a negative probability of disease, which a carefully written regression program should recognize as an error, thus causing the calculations to cease.

Just because the linear odds regression model can give inadmissable values is no reason to necessarily abandon it; in some instances, this model can provide a good description of data over the range of values observed for the regressors. To make sure that a regression package does not stop because values are out of range, one can try forcing the probability of disease to be some small arbitrary number when it is negative, so that an error is never produced by the program. While this can avoid errors recognized by the computer, it does not always eliminate the problem: for this model, the tangent plane at the peak may not be horizontal which the program recognizes when the gradient vector is **0**. The relationship between the linear predictor and the probability of disease takes the form shown by the line in Figure 6–4, which has a sharp corner at the origin, thus violating a fundamental assumption used in deriving many asymptotic results, such as variance estimators, significance tests, confidence intervals and other basic summaries of the regression model. In fact, the maximum of the likelihood may lie along a sharp cusp that is not smooth, which can re-

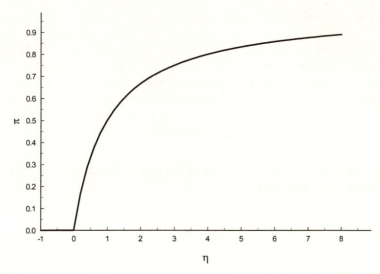

Figure 6–4 The relationship between the linear predictor and the probability of disease for the linear odds model.

sult in an algorithm endlessly jumping between two or more values rather that converging to a single solution.

Example 6–2   Thomas (8,9) presents the data shown in Table 6–1 on the association between asbestos exposure and lung cancer incidence. A plot of the log odds against asbestos exposure is shown in Figure 6–5, along with the fitted line from a linear logistic model. Notice the systematic departure from the regression line, in

Table 6–1. Data on the association between risk of lung cancer and asbestos exposure (9)

| Asbestos exposure* | Disease status (no. of subjects) | | Odds ratio |
	Healthy	Lung cancer	
0–6*	285	43	1.000
6–10	62	10	1.069
10–30	166	24	0.958
30–100	211	37	1.162
100–300	168	31	1.223
300–600	95	27	1.884
600–1000	50	18	2.386
1000–1500	19	10	3.488
1500–2000	8	6	4.971
2000–∞	11	9	5.423

* Reference group for calculating odds ratios.

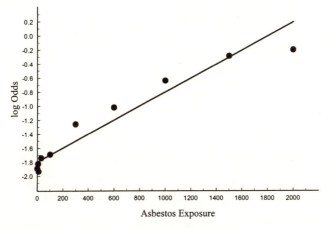

Figure 6–5 Plot of the log odds for lung cancer against asbestos exposure using the data in Table 6–1.

that the middle points consistently lie above while those at the extremes lie below the line. Alternatively, consider the plot using the untransformed odds ratio shown in Figure 6–6, which has largely eliminated the systematic departure from the underlying model. In Chapter 7, we consider the question of selecting transformations in greater detail, but let us now fit a linear odds model using the methods under discussion.

As with the linear logistic model, the distribution of the response is binary, so our choice of a distribution for error is still the binomial. However, the link function and the corresponding inverse and/or derivative that are required for fitting the data are shown in Table A5–1. A summary of the results from fitting these data are shown in Figure 6–7. The overall fit appears to be very good indeed, with both

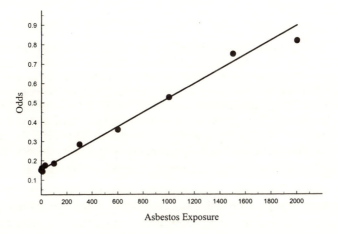

Figure 6–6 Plot of the odds for lung cancer against asbestos exposure using the data in Table 6–1.

```
Criteria For Assessing Goodness Of Fit

Criterion              DF         Value       Value/DF

Scaled Deviance        8          0.5016       0.0627
Pearson Chi-Square     8          0.5024       0.0628
Log Likelihood         .         -565.1120        .



Analysis Of Parameter Estimates

Parameter    DF    Estimate     Std Err    ChiSquare   Pr>Chi

INTERCEPT    1       0.1529      0.0151     102.8317    0.0001
X            1       0.0004      0.0001      15.5714    0.0001



CASE      NUM     Pred      Xbeta      Std      Resraw      Reschi      Resdev

 43       328    0.1326    0.1529     0.0151    -0.4981    -0.0811     -0.0812
 10        72    0.1343    0.1551     0.0149     0.3309     0.1144      0.1138
 24       190    0.1354    0.1566     0.0147    -1.7272    -0.3662     -0.3698
 37       248    0.1409    0.1641     0.0142     2.0484     0.3738      0.3708
 31       199    0.1597    0.1901     0.0144    -0.7874    -0.1524     -0.1529
 27       122    0.2092    0.2645     0.0265     1.4792     0.3293      0.3270
 18        68    0.2733    0.3762     0.0527    -0.5868    -0.1597     -0.1602
 10        29    0.3443    0.5250     0.0897     0.0165     0.006450    0.006450
  6        14    0.4156    0.7110     0.1364     0.1822     0.0988      0.0986
  9        20    0.4729    0.8971     0.1834    -0.4575    -0.2049     -0.2051
```

Figure 6–7 Summary of the results from fitting a linear odds model to the data in Table 6–1.

the scaled deviance and the Pearson chi-square taking values of about 0.5 with 8 df. Likewise, none of the residuals is large, nor do they exhibit a systematic pattern that might suggest that the model was inappropriate for this range of exposures. Hence, we can conclude that this model gives an adequate description of these data. Our estimate of the effect of asbestos is that for each unit increase in the level of asbestos exposure, the odds for lung cancer increases by 0.0004 (SE = 0.0001). The single-digit accuracy of the result arises because of the units selected for exposure. If we choose instead to code these in 100s of units, our estimate of effect is 0.0372 (SE = 0.0094), providing an estimate of the change in the odds for disease per 100 units change in exposure. Under the circumstances, it makes more sense to discuss risk in terms of larger changes in exposure.

Odds power family of models. We have considered two models for the odds, but let us now consider a power family, which allows us to test whether either model yields a significant improvement in fit, as well as the possibility of estimating a maximum likelihood estimate for the power transformation. The link function for our model involves powers of the odds ratio,

$$\eta = g(\pi) = \left(\frac{\pi}{1-\pi}\right)^{\gamma} \qquad \text{if } \gamma \neq 0$$

$$= \log\left(\frac{\pi}{1-\pi}\right) \qquad \text{if } \gamma = 0$$

and the corresponding inverse link is shown in Table A5–1. We now consider an example in which we fit data this model to data.

Example 6–2 (continued)   Let us return to the data in Table 6–1, only this time let us try to fit the odds power model. If we specify the value of γ, we can use standard software to find the maximum likelihood estimators, as well as the corresponding maximum of the log likelihood. Figure 6–8 shows a plot of this profile log-likelihood against γ. While the maximum likelihood estimator for γ is 1.18945, the difference between its maximum log likelihood and that obtained under the linear logistic model ($\gamma = 0$) can be used to construct a test of whether the linear logistic model results in significantly worse fit, H_0: $\gamma = 0$, $\Delta G^2 = 2[-565.0855 - (-566.5365)] = 2.902$, which can be compared to a chi-square distribution with 1 df. Hence, both the linear logistic and the linear odds models are well within the

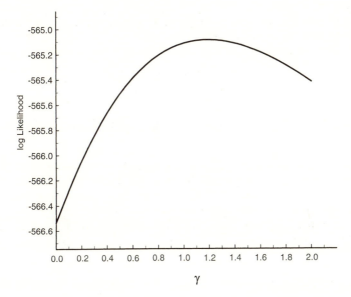

Figure 6–8 Profile log likelihood for the power parameter resulting from fitting the data in Table 6–1.

Table 6–2. Summary of parameters from alternative models for the data in Table 6–1

Parameter	Estimate	SE	W^2	p value
LOGIT				
Intercept	−1.7974	0.0850	446.73	<.0001
Asbestos/100	0.0994	0.0177	31.44	<.0001
$G^2 = 3.35$; $\chi^2 = 3.41$; df $= 8$				
LINEAR				
Intercept	0.1529	0.0151	102.83	<.0001
Asbestos/100	0.0372	0.0094	15.57	<.0001
$G^2 = 0.50$; $\chi^2 = 0.50$; df $= 8$				
LINEAR POWER				
Intercept	0.1058	0.0127	69.32	<.0001
Asbestos/100	0.0354	0.0094	14.16	.0002
$G^2 = 0.45$; $\chi^2 = 0.45$; df $= 8$				
LINEAR POWER WITH CORRECTED VARIANCE				
Intercept	0.1058	0.1749	0.36	.5453
Asbestos/100	0.0354	0.0144	6.03	.0141
$G^2 = 0.45$; $\chi^2 = 0.45$; df $= 7$				

W^2 = Wald statistic.

confidence limits for our estimate of γ. Table 6–2 summarizes the parameter estimates obtained under three models implied by this family of functions. While the estimates vary considerably, the significance of the trend with level of exposure is very strong in all cases.

By employing the method described in Appendix 5, we can obtain the standard error of our estimate of γ, 0.84638. The covariance matrix for the regression parameters that does not allow for the fact that we have estimated γ is

$$\begin{bmatrix} 0.0001615 & -0.000044 \\ -0.000044 & 0.0000884 \end{bmatrix}$$

but if we calculate the corrected matrix, using the procedure described in Appendix 5, we obtain

$$\begin{bmatrix} 0.0305983 & 0.0018629 \\ 0.00189629 & 0.0002079 \end{bmatrix}$$

which is considerably larger. Table 6–2 shows that even though we maintain the significance of the association between asbestos exposure and risk of lung cancer, the p value is considerably larger than before.

Problems in model fitting

The examples we have considered up to this point are ideal in that the maximum likelihood estimates exist because the likelihood surface exhibits

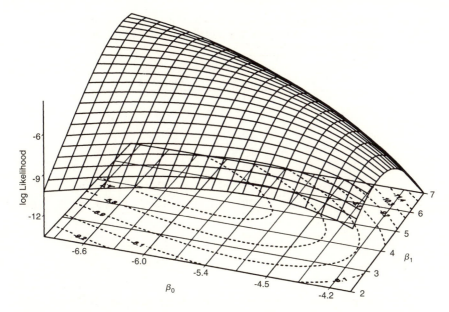

Figure 6–9 Likelihood surface for the linear logistic model using the data on psittacosis among mink room workers shown in Table 3–8.

a unique mode. But we also need to look out for instances in which there are no maximum likelihood estimates so that we may understand the behavior we might expect to observe in these cases. The following two examples illustrate instances in which the log likelihood does not have a peak; rather, it describes a ridge that extends to infinity.

Example 6–3 Let us consider once again the data on the incidence of psittacosis among mink room workers, as shown in Table 3–8. We have already noted that the odds ratio is not defined, and the corresponding log likelihood surface for these data, if we represent working area by $x = 1$ for those in the mink room and 0 otherwise, is shown in Figure 6–9. In this case, the surface continues to increase along a ridge as $\beta \to \infty$ and $\alpha \to -\infty$. If we recall that β gives the log odds ratio in this instance, this is consistent with our calculations in Chapter 3, but because the software employs an iterative algorithm to climb the log-likelihood mountain, it never finds a peak within the restricted number of steps but keeps wandering out to infinity. Typically, we are warned with the message that the algorithm "failed to converge," but occasionally some software packages do not pick up this difficulty; hence, we should always regard very large parameters with suspicion and investigate further to determine whether, in fact, the estimates exist. If the algorithm is in the process of diverging when it stops, we cannot trust the resulting output.

Table 6–3. Hypothetical data in which maximum likelihood estimators for unadjusted log odds ratios exist while the adjusted estimators do not

Exposure		Healthy	Diseased	Total
χ_A	χ_B			
0	0	13	12	25
0	1	0	25	25
	+	13	37	50
1	0	25	0	25
1	1	10	15	25
	+	35	15	50
+	0	38	12	50
+	1	10	40	50
	+	48	52	100

This is a special case of a more general situation in which the linear logistic model parameters are infinite, which suggests that there is a particular level of the covariate that identifies all diseased (or healthy) individuals. A similar phenomenon can be observed for a continuous regressor variable if a level of the covariate exists that separates diseased from healthy individuals. The likelihood surface in these instances will likewise exhibit this characteristic ridge, and the parameter estimates will diverge to $\pm\infty$. We can easily recognize that parameters will diverge when a univariate analysis of the unadjusted logistic regression parameter is $\pm\infty$, but divergence can also occur in more subtle ways when we are conducting a multivariable analysis. The following example illustrates such an instance in which the maximum likelihood estimates do not exist, even though the univariate values are defined. Unfortunately, a general rule is not known for identifying when the algorithm will diverge; hence, we must always be careful to look for signs that the algorithm is having difficulty in finding a maximum of the log likelihood.

Example 6–4   Table 6–3 shows a hypothetical set of data dealing with the effect of exposure to two putative risk factors, which we will refer to as A and B. When we attempt to fit a linear logistic model, it becomes apparent that the parameters are once again diverging. Because the model now involves three parameters, it is not possible to plot the likelihood surface because there are now four dimensions to be considered, but in Figure 6–10 we see the profile likelihood surface on the plane for the risk factor effects, β_A and β_B. Once again, the highest points on the surface lie along a ridge that increases as $\beta_A \to -\infty$ and $\beta_B \to +\infty$. This is not readily apparent if we determine the marginal or unadjusted associations with disease

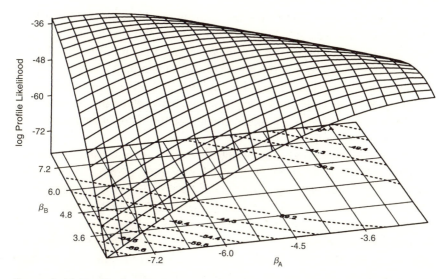

Figure 6-10 Profile log likelihood surface for the hypothetical data shown in Table 6-3.

by combining data over one of the factors, in that the odds ratios for each factor is finite,

$$\hat{\beta}_{A,unadj} = \log[(13)(15)/(37)(35)] = -1.8933$$

and

$$\hat{\beta}_{B,unadj} = \log[(38)(40)/(12)(10)] = 2.5390$$

However, the log odds ratio for A when $X_B = 0$ is $\log[(13)(0)/(12)(25)] \to -\infty$, which is also the case for $X_B = 1$, and, likewise, the estimated stratum-specific log odds ratio for β_B is estimated to be $+\infty$. The iterative algorithms used by software to find the maximum likelihood estimates will attempt to approach these values, but the ultimate result will obviously be a diverging process.

Summary

In this chapter, we have considered the problem of fitting binary response models to data in which there are multiple regressor variables that may be either discrete or continuous in nature. The linear logistic model, the most commonly used model for this type of response, provides estimates of parameters that are assumed to have linear effects on the log odds ratio, thus yielding values that can be interpreted as log odds ratios. We have also considered the more flexible generalized linear models family that can readily be adapted for fitting many alternative forms for the relationship between exposure and disease outcome. The particular models that were specifically described were as follows: the log-linear hazard, the probit model, the linear odds model, and the linear power of the odds model. Each model can be characterized by identifying the outcome as having a binomial distribution and by specifying the link function that relates the mean or the probability of disease with a linear portion of the model that depends on the regressor variables.

The linear power odds model introduced an unknown parameter that could not be included as one of the usual regression parameters in the linear predictor. However, the approach we have described was readily modified to include such terms in a generalized conditionally linear model. While this approach can easily be employed for a single nonlinear parameter, the particular approach we have used here quickly becomes more difficult to apply when we include additional parameters. However, we have seen that if we are trying to estimate the nonlinear parameter from our data, it is essential to introduce an appropriate adjustment for the covariance matrix; otherwise, we can seriously underestimate the variance.

While the class of models we have seen here is very rich, it must be said that in particular problems there may be models for a set of data that are not linearizable and thus do not belong to this class. These can arise from theoretical considerations of the underlying disease process in situations where we have extensive knowledge of the underlying biology. However, we do have a very flexible tool for describing binary response data that offers a practical way of fitting models to data and obtaining good estimates of the parameters.

Each of the models considered in this chapter required that we use the link function to arrive at the linear part of the model; that is, we transformed the response. In Chapter 7, we consider, among other things, taking transformations of the regressor variables, which extends still further the types of models we can employ. This methodology is extended still further by introducing the effect of risk factors as unspecified functions, described in Chapter 11. Hence, we have only just begun to explore the alternative ways of summarizing binary response data that are available to us. In subsequent chapters, we will also see how these approaches can be applied in situations that include the element of time in determining the response.

Exercises

6.1. The data in the following table are from a clinical trial in which an oral agent used to lower blood sugar was compared to a placebo in the treatment of adult-onset diabetes (10, 11). The outcome of interest in this analysis is death from cardiovascular disease (CHD), which is one of the most common complications of this disease.

		Male		Female	
Age	Treatment	No. patients	No. CHD deaths	No. patients	No. CHD deaths
≤ 53	Placebo	28	1	85	1
	Oral agent	26	5	71	1
>53	Placebo	35	6	58	2
	Oral agent	37	6	70	14

a. The Mantel–Haenszel test provides a score statistic for testing the association between CHD death and treatment, adjusting for gender and age. From the perspective of model fitting, calculate the identical test using:
   i. The Wald statistic
   ii. The likelihood ratio statistic
b. Estimate the adjusted odds ratios for treatment and CHD, using the model fitted in (a).
c. Test for a modification of the effect of treatment by sex.

6.2. Repeat Exercise 6.1 using the log-linear hazard (complementary log-log) model. How do the results compare? Why?

6.3. Return to the data from the case-control study of the relationship between epithelial ovarian cancer and the use of combination oral contraceptives in Exercise 3.4 of Chapter 3.

a. Find the maximum likelihood estimate of the overall log odds ratio for the oral contraceptive ovarian cancer association adjusted for age, and provide a 90% confidence interval for your estimate.
b. Give an overall Wald test for the association.
c. Give an overall likelihood ratio test of the association.

6.4. The data in this exercise are from a case-control study of esophageal cancer conducted in Ille-et-Vilaine, Brittany (12). The cases were 200 males diagnosed with esophageal cancer in one of the regional hospitals between January 1972 and April 1974. Controls were from a sample of 775 adult males drawn from electoral lists. Each subject was given a dietary interview, which contained questions on their consumption of tobacco and alcohol. The data, provided as a sequence of five numbers, are coded as follows (available on the website http://gisserver.yale.edu/holford/examples):

Age: 1 = 25–34; 2 = 35–44; 3 = 45–54; 4 = 55–64; 5 = 65–74; 6 = 75+
Alcohol (g/day): 1 = 0–39; 2 = 40–79; 3 = 80–119; 4 = 120+

Tobacco (g/day): $1 = 0-9$; $2 = 10-19$; $3 = 20-29$; $4 = 30+$

Number of cases

Number of controls

a. Estimate the odds ratio for disease for each of the factors, adjusting for the others by using a linear logistic model.

b. For each of the factors, test whether there is a significant departure from a linear trend, and propose an effective way of providing a succinct description of the effect of that variable on the risk of esophageal cancer.

c. Find the best-fitting model for these data, and summarize your conclusions.

References

1. Mantel N, Haenszel W. Statistical aspects of the analysis of data from retrospective studies of disease. *Journal of the National Cancer Institute* 1959;22: 719–748.

2. McCullagh P, Nelder JA. *Generalized Linear Models*. London: Chapman and Hall, 1989.

3. Cox DR. Regression models and life-tables (with discussion). *Journal of the Royal Statistical Society, Series B* 1972;34:187–220.

4. Bliss CI. The method of probits. *Science* 1934;79:38–39.

5. Bliss CI. The method of probits—a correction. *Science* 1934;79.

6. Finney DJ. *Probit Analysis* (3rd ed.). Cambridge: Cambridge University Press, 1971.

7. SAS Institute Inc. *SAS/STAT User's Guide*, (Version 6). Cary, NC: SAS Institute, 1989.

8. Liddell FDK, McDonald JC, Thomas DC. Methods of cohort analysis: appraised by application to asbestos mining. *Journal of the Royal Statistical Society, Series A* 1977;140:469–491.

9. Thomas DC. General relative risk models for survival time and matched case-control analysis. *Biometrics* 1981;37:673–686.

10. University Group Diabetes Program. A study of the effects of hypoglycemic agents on vascular complications in patients with adult onset diabetes: I. Design, methods, and baseline results; II. Mortality results. *Diabetes* 1970;12, Suppl. 2:747–830.

11. Committee for the Assessment of Biometric Aspects of Controlled Trials of Hypoglycemic Agents. Report of the Committee for the Assessment of Biometric Aspects of Controlled Trials of Hypoglycemic Agents. *Journal of the American Medical Association* 1975;231:583–608.

12. Breslow NE, Day NE. *Statistical Methods in Cancer Research*. Lyon: International Agency for Research on Cancer, 1980.

7

Defining Regressor Variables

The successful use of models in the conduct of statistical inference in epidemiology depends on the appropriate specification of the exposure-response relationship. In Chapter 6, the particular models described involved the probability of disease developing within a specified period of time. The power of these models can be enhanced by the careful choice of regressor variables, which are discussed in some detail in this chapter. Hypotheses of interest in an epidemiologic study can sometimes be fairly complex, but the concept of a general linear hypothesis provides a flexible and powerful tool that can address many different questions when one wishes to compare various risk groups. Questions of particular interest may include the comparison of specific subgroups and investigations into the adequacy of the model. The latter includes analyses of the homogeneity of the association between a risk factor and the response among subgroups of the study population. Effects that are not homogeneous can be especially useful when trying to understand the etiology of a disease because they sometimes provide clues to the underlying causal mechanisms. In addition, nonhomogeneous effects can sometimes be used to devise more focused and cost-effective strategies for disease prevention, by pointing out populations that may be targets for prophylaxis.

A genuine concern when one is analyzing continuous variables is the values that should be included in the model. In Chapter 6, alternative transformations for the odds of disease were considered, and in much the same way we can also consider alternative transformations of the regressor variables. In this chapter we discuss a strategy for selecting a transformation for either the regressor variables or the response.

Categorical Variables

At the most basic level, categorical variables (sometimes called nominal variables) are those that describe named groups, and they are not meant to imply anything resembling a natural order. In Chapter 3, we considered an example where the nominal categories were exposed and not exposed to cigarette smoke. In this instance, it was natural to consider the unexposed as the reference category, and the purpose of the analysis would be to estimate disease risk of those exposed relative to those unexposed. However, the choice of a comparison group may be completely arbitrary, such as an analysis of the effect of gender. In this analysis, it is just as logical to compare the risk for men with women as it is to compare women with men, and no confusion arises, as long as the comparison is clearly specified when the results are presented.

Nominal variables may also have more than two levels, such as the analysis of the effect of ethnicity on disease risk, where the categories might be loosely referred to as European, African American, Native American, Asian, and Hispanic. Once again, the choice of a reference category is completely arbitrary, although it is usually not practical to select a small group as the reference because all of the resulting estimates of risk become imprecise.

The next order of complexity for categorical variables involves a natural ordering in the groups, but one may not wish to force that order to have a specific mathematical effect on the response, at least not at an early stage of the analysis. For example, stage of disease is often useful in evaluating prognosis in cancer, and one scheme is to classify tumors as local, regional, and remote. While these categories indicate progressive degrees of tumor invasion into surrounding tissue, there is generally not a sound basis for defining a specific mathematical form for the effect on the response.

Finally, categories are occasionally formed from variables that are intrinsically continuous. If one is analyzing the effect of duration of use of oral contraceptives, the categories might be none (0 years), less than 1 year, 1–2 years, 3–5 years, and greater than 5 years. While there is a specific numerical quantity underlying these categories, one might wish initially to allow that effect on risk to emerge from the analysis rather than force a specific relationship. For instance, is it reasonable to extrapolate a trend among oral contraceptive users to obtain estimates of risk for non-users? Women who do not use oral contraceptives may make that decision for a variety of reasons that could be related to their risk of disease and have nothing to do with the constituents of the pill, including a desire to become pregnant or sexual inactivity for either voluntary or physiological reasons. The methods described in this section will allow the pattern to emerge from the data, and one can also test for whether there is a statistically significant departure from a specified model. In this example, there is clearly more detailed information on duration of use that could have been obtained, but this has been lost by forming the categories. In Chapter 12, we shall describe other alternatives being developed that are even more flexible in estimating the exposure–response relationship, methods that do not require identification of a specific parametric form. After one is satisfied with the specification for the regressor variables, a final run that includes these variables provides an overall summary of the results.

Two coding schemes for categorical variables are commonly used: 0 1 coding and -1 0 1 coding. To obtain estimates of the adjusted odds ratio and the adjusted hazard ratio, it is often easier to use a 0 1 coding. However, not all statistical packages have adopted this convention, so it is necessary to become familiar with both approaches if one is to use the default parameterization offered by the software. To interpret the parameters, one must have a particular model in mind because the interpretation often arises from an evaluation of a change in the linear predictor for the exposure and the reference group, $\eta_1 - \eta_0$. For the linear logistic model, the change represents the log odds ratio:

$$\eta_1 - \eta_0 = \log\left(\frac{P(X_1) \cdot [1 - P(X_0)]}{[1 - P(X_1)] \cdot P(X_0)}\right)$$

Likewise, for the linear odds model, the change in the linear predictor represents a difference in the odds for disease:

$$\eta_1 - \eta_0 = \frac{P(X_1)}{1 - P(X_1)} - \frac{P(X_0)}{1 - P(X_0)}$$

If the log-linear hazard or complementary log-log model for proportions is used, the change in the linear predictor represents a change in the log hazard ratio:

$$\eta_1 - \eta_0 = \log\left[\frac{\lambda_0(t) \cdot \exp(X_1\beta)}{\lambda_0(t \cdot \exp(X_0\beta)}\right]$$

Similar interpretations could be used for the more complex models, such as the power models, but these do not correspond to some of the more commonly used measures of association between exposure and disease, so they will not be discussed in detail.

0 1 coding

One approach to coding is to let a variable take the value 1 when a particular level is observed and 0 otherwise. In the instance of cigarette smoking, we could define

$$X_1 = 0 \qquad \text{if not exposed}$$
$$= 1 \qquad \text{if exposed}$$

Comparing an exposed group with a group that is unexposed but identical with respect to all other factors in the model results in a change in the linear predictor given by

$$\eta_1 - \eta_0 = (1 - 0)\beta_1 + (X_2 - X_2)\beta_2 + (X_3 - X_3)\beta_3 + \cdots + (X_p - X_p)\beta_p$$
$$= \beta_1$$

Thus, the regression coefficient, β_1, represents the change holding all other variables in the model constant, which is often stated as "the effect of cigarette smoking adjusted for the other factors in the model." This coefficient would represent an adjusted log odds ratio if it appeared in the linear logistic model; an adjusted odds difference in a linear odds model, and an adjusted log hazard ratio in a log-linear hazards model.

If three categories are represented by a particular factor, then these are represented in the regression model by including additional 0 1 regressor variables. In general, a factor that had k levels would require one fewer regressor variables than the number of levels, $k - 1$, in the regression model. For example, if the factor under consideration is the extent of disease, $k = 3$ levels, then one might define two $(3 - 1)$ regressor variables, as follows:

(0) Local: $X_1 = 0, X_2 = 0$
(1) Regional: $X_1 = 1, X_2 = 0$
(2) Remote: $X_1 = 0, X_2 = 1$

If (0) local is the reference level and one wishes to compare the risk of (1) regional to it holding all other factors constant,

$$\eta_1 - \eta_0 = (1 - 0)\beta_1 + (0 - 0)\beta_2 + 0\beta_3 + 0\beta_4 + \cdots$$
$$= \beta_1$$

Similarly, the comparison of (2) remote to (0) local is given by

$$\eta_2 - \eta_0 = (0 - 0)\beta_1 + (1 - 0)\beta_2 + 0\beta_3 + 0\beta_4 + \cdots$$
$$= \beta_2$$

A general rule to use when interpreting the regression coefficients from a 0 1 coding is the following: The regression coefficients give the risk for the particular category using the level with all zeros as the reference.

While the simplest interpretation of parameters obtained using this coding scheme arises from a comparison with the level with all zeros, other comparisons can also be made. To understand these comparisons, one can once again make use of the change in the linear predictors. For example, to compare (2) remote with (1) regional in the preceding illustration, the difference in linear predictors becomes

$$\eta_2 - \eta_1 = (0 - 1)\beta_1 + (1 - 0)\beta_2 + 0\beta_3 + 0\beta_4$$
$$= \beta_2 - \beta_1 \tag{7.1}$$

which involves more than one regression parameter. This modest complication is not difficult to deal with if one is only interested in a point estimate of risk. However, to calculate the standard error for this estimate, one must use not only the standard error for both parameters but also their covariance. A general expression for the variance of a linear function of random variables, in this case regression parameters, is given by

$$\text{Var}(\textstyle\sum_i c_i \cdot \hat{\beta}_i) = \textstyle\sum_i c_i^2 \, \text{Var}(\hat{\beta}_i) + 2 \textstyle\sum_{i,j<i} c_i c_j \, \text{Cov}(\hat{\beta}_i, \hat{\beta}_j) \tag{7.2}$$

For the estimate of the difference in linear predictors considered in equation 7.1, the constants are $c_1 = -1$ and $c_2 = 1$. Thus, the standard error would be computed by

$$\text{Var}(\hat{\beta}_2 - \hat{\beta}_1) = \text{Var}((-1)\cdot\hat{\beta}_1 + (1)\cdot\hat{\beta}_2)$$
$$= (-1)^2\text{Var}(\hat{\beta}_1) + (1)^2\text{Var}(\hat{\beta}_2) + 2(-1)(1)\text{Cov}(\hat{\beta}_1,\hat{\beta}_2)$$
$$= \text{Var}(\hat{\beta}_1) + \text{Var}(\hat{\beta}_2) - 2\text{Cov}(\hat{\beta}_1,\hat{\beta}_2)$$

Example 7–1   Petrakis et al. (1), in an earlier study, demonstrated that fluid secreted from some adult nonlactating women's breasts could be readily aspirated for a potential cancer screening test. To assess the usefulness of the test, they were interested in learning whether the distribution of women who secreted fluid, so-called secretors, was related to factors that are known to be related to breast cancer. This could provide leads for understanding the biology of breast cancer, and further cytological and biochemical analysis of the breast fluid might help identify women at high risk for developing breast cancer. As part of that study, the investigators reported the data shown in Table 7–1, which gives the number of secretors and the total number sampled broken down by age and four ethnic groups: white, black, Chinese, and Latin American.

   For now, we will treat age as a categorical variable, even though it is obviously derived from a continuous variable. Alternative approaches for dealing with age are considered in more detail in the following section, "Deviations from the Model." Because there are four ethnic groups considered in this analysis, $4 - 1 = 3$ regressor variables must be created to completely describe all the categories. In this situation the choice of a reference level is clearly arbitrary, but suppose the white group is selected, because it is by far the largest group represented in the study,

Table 7–1. Number of women who yielded breast fluid by age and ethnic group (1)

	White		Black		Chinese		Latin American	
Age	No. of secretors	No. studied	No. of secretors	No. studied	No. of secretors	No. studied	No. of secretors	No. studied
<20	9	32	2	13	1	1	1	1
20–29	208	424	25	62	11	48	7	13
30–39	428	607	55	102	29	78	32	45
40–49	580	819	83	114	40	94	35	56
50–59	361	628	50	98	7	47	18	30
≥60	138	337	23	66	7	61	3	9

thus providing a good opportunity for the most stable estimates of risk. A 0 1 coding might result in the creation of the regressor variables, (X_1, X_2, X_3), shown in Table 7–2. Fitting a linear logistic model to these data, including age as a similarly coded categorical variable, gave the likelihood ratio statistic, $G^2 = 21.61$ with 15 df ($p = .117$), which indicates that the model is giving an adequate description of the data, as the test for goodness of fit cannot be rejected. The estimates of the regression parameters for the ethnicity variables (the age parameters included in the model are not displayed in this table), as well as their variances and covariances, are also displayed in Table 7–2. Only the lower left triangle is shown as the covariance matrix is symmetric, i.e., $\text{Cov}(\hat{\beta}_i, \hat{\beta}_j) = \text{Cov}(\hat{\beta}_j, \hat{\beta}_i)$.

The estimate of the age-adjusted odds ratio for the comparison of the black group with the white group is $\exp\{-0.304\} = 0.738$, with 95% confidence limits

$$\exp\{-0.304 \pm (1.96)\sqrt{(0.01098)}\} = (0.601, 0.906)$$

which indicates that a smaller proportion of black women than white women are secretors. Similarly, a comparison of Chinese to whites yields an age-adjusted odds ratio of $\exp\{-1.385\} = 0.250$ with 95% confidence limits

$$\exp\{-1.385 \pm (1.96)\sqrt{(0.01723)}\} = (0.194, 0.324)$$

Table 7–2. Coding for ethnicity, the corresponding linear logistic model parameters, and the variance-covariance matrix for a 0 1 coding using the data in Table 7–1

Source	X_1	X_2	X_3
ETHNIC GROUP			
White	0	0	0
Black	1	0	0
Chinese	0	1	0
Latin American	0	0	1
COEFFICIENTS	−0.30434	−1.38546	−0.08651
VARIANCE-COVARIANCE			
X_1	0.010982		
X_2	0.001561	0.017227	
X_3	0.001563	0.001675	0.030597

which indicates an even lower proportion of secretors among Chinese than whites. Finally, Latin Americans compared to whites have an age-adjusted odds ratio of $\exp\{-0.087\} = 0.917$ with 95% confidence limits

$$\exp\{-0.087 \pm (1.96)\sqrt{(0.03059)}\} = (0.651, 1.291)$$

which does not suggest much of a difference at all.

Should one wish to compare blacks with Latin Americans, the age-adjusted odds ratio is given by $\exp\{-0.304 - (-0.087)\} = 0.805$. The standard error of the log odds ratio is given by

$$SE(\hat{\beta}_1 - \hat{\beta}_3) = \sqrt{(0.01098) + (0.03059) - 2(0.00156)}$$

$$= 0.1961$$

and the 95% confidence interval is

$$\exp\{[-0.304 - (-0.087)] \pm (1.96)(0.1961)\} = (0.548, 1.182)$$

This example illustrates that when several categories are under investigation, they do not necessarily form indistinguishable groups, as Latin Americans are not clearly different from either the whites or the blacks in terms of whether they are secretors. The relatively small number of subjects in the Latin American group resulted in less precision in the estimates of the odds ratio that involved this group.

It is important to keep in mind that if the reference group is not coded so as to have all the regressors equal to zero in a 0 1 coding scheme, it will be necessary to include the relevant covariance terms when computing the standard error. Hence, the judicious choice of coding for the reference group at the beginning of the analysis can result in the direct application of single-regression parameters and their standard errors when summarizing the results, which can be a considerable simplification.

−1 0 1 coding

An alternative to the coding scheme discussed in the preceding section is to adopt the approach used in the development of the analysis of variance. For the analysis of the two-level exposure to cigarettes discussed earlier, this alternative would use the regressor variable

$$X_1 = -1 \qquad \text{if not exposed}$$

$$= 1 \qquad \text{if exposed}$$

Evaluating the change in the linear predictor when one compares exposed to unexposed, holding all other factors constant, yields

$$\eta_1 - \eta_0 = ([1 - (-1)]\beta_1 + (X_2 - X_2)\beta_2 + (X_3 - X_3)\beta_3 + \cdots$$

$$= 2\beta_1$$

Hence, to find the adjusted log odds ratio from the regression coefficients of a linear logistic model, one must multiply the parameter estimate by 2. In calculations that require the standard error, one must also multiply the standard error for the regression coefficient by the same factor, 2.

This approach to coding categorical variables extends to the analysis of a factor with more than two levels, and in general for a k-level categorical variable, $k - 1$ regressor variables are required, just as the preceding section discussion. In the case of the three-category cancer stage example discussed above, this coding scheme could use the two regressor variables:

(0)   Local: $X_1 = -1, X_2 = -1$
(1)   Regional: $X_1 = 1, X_2 = 0$
(2)   Remote: $X_1 = 0, X_2 = 1$

To compare (1) regional with (0) local, the difference in the linear predictor holding all other variables constant is

$$\hat{\eta}_1 - \hat{\eta}_0 = [1 - (-1)]\,\hat{\beta}_1 + [0 - (-1)]\,\hat{\beta}_2$$
$$= 2\hat{\beta}_1 + \hat{\beta}_2$$

with the standard error given by

$$\mathrm{SE}(\hat{\eta}_1 - \hat{\eta}_0) = \sqrt{2^2\,V(\hat{\beta}_1) + V(\hat{\beta}_2) + 2\cdot 1\cdot 2\cdot \mathrm{Cov}(\hat{\beta}_1,\hat{\beta}_2)}$$

Likewise, the (2) remote with (0) local comparison leads to

$$\hat{\eta}_2 - \hat{\eta}_0 = [0 - (-1)]\,\hat{\beta}_1 + [1 - (-1)]\,\hat{\beta}_2$$
$$= \hat{\beta}_1 + 2\hat{\beta}_2$$

with the standard error given by

$$\mathrm{SE}(\hat{\eta}_2 - \hat{\eta}_0) = \sqrt{V(\hat{\beta}_1) + 2^2\,V(\hat{\beta}_2) + 2\cdot 1\cdot 2\cdot \mathrm{Cov}(\hat{\beta}_1,\hat{\beta}_2)}$$

The simplicity of focusing on a single regression parameter to evaluate the adjusted estimate of risk is not possible when one uses the $-1\ 0\ 1$ coding for more than two levels, as it was for the $0\ 1$ coding. This can complicate considerably the computation of the estimates themselves, as well as their standard errors. For more than three levels, this calculation can be even more complex, as seen in Example 7–1.

Example 7–1 (continued)   In the preceding section, the data from the report by Petrakis et al. (1) was analyzed by using a $0\ 1$ coding. For comparison, consider a $-1\ 0\ 1$ coding, such as that shown in Table 7–3. The fitted values are, of course,

Table 7–3. Coding for ethnicity, the corresponding linear logistic model parameters, and the variance-covariance matrix for a -1 0 1 coding using the data in Table 7–1

Source	X_1	X_2	X_3
ETHNIC GROUP			
White	−1	−1	−1
Black	1	0	0
Chinese	0	1	0
Latin American	0	0	1
COEFFICIENTS	0.139734	−0.941385	0.357568
VARIANCE-COVARIANCE			
X_1	0.008204		
X_2	−0.002806	0.01127	
X_3	−0.006147	−0.007624	0.017955

identical to the results in the previous section, where the likelihood ratio statistic was $G^2 = 21.61$ with 15 df ($p = .117$). However, the regression parameter estimates and the corresponding variance and covariance terms, as shown in Table 7–3, are quite different. To translate these parameters into estimates of age-adjusted odds ratios, we must consider the difference in the linear predictors implied by the comparison. For instance, if one wishes to compare black and white women, the difference in linear predictors is

$$[1\beta_1 + 0\beta_2 + 0\beta_3 + \cdots] - [(-1)\beta_1 + (-1)\beta_2 + (-1)\beta_3 + \cdots]$$
$$= [1 - (-1)]\beta_1 + [0 - (-1)]\beta_2 + [0 - (-1)]\beta_3 \qquad (7.3)$$
$$= 2\beta_1 + \beta_2 + \beta_3$$

which involves all three regression parameters. The estimate of the adjusted odds ratio for these data is $\exp\{2(0.1397) + (-0.9414) + (0.3576)\} = \exp\{-0.304\}$, which is identical to the result computed using the 0 1 coding. Using equation 7.2 to find the variance of the linear combination of parameter estimates shown in equation 7.3, we obtain the variance of the log odds ratio to be

$$\begin{aligned} \text{Var}(2\hat{\beta}_1 + \hat{\beta}_2 + \hat{\beta}_3) = &\ (2^2)(0.00820) + (0.01127) + (0.01795) \\ &+ 2(2)(1)(-0.00281) + 2(2)(1)(-0.00615) \\ &+ 2(1)(1)(0.00762) \\ = &\ 0.01094 \end{aligned}$$

which is, once again, identical to the variance found in the discussion in the preceding section, except for rounding error. The 95% confidence limits for this estimate are given by

$$\exp\{-0.304 \pm (1.96)\sqrt{(0.01094)}\} = (0.601, 0.906)$$

This example illustrates that, while it is feasible to use this particular coding scheme to obtain estimates of the adjusted hazard ratio when there are more than two levels of a categorical variable, the calculations are not as simple as those that can be obtained from 0 1 coding, especially when a single reference group is chosen in advance. It was noted at the beginning of this section that this particular coding scheme arose from work on the analysis of variance, and in that context it gave rise to an estimate of the of the difference between the mean for a particular category and the mean of all the separate category means—that is, the grand mean. In addition, the use of this coding scheme resulted in some simplification in the calculations. Unfortunately, in the context of epidemiologic studies, the comparison of a particular group with some average group is not of particular interest. Hence, the regression parameter estimates that correspond to these regressor variables are not as useful by themselves, and the computational advantage for a well-designed computer program is small when compared to the additional human effort needed to understand the results. When using a computer program that uses a $-1\ 0\ 1$ coding scheme as the default, one might consider defining their own regressor variables to obtain point and interval estimators of hazard ratios and odds ratios.

Deviations from the model

Treating a factor that has ordered levels as if it were a nominal categorical variable makes no assumption about the way in which that variable might influence the response. The categories are simply named groups, and it is not implied by the parameterization of the model that an increase in the level of the variable implies anything about the corresponding change in the response. A disadvantage in this lack of specificity is that it usually results in a loss of power, when compared to a model that is appropriate for the data. Nevertheless, it is often the case that one is uncertain as to the actual form for the model, so that an analysis that inappropriately specifies a unique mathematical equation to describe a relationship can yield misleading conclusions. A useful strategy when trying to find a good model to describe a set of data is to compare the fit of a particular model of interest with the fit of one that uses a dummy variable treatment of the categories.

As a first step in evaluating possible forms for the effect of a continuous variable, it is useful to draw a graph showing the relationship between the categories and the response to be fitted. If the linear logistic model is being considered, then such a plot would use the log odds ratio for the vertical axis and a midpoint of the exposure category for the horizontal axis. This graph can be used to decide whether (a) a particular model is at all realistic, (b) a more complex model is needed, or (c) a transformation of the factor should be considered.

The comparison of the fit of two models can also be used in a more formal way to obtain a likelihood ratio test of whether there is a significant departure from the trend implied by the more restrictive mathematical equation. This is a goodness-of-fit test that looks specifically at the fit as it applies to the particular variable of interest. To construct this test, one must obtain the likelihood ratio goodness-of-fit statistic for two models: one that uses the specific mathematical equation to describe the effect of the variable G_0^2; and one that is identical to the first, except that the factor under investigation is treated as a nominal categorical variable, G_1^2. The improvement in fit that results from using the categorical analysis $\Delta G^2 = G_0^2 - G_1^2$ is compared to a chi-square distribution, with degrees of freedom equal to the difference in the degrees of freedom for the two models, $\Delta df = df_0 - df_1$. An equivalent way of computing the degrees of freedom is to use Δdf = (number of categories $-$ 1) $-$ (number of parameters for factor).

A limitation of this test in assessing goodness of fit arises when there is a large number of categories, resulting in a large number of degrees of freedom associated with the categories. As noted in other contexts, a test with many degrees of freedom may not have the specificity needed to show statistical significance in a particular set of data, especially if the total sample size is not large. In addition, one must question a model that uses nearly as many parameters as the nominal treatment, because very little data reduction is being achieved and it is known that the effect of the k nominal categories can be fitted exactly with $(k - 1)$ regression parameters. Hence, this goodness-of-fit statistic must be used in combination with other approaches to evaluating the fit of the model, including graphical displays that might suggest reasonable alternative models.

Example 7–1 (continued)   In the two preceding sections, we fitted a linear logistic model to the data shown in Table 7–1, treating both age and ethnic group as nominal variables. Up to this point, we have concentrated on the effect of ethnicity, which is truly a categorical variable. Using these same methods, we can estimate the ethnicity-adjusted log odds ratios for age, arbitrarily using the ≥60-year age group as the reference. These estimates are displayed in Table 7–4 and are plotted against the midpoint of the age interval in Figure 7–1. The graph is striking in that it suggests that the trend in risk steadily increases for the first four age intervals, and then drops for the two oldest age groups.

The simplest model that might be used to describe the effect of age is one that assumes that there is a linear trend in the log odds ratio. This can be incorporated into the model by using the midpoint of the age intervals—15, 25, 35, 45, 55, and 65. Because these points are equally spaced, we can represent them in an equivalent manner by simply using the integers, $X = 1, 2, \ldots, 6$, keeping in mind that a unit change in X represents a 10-year difference in age. As shown in Table 7–5,

Table 7-4. Estimates of the log odd ratio for nominal and polynomial models, using age 25 as the reference for the data in Table 7-1

| X | Age | Nominal | Polynomial | | | |
			Linear	2nd-order	3rd-order	4th-order
1	<20	−0.475	0.414	−0.618	−1.014	−0.471
2	20–29	0.360	0.331	0.583	0.518	0.359
3	30–39	1.204	0.248	1.245	1.240	1.206
4	40–49	1.317	0.166	1.369	1.297	1.316
5	50–59	0.673	0.083	0.954	0.836	0.674
6	≥60	0.000	0.000	0.000	0.000	0.000

this results in a regression parameter for age of −0.0827, which suggests a decreasing trend with age. To determine the statistical significance of this parameter, we can compare the scaled deviance for the model with no age variable (i.e., only the variables for ethnicity), $G^2(0) = 230.91$, df = 20, to the scaled deviance that includes a linear effect of age, shown in Table 7–5. This results in the likelihood ratio test of linear trend, $\Delta G^2 = 230.91 - 220.95 = 9.96$, df = 20 − 19 = 1 ($p = .002$), indicating fairly strong evidence for a decreasing trend with age.

The model that implies a linear trend with age implies that the log odds ratio comparing X with the ≥60 year age group ($X = 6$), holding all other variables constant, is given by $\eta(X) - \eta(6) = (X - 6) \beta_1$. These estimates of the log odds ratio are shown in the "Linear" column of Table 7–4 and are displayed by the dotted line in Figure 7–1. Clearly, this does not appear to give a good description of the

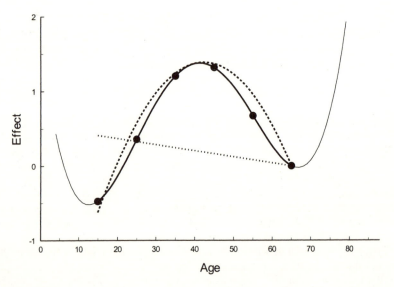

Figure 7–1 Plot of estimated age effects for the data in Table 7–1 using dummy variables (*dots*), linear trend (*dotted line*), quadratic trend (*broken line*), and fourth-order polynomial (*solid line*).

Table 7–5. Regression parameters and likelihood ratio statistics for polynomial models of the effect of age, using the data in Table 7–1

X	Linear	2nd-order	3rd-order	4th-order
REGRESSION PARAMETERS				
X	-0.0827	2.009	3.013	-2.113
X^2		-0.269	-0.550	1.837
X^3			0.024	-0.433
X^4				0.0307
LIKELIHOOD RATIO STATISTICS				
G^2	220.95	32.30	29.89	21.61
df	19	18	17	16

effect of age. To test whether the departure from this model is statistically significant, one can compare the scaled deviance for the linear age model with the scaled deviance for the model that uses age as a nominal categorical variable, G^2(nominal) = 21.61, df = 15, giving

$$\Delta G^2(\text{Departure from linear}) = 220.95 - 21.61 = 199.34$$

$$\Delta df = 19 - 15 = 4$$

($p < .001$). Hence, there is very strong evidence, indeed, that the trend is not linear, and an alternative model must be found.

An alternative to an effect that is linear is to consider a polynomial model—to include increasing powers of age in the model, $\eta = \beta_0 + X \beta_1 + X^2 \beta_2 + X^3 \beta_3 + \cdots$ Once again, the change in the linear predictor can be used to determine the model's estimate of the log odds ratio, which if $X = 6$ is the reference becomes $\eta(X) - \eta(6) = (X - 6) \beta_1 + (X^2 - 6^2) \beta_2 + (X^3 - 6^3) \beta_3 + \cdots$

For a second-order polynomial, a quadratic effect of age, the estimates of the regression coefficients for X and X^2 are shown in the third column of Table 7–5. We might expect this equation to give a reasonable description of the data because it can increase and then decrease, which is roughly the overall observed pattern. Figure 7–1 shows the pattern of the adjusted odds ratio described by the fitted second-order model, and it indeed represents a great improvement over the first model, resulting in an improvement in the scaled deviance of

$$\Delta G^2 = 220.95 - 32.30 = 188.65$$

$$\Delta df = 19 - 18 = 1$$

which is highly significant. However, the test for whether there is still significant departure from this model can be obtained by comparing G^2 of this model with the nominal model

$$\Delta G^2 = 32.30 - 21.61 = 10.69$$

$$\Delta df = 18 - 15 = 3$$

($p = .014$), which suggests that there indeed remains a significant portion of the age pattern that is not explained by this model. In fact, an inspection of Figure 7–1 reveals that the second-order polynomial model was not flexible enough to reach the peak while still fitting the remaining points.

Adding the term X^3 to the model, improves the fit by

$$\Delta G^2 = 32.30 - 29.89 = 2.41$$

$$\Delta df = 18 - 17 = 1$$

($p = .121$) which is not significant, while the lack of fit remains statistically significant

$$\Delta G^2 = 29.89 - 21.61 = 8.28$$

$$\Delta df = 17 - 15 = 2$$

($p = .016$). The fourth-order model that adds X^4, results in further improvement in the likelihood ratio statistic

$$\Delta G^2 = 29.89 - 21.61 = 8.28$$

$$\Delta df = 17 - 16 = 1$$

($p = .004$) that is highly significant, and there is essentially nothing left to explain by adding a possible fifth term. The fit of this model to the nominal representation of age is shown by the heavy solid line in Figure 7–1, indicating that the fit is very good indeed.

Three additional points may be gleaned from this analysis of the effect of age. First, the linear parameter was estimated to be negative, even though a visual inspection of the data would suggest a slightly greater inclination to increase with age rather than decrease. This is because the maximum likelihood estimation effectively gives greater weight to the groups that are more precisely determined, which is heavily influenced here by the greater number of women in the oldest age group than in the youngest. Second, the use of the fourth-order polynomial has resulted in the reduction of only one parameter, when compared to the nominal model, which has not provided much of an improvement in parsimony. However, it does have some advantage in that we can now proceed to use the fourth-order polynomial with actual ages and not just the categories displayed in Table 7–1. Third, great care should be taken when extending a model that gives an excellent fit beyond the range of observation, especially for fairly complex models like a high-order polynomial. Figure 7–1 shows a graph of this fourth-order polynomial extended to younger and older ages, indicating an upturn in both instances. This pattern would not seem to be biologically plausible, so that one should limit the use of the model to the observed age range of 15 to 65.

Threshold and other models for trend

The use of coded variables can also be extended in ways that allow for the fitting of models with a dose threshold, so that doses below a particular level produce no effect on the response while higher doses may indeed produce an effect. Suppose, for example, that one is studying the association between duration of oral contraceptive use and risk of heart disease. One equation might imply a linear trend for the log hazard that begins to increase once a woman starts to use the pill, so that the log hazard ratio for a woman using oral contraceptives for X months compared with a non-users ($X = 0$) is given by

$$\log\left(\frac{\lambda_0(t)\,\exp\{X\cdot\beta\}}{\lambda_0(t)\,\exp\{0\cdot\beta\}}\right) = X\beta$$

As an alternative, we can consider a model in which there is no effect of oral contraceptive use for the first 6 months, so that the log hazard ratio remains at 0 until a 6-month lag period has passed. We can accomplish this by defining a regressor variable:

$$X_1 = 0 \qquad \text{if } Z \le 6 \text{ months}$$
$$\quad = (Z - 6) \qquad \text{if } Z > 6 \text{ months}$$

where Z represents months of use. Figure 7–2 displays the trend implied by a model in which X_1 alone is included by a broken line. Those using oral contraceptives for fewer than 6 months would be expected to have a disease risk that is the same as nonusers. An additional regressor variable

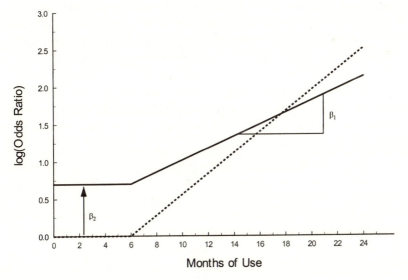

Figure 7–2 Hypothetical threshold models for the effect of oral contraceptive use: no difference at 0 month use (*broken line*), and a positive initial difference (*solid line*).

is required if one wishes the model to distinguish between users and nonusers,

$$X_2 = 0 \quad \text{if not a user of oral contraceptives}$$

$$= 1 \quad \text{if a user of oral contraceptives}$$

When both of these regressor variables are included in a model, the trend in the log odds ratio, using nonusers as the reference, becomes

$$X_1\beta_1 + X_2\beta_2 = 0 \qquad \text{if a nonuser}$$

$$= \beta_2 \qquad \text{if a user for } Z \leq 6 \text{ months}$$

$$= \beta_2 + (Z - 6)\beta_1 \qquad \text{if a user for } Z > 6 \text{ months}$$

which is shown as a solid line in Figure 7–2.

In the threshold models considered thus far, we have assumed that the breakpoint is known—6 months in the specific example considered. Often, we need to estimate this point as well, so that it becomes another parameter in our model. Unfortunately, when the threshold point is a parameter to be estimated along with the other regression parameters, the model is no longer a generalized linear model. We can try various values for the breakpoint and choose the one that maximizes the log likelihood, thus providing a maximum likelihood estimate. But the fact that we have estimated the breakpoint also influences the precision of the other regression parameters, which actually raises some fairly subtle problems when making inferences.

A variation of the approach just described is an analysis that considers the question of whether one or more points fit into the overall trend under consideration. If the dose–response relationship is assumed to be linear, then a particular model may represent the dose, Z, by the regressor variable $X_1 = Z$. Suppose that a question is raised as to whether a particular dose, Z_0, deviates significantly from this linear trend. One approach to addressing this question is to let

$$X_2 = 1 \qquad \text{if } Z = Z_0$$

$$= 0 \qquad \text{otherwise}$$

The linear predictor would be given by

$$X_1\beta_1 + X_2\beta_2 = Z\beta_1 + \cdots \qquad \text{if } Z \neq Z_0$$

$$= Z\beta_1 + \beta_2 + \cdots \qquad \text{if } Z = Z_0$$

The parameter β_2 estimates the deviation of the dose Z_0 from the remaining dose–response relationship, and a test of $H_0: \beta_2 = 0$ would indicate whether that deviation was statistically significant. The following example illustrates how this approach can be applied.

Example 7–2 Let us consider data from a large postal survey conducted to study lung disease, the results of which are shown in Table 7–6 (2). We wish to explore the association between cigarette smoking and the prevalence of symptoms defined as "persistent cough and phlegm production." The table gives a breakdown of the data by age, sex, and cigarette smoking history, which is classified as nonsmoker, ex-smoker, fewer than 20 cigarettes per day, 20 cigarettes per day, and more than 20 cigarettes per day. Some subjects did not respond to the smoking question or they did not fit into one of these smoking categories. Thus, they are excluded from further consideration in this analysis.

Sex of the subject is clearly a nominal variable, and age is a categorization of a continuous variable that might have a linear trend. Table 7–7 summarizes scaled deviances related to each of these factors, indicating that both sex and age have a highly significant association with persistent cough and phlegm production and that the effect of age is well described by a linear trend.

Cigarette smoking was the factor of primary interest in the study. There is clearly a natural progression in these categories, in that ex-smokers may be thought of as having greater exposure than nonsmokers, current smokers greater than ex-smokers, and so on. Because of this progression, a plausible parameterization of the model might be to introduce a linear trend in the log odds ratio, using the regressor variable:

$$X_L = 1 \quad \text{if nonsmoker}$$
$$= 2 \quad \text{if ex-smoker}$$
$$= 3 \quad \text{if smoked} <20 \text{ cigarettes per day}$$
$$= 4 \quad \text{if smoked 20 cigarettes per day}$$
$$= 5 \quad \text{if smoked} >20 \text{ cigarettes per day}$$

Table 7–6. Number of respondents reporting the symptom "persistent cough and phlegm production" by age, sex, and smoking status (2)

Cigarette smoking	35–44 n	35–44 No. with symptoms	45–55 n	45–55 No. with symptoms	55–64 n	55–64 No. with symptoms
MALES						
Nonsmoker	227	16	200	12	171	19
Ex-smoker	303	21	358	39	335	50
<20 per day	521	78	488	107	490	147
20 per day	191	44	204	57	149	48
>20 per day	148	40	136	52	121	51
Not known	79		81		89	
FEMALES						
Nonsmoker	500	15	637	25	925	46
Ex-smoker	127	4	128	10	94	7
<20 per day	602	54	472	61	306	49
20 per day	128	20	122	33	77	24
>20 per day	22	5	39	10	7	3
Not known	164		174		182	

Table 7–7. Summary analysis of likelihood ratio statistics for the data in Table 7–6

Model	df	G^2	Δdf	ΔG^2	Effect
(1) Sex, Age, Smoke	22	16.50			
(2) Age, Smoke	23	78.28	1	61.78	Sex $\mid$ Age, Smoke (2)–(1)
(3) Sex, Smoke	24	93.06	2	76.56	Age $\mid$ Sex, Smoke (3)–(1)
(4) Sex, Age (linear), Smoke	23	17.12	1	0.62	Deviations (4)–(1)
			1	75.94	Linear age (3)–(4)
(5) Sex, Age	26	402.18	4	385.68	Smoke $\mid$ Age, Sex (5)–(1)
(6) Sex, Age, X_L, X_1, X_2	23	17.70	1	1.20	Deviations (6)–(1)
(7) Sex, Age, X_L	25	31.63	2	13.93	$X_1 X_2 \mid X_L$ (7)–(6)
(8) Sex, Age, X_1, X_2	24	72.24	1	54.54	$X_L \mid X_1 X_2$ (8)–(6)

This particular parameterization is questionable in other respects, however, because the first two levels do not have the same quantitative basis as the last three. For instance, is it reasonable to say that the difference between ex-smokers and non-smokers is comparable to the difference between smokers of 20 and >20 cigarettes?

To determine whether the first two smoking categories depart significantly from the trend implied by current smokers, one can introduce two regressor variables:

$$X_1 = 1 \quad \text{if nonsmoker}$$
$$= 0 \quad \text{otherwise}$$
$$X_2 = 1 \quad \text{if ex-smoker}$$
$$= 0 \quad \text{otherwise}$$

Considering the combined effect of these three smoking variables on the linear predictor for the logistic regression model, we obtain the following results for each of the five categories:

$$\beta_0 + X_L \beta_L + X_1 \beta_1 + X_2 \beta_2 = \beta_0 + 1\beta_L + \beta_1 \quad \text{if nonsmoker}$$
$$= \beta_0 + 2\beta_L + \beta_2 \quad \text{if ex-smoker}$$
$$= \beta_0 + 3\beta_L \quad \text{if } <20 \text{ cigarettes}$$
$$= \beta_0 + 4\beta_L \quad \text{if } 20 \text{ cigarettes}$$
$$= \beta_0 + 5\beta_L \quad \text{if } >20 \text{ cigarettes}$$

This model implies a linear trend among the current smokers, and β_1 and β_2 give the departure from the trend for nonsmokers and ex-smokers, respectively. A graphical display of what this analysis is trying to achieve is shown in Figure 7–3, which gives the log odds ratio for the effect of smoking using nonsmokers as the reference. The solid line shows the linear trend for current smokers, and the question to be considered is whether this can reasonably be extended, as shown by the broken line.

Table 7–7 summarizes the statistical significance of the association between cigarette smoking and disease. The overall test for an association with smoking, treated

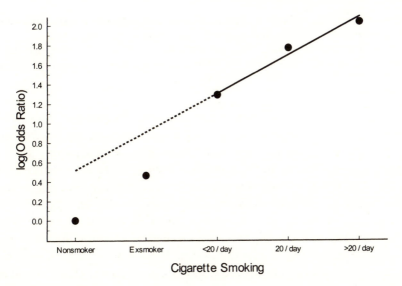

Figure 7–3 Log odds ratios for the effect of cigarette smoking using data from Table 7–6 using dummy variable (*dots*) and linear trend among smokers (*solid and broken lines*).

as a nominal categorical variable, is highly significant, $\Delta G^2 = 385.68$, $\Delta df = 4$ ($p \ll .001$), but can we obtain a more concise description of a trend? Fitting a model that implies a linear trend among current smokers but not former smokers results in a model that fits well, $G^2(X_L, X_1, X_2) = 17.70$, df $= 23$ ($p = .774$), and there is no significant deviation between this model and the full nominal model for smoking, $\Delta G^2 = 1.20$, $\Delta df = 1$ ($p = .273$). Evaluating the change in the likelihood ratio statistic that results from dropping X_1 and X_2 from the model tests whether the first two smoking categories show significant departure from an overall linear trend:

$$\Delta G^2(X_1, X_2 \mid X_L) = G^2(X_L) - G^2(X_L, X_1, X_2)$$

$$= 31.63 - 17.70$$

$$= 13.93$$

$\Delta df = 25 - 23 = 2$ ($p < .001$). Hence, there is strong evidence that nonsmokers and ex-smokers do not fit with the linear trend among smokers, even though we can readily see a consistent progression in disease risk in Figure 7–3.

A final question that can be addressed using this model is whether the linear trend is significant among current smokers. This can be addressed by testing H_0: $\beta_L = 0$ with β_1 and β_2 included in the model. The likelihood ratio statistic of this null hypothesis is given by

$$\Delta G^2(X_L \mid X_1, X_2) = G^2(X_1, X_2) - G^2(X_L, X_1, X_2)$$

$$= 72.24 - 17.70$$

$$= 54.54$$

$\Delta df = 24 - 23 = 1$ ($p \ll .001$). Hence, it is not feasible to further reduce the number of parameters in the model to describe the effect of smoking.

As a final summary model for these data, we can include the effect for sex, a linear trend for age, and a linear trend for current smokers only using X_L X_1 and X_2. This model gives a good fit to the data, $G^2 = 18.35$, df = 24 ($p = .786$).

When determining whether a particular dose deviates from the overall trend, special consideration is necessary if that dose was not selected before looking at the results. When one visually inspects departure from a model, it is only natural to focus on the extreme points of departure from the fitted values. If many doses are considered, then it is more likely that some values will achieve statistical significance, so that an adjustment is appropriate. When deviant doses are not selected a priori, then the Bonferroni adjustment is appropriate when trying to determine statistical significance. Suppose that one out of N dose levels is selected because it has the largest departure from the model, then a good approximation to an α-level significance test is obtained by choosing as the critical value α/N. Hence, if 10 doses are considered and one is interested in significance at the .05 level, then the critical value using the Bonferroni method is $0.05/10 = 0.005$.

Interactions and parallelism

A question that is often raised in the analysis of a substantial set of data is whether the effect is consistent among different subgroups of the population, which is sometimes referred to as *effect modification*. When the factor under consideration is continuous, the effect is usually described in terms of a dose–response relationship, so that the issue of homogeneity of effect may be raised in this context as a question of whether the dose–response curves are parallel. Both of these issues can be addressed in the context of regression models through the use of interaction terms, which are carefully constructed variables to be included in the model.

One limitation present in an analysis of effect modification or parallelism must be emphasized at the outset: it can readily depend on the scale of measurement for the response. This issue was considered to some extent in Chapter 2, with a hypothetical example of two factors with two levels each. In that example, one scale suggested that the effect was lowered by the presence of the second factor, and another scale suggested that it was raised. Because the correct model is not known for most diseases, we must adopt the pragmatic view of using these models for descriptive purposes and not as definitive indications of causal mechanisms. The results of a model that gives a good description of the association between factors and disease can be used in a variety of ways, including projections of the effect of adopting various disease-prevention strategies. The limitation primarily effects the interpretation of individual regression parameters in the model, not the quantitative description of the exposure–response relationship.

Interaction regressor variables are constructed by taking the product of two or more main effects that are already in the model. For a nominal factor, we can introduce a regressor variable that uses a 0 1 coding scheme. If we are considering the effect of exposure to a putative risk in men and women, then two variables may be used for the main effects, in the case of exposure (E)

$$X_E = 0 \quad \text{if unexposed}$$
$$= 1 \quad \text{if exposed}$$

and for sex (S)

$$X_S = 0 \quad \text{if a man}$$
$$= 1 \quad \text{if a woman}$$

The interaction variable is defined as the product of these two regressor variables, i.e.,

$$X_{ES} = X_E X_S = 1 \quad \text{if exposed woman}$$
$$= 0 \quad \text{otherwise}$$

There are four combinations of exposure and gender in this particular example, and the linear predictor is given by

$$\eta = X_E \beta_E + X_S \beta_S + X_{ES} \beta_{ES} + \text{(terms independent of E and S)}$$

Let unexposed men be the reference group, so that the change in linear predictors becomes

$$(X_E - 0)\beta_E + (X_S - 0)\beta_S + (X_{ES} - 0)\beta_{ES}$$
$$= 0 \qquad \text{if unexposed men}$$
$$= \beta_E \qquad \text{if exposed men}$$
$$= \beta_S \qquad \text{if unexposed women}$$
$$= \beta_E + \beta_S + \beta_{ES} \qquad \text{if exposed women}$$

Under this parameterization, $\beta_E - 0 = \beta_E$ gives the effect of exposure in men, but for women the effect is $(\beta_E + \beta_S + \beta_{ES}) - \beta_S = \beta_E + \beta_{ES}$. Hence, the regression parameter for the interaction variable, β_{ES}, estimates the difference between the effect in women and the effect in men, adjusted for any other parameters that may be included in the model.

If a -1 1 coding is used instead of the 0 1 as described, then

$$X_E' = -1 \qquad \text{if unexposed}$$
$$= 1 \qquad \text{if exposed}$$

and

$$X_S' = -1 \qquad \text{if a man}$$
$$= 1 \qquad \text{if a woman}$$

The exposure–sex interaction is once again created by taking the product of these two regressor variables,

$$X_{ES}' = X_E' \, X_S' = 1 \qquad \text{if unexposed man or exposed woman}$$
$$= -1 \qquad \text{if exposed man or unexposed women}$$

Ignoring the terms in the expression that do not involve exposure or sex, we can obtain the components of the linear predictor that define these four categories

$$\eta = X_E' \, \beta_E' + X_S' \, \beta_S' + X_{ES}' \, \beta_{ES}'$$
$$= -\beta_E' - \beta_S' + \beta_{ES}' \qquad \text{if unexposed man}$$
$$= \beta_E' - \beta_S' - \beta_{ES}' \qquad \text{if exposed man}$$
$$= -\beta_E' + \beta_S' - \beta_{ES}' \qquad \text{if unexposed woman}$$
$$= \beta_E' + \beta_S' + \beta_{ES}' \qquad \text{if exposed woman}$$

The effect of exposure in women is $2(\beta_E' + \beta_{ES}')$, and likewise for men it is $2(\beta_E' - \beta_{ES}')$, so that the average for the two sexes is $2\beta_E'$. For this coding scheme, the interaction, β_{ES}', can be interpreted as the difference between the average effect for men and women and the effect for women. If these linear predictors were means, as they are for an analysis of variance, then it is easier to interpret the regression parameters that result from this coding, but in most models used in epidemiology they are not. Hence, for ease of interpretation, the parameters from the 0 1 coding are somewhat simpler to use than a -1 1 coding.

Example 7–2 (continued)   Returning once again to the data from the postal survey investigating the association between cigarette smoking and disease, we consider the question of whether the effect of age is the same for men and women, using the final model as the reference point. One approach would be to consider separate age trends for men and women:

$$X_M = \text{age index} \qquad \text{if man}$$
$$= 0 \qquad\qquad \text{otherwise}$$

and

$$X_W = \text{age index} \qquad \text{if woman}$$
$$= 0 \qquad\qquad \text{otherwise}$$

The resulting regression parameters for these two variables are

$$\begin{pmatrix} \beta_M \\ \beta_W \end{pmatrix} = \begin{pmatrix} 0.3761 \\ 0.3298 \end{pmatrix}$$

with the covariance matrix

$$\begin{pmatrix} \text{Var}(\hat{\beta}_M) & \text{Cov}(\hat{\beta}_M, \hat{\beta}_W) \\ \text{Cov}(\hat{\beta}_M, \hat{\beta}_W) & \text{Var}(\hat{\beta}_W) \end{pmatrix} = \begin{pmatrix} 0.002657 & 0.000007 \\ 0.000007 & 0.005028 \end{pmatrix}$$

The difference between women and men is estimated by $0.3298 - 0.3761 = -0.0463$, with a variance estimated by

$$\text{Var}(\hat{\beta}_M) + \text{Var}(\hat{\beta}_W) - 2 \cdot \text{Cov}(\hat{\beta}_M, \hat{\beta}_W) = 0.002657 + 0.005028 - 2 \cdot (0.000007)$$
$$= 0.007671 = (0.08758)^2$$

Hence, a Wald test of equality of the two slopes is given by

$$W = \frac{-0.0463}{0.08758} = -0.53$$

which is not statistically significant when compared to a standard normal deviate ($p = .597$).

An alternative treatment of this question is to introduce an interaction term into a model that includes main effects for age and gender:

$$X_{AS} = \text{age index} \qquad \text{if woman}$$
$$= 0 \qquad\qquad \text{otherwise}$$

The corresponding regression parameter is -0.04635 (SE $= 0.08759$), which is identical to our previous results.

The likelihood ratio test is sometimes useful as an alternative to the Wald statistic, especially when one is dealing with more than one parameter at a time. For this example, we would compare the scaled deviance for the model that includes the interaction term with one that does not, $\Delta G^2 = 18.35 - 18.07 = 0.28$, with $\Delta df = 24 - 23 = 1$ ($p = .597$), giving essentially the same conclusion as before.

Interactions are not only useful when one is dealing with nominal variables, but they also can provide interesting results when used with continuous variables. For example, suppose that X_E represents the actual level of exposure to a particular risk factor, and X_A is age. The product of these two variables is defined as $X_{EA} = X_E X_A$ and the linear predictors becomes

$$\eta = X_E \beta_E + X_A \beta_A + X_E X_A \beta_{EA}$$
$$= X_A \beta_A + X_E (\beta_E + X_A \beta_{EA})$$

Hence, the slope for the exposure trend is $(\beta_E + X_A \beta_{EA})$ which depends on age, X_A. In this instance, the slope itself is a linear function of age, with the slope given by the interaction term, β_{EA}. A test of H_0: $\beta_{EA} = 0$, indicates whether there is a significant departure from a dose–response relationship that is independent of age.

Testing Linear Hypotheses

The simple comparison of two groups does not always offer sufficient flexibility for addressing some scientific questions. In an example discussed in the preceding section, the question of ethnicity was considered in a particular study. Suppose one considers another study in which ethnicity is related to risk of malignant melanoma, where a subject's ethnic group is defined in terms of the country of birth. For the purpose of discussion, let the countries be England, France, Italy, China, and Japan. Let the effects for these five countries be represented by the vector $\boldsymbol{\theta}' = (\theta_1 \, \theta_2 \, \theta_3 \, \theta_4 \, \theta_5)$. One question that the investigator may wish to address is whether the risk of melanoma is identical for the three European countries—that is, H_0: $\theta_1 = \theta_2 = \theta_3$, or, equivalently,

$$H_0: \theta_1 - \theta_3 = \theta_2 - \theta_3 = 0 \tag{7.4}$$

Hypotheses like the one shown in equation 7.4 are described in general terms as linear hypotheses, which take the form H_0: $\sum_i c_{ij} \cdot \theta_i = 0$ (for all i), where c_{ij} are specified constants. Sometimes it is convenient to write this expression in terms of a contrast matrix, where the elements of the matrix are the constants c_{ij}:

$$\mathbf{c_\theta} = \begin{pmatrix} c_{11} & c_{12} & \cdots & c_{1p} \\ c_{21} & c_{22} & \cdots & c_{2p} \\ \cdot & \cdot & \cdots & \cdot \\ c_{r1} & c_{r2} & \cdots & c_{rp} \end{pmatrix}$$

which is a matrix of full row rank. The general linear hypothesis becomes

$$H_0: \mathbf{c_\theta} \cdot \boldsymbol{\theta} = 0 \tag{7.5}$$

In the melanoma example in which the European countries are to be compared, $\mathbf{c_\theta}$ may be given as

$$\mathbf{c_\theta} = \begin{pmatrix} 1 & 0 & -1 & 0 & 0 \\ 0 & 1 & -1 & 0 & 0 \end{pmatrix}$$

so that the linear contrast becomes

$$\mathbf{c_\theta} \cdot \boldsymbol{\theta} = \begin{pmatrix} \theta_1 - \theta_3 \\ \theta_2 - \theta_3 \end{pmatrix}$$

and the test of the linear hypothesis, $H_0: \mathbf{c_\theta} \cdot \boldsymbol{\theta} = 0$, is identical to that shown in equation 7.4.

When applying contrasts to parameters that have had linear constraints applied, such as those implied by a particular coding scheme, we must take the additional step of evaluating the appropriate contrast for the regression parameters. Suppose that we consider once again the case of five groups, and a regression analysis that has used a 0 1 coding scheme, using Group 1 as the reference. This can be represented as a design matrix with five rows, one for each group, and four columns for the $5 - 1 = 4$ regressor variables:

$$\mathbf{X} = \begin{pmatrix} 0 & 0 & 0 & 0 \\ 1 & 0 & 0 & 0 \\ 0 & 1 & 0 & 0 \\ 0 & 0 & 1 & 0 \\ 0 & 0 & 0 & 1 \end{pmatrix} \tag{7.6}$$

Each column has a corresponding regression parameter, $\boldsymbol{\beta}' = (\beta_1, \beta_2, \beta_3, \beta_4)$. The group effects can now be estimated in terms of the regression parameters,

$$\boldsymbol{\theta} = \mathbf{X}\boldsymbol{\beta} = \begin{pmatrix} 0 \\ \beta_1 \\ \beta_2 \\ \beta_3 \\ \beta_4 \end{pmatrix}$$

where $\boldsymbol{\beta}$ represents the column vector of regression parameters that correspond to the columns of $\mathbf{X}$. The linear constraint on the group effects is given by $\mathbf{c}_\theta \boldsymbol{\theta} = \mathbf{c}_\theta \mathbf{X} \boldsymbol{\beta}$. Hence, if we wish to find the contrast, $\mathbf{c}_\theta$, on the group effects, $\boldsymbol{\theta}$, we need to evaluate the linear contrast $\mathbf{c}_\beta = \mathbf{c}_\theta \mathbf{X}$ on the regression parameters, $\boldsymbol{\beta}$.

To illustrate the effect on the contrast $\mathbf{c}_\theta = (0\ 1\ -1\ 0\ 0)$ that was used to test the hypothesis H_0: $\theta_2 - \theta_3 = 0$, this corresponds to the contrast

$$\mathbf{c}_\theta \mathbf{X} = (0\ 1\ -1\ 0\ 0) \cdot \begin{pmatrix} 0 & 0 & 0 & 0 \\ 1 & 0 & 0 & 0 \\ 0 & 1 & 0 & 0 \\ 0 & 0 & 1 & 0 \\ 0 & 0 & 0 & 1 \end{pmatrix} \tag{7.7}$$

$$= (1\ -1\ 0\ 0)$$

on the regression parameters. Similarly, the contrast $\mathbf{c} = (2\ -1\ -1\ 0\ 0)$ becomes

$$\mathbf{c}_\theta \mathbf{X} = (2\ -1\ -1\ 0\ 0) \cdot \begin{pmatrix} 0 & 0 & 0 & 0 \\ 1 & 0 & 0 & 0 \\ 0 & 1 & 0 & 0 \\ 0 & 0 & 1 & 0 \\ 0 & 0 & 0 & 1 \end{pmatrix}$$

$$= (-1\ -1\ 0\ 0)$$

when evaluated for the regression parameters. This particular illustration demonstrates that while the sum of the contrast constants is zero for a contrast on the effects, $\sum_i c_{\theta i} = 0$, this is not necessarily true for the contrast on the regression parameters.

One can see the importance of taking into account the coding scheme, by comparing the contrast for the 0 1 coding given in equation 7.7 with the contrast for a −1 0 1 coding. Suppose that $\mathbf{X}$ is defined to be

$$\mathbf{X} = \begin{pmatrix} -1 & -1 & -1 & -1 \\ 1 & 0 & 0 & 0 \\ 0 & 1 & 0 & 0 \\ 0 & 0 & 1 & 0 \\ 0 & 0 & 0 & 1 \end{pmatrix} \tag{7.8}$$

Then the previous contrast among the corresponding regression parameters becomes

$$\mathbf{c}_\theta\mathbf{X} = (2 \ -1 \ -1 \ 0 \ 0) \cdot \begin{pmatrix} -1 & -1 & -1 & -1 \\ 1 & 0 & 0 & 0 \\ 0 & 1 & 0 & 0 \\ 0 & 0 & 1 & 0 \\ 0 & 0 & 0 & 1 \end{pmatrix} \tag{7.9}$$

$$= (-3 \ -3 \ -2 \ -2)$$

which is, once again, very different from the comparison in equation 7.7, indicating the importance of the coding in defining contrasts for regression parameters. It is interesting to note that in this example, the appropriate contrast involves all four regression parameters, even though only the first three groups are being compared.

Wald tests for linear hypotheses

In Chapter 3, we calculated the Wald test using maximum likelihood estimates of the parameters and the corresponding covariance matrix. If one is analyzing maximum likelihood estimates of the regression parameters, $\hat{\beta}$, then the invariance property (3) implies that the maximum likelihood estimate of a contrast, $\mathbf{c}_\beta$, on those parameters is given by $\mathbf{c}_\beta\hat{\beta}$. Because this is a linear function of the estimates, the covariance matrix may be computed using the quadratic form,

$$\mathrm{Var}(\mathbf{c}_\beta\hat{\beta}) = \mathbf{c}_\beta\mathrm{Var}(\hat{\beta})\mathbf{c}_\beta'$$

For large samples, the linear contrast has a multivariate normal distribution, with a mean given by $\mathbf{c}_\beta\beta$.

To test the null hypothesis, $H_0: \mathbf{c}_\beta\beta = \mathbf{c}_\beta\beta_0$ using a Wald test, one must use the quadratic form,

$$\begin{aligned} W^2 &= (\mathbf{c}_\beta\hat{\beta} - \mathbf{c}_\beta\beta_0)' \cdot \mathrm{Var}(\mathbf{c}_\beta\hat{\beta})^{-1} \cdot (\mathbf{c}_\beta\hat{\beta} - \mathbf{c}_\beta\beta_0) \\ &= (\mathbf{c}_\beta\hat{\beta} - \mathbf{c}_\beta\beta_0)' \, [\mathbf{c}_\beta\mathrm{Var}(\hat{\beta})\mathbf{c}_\beta']^{-1}(\mathbf{c}_\beta\hat{\beta} - \mathbf{c}_\beta\beta_0) \end{aligned} \tag{7.10}$$

which has an asymptotic chi-square distribution with degrees of freedom equal to the number of rows in c_β. For the null hypothesis that the contrast is zero, $H_0: c_\beta\beta = 0$, the Wald test simplifies to

$$W^2 = (c_\beta\hat{\beta})'[c_\beta \mathrm{Var}(\hat{\beta})c_\beta']^{-1}\hat{\beta}c_\beta \qquad (7.11)$$

Example 7–1 (Continued)   To illustrate the use of linear contrasts and the construction of Wald tests, consider again the first example which involved an analysis of the age and ethnic effects on yield of breast fluid. Suppose that we are interested in testing whether there are significant differences among the non-Asian groups—a comparison of whites, blacks, and Latin Americans. This can be constructed by considering the contrasts comparing blacks to whites and Latin Americans to whites:

$$c_\theta = \begin{pmatrix} -1 & 1 & 0 & 0 \\ -1 & 0 & 0 & 1 \end{pmatrix}$$

When a 0 1 coding is used, the contrast among the regression coefficients is

$$c_\beta = c_\theta X$$

$$= \begin{pmatrix} -1 & 1 & 0 & 0 \\ -1 & 0 & 0 & 1 \end{pmatrix} \cdot \begin{pmatrix} 0 & 0 & 0 \\ 1 & 0 & 0 \\ 0 & 1 & 0 \\ 0 & 0 & 1 \end{pmatrix} \qquad (7.12)$$

$$= \begin{pmatrix} 1 & 0 & 0 \\ 0 & 0 & 1 \end{pmatrix}$$

Hence, the estimate of the contrasts becomes

$$c_\beta\hat{\beta} = \begin{pmatrix} 1 & 0 & 0 \\ 0 & 0 & 1 \end{pmatrix} \cdot \begin{pmatrix} -0.30434 \\ -1.38546 \\ -0.08651 \end{pmatrix}$$

$$= \begin{pmatrix} -0.30434 \\ -0.08651 \end{pmatrix}$$

and the corresponding covariance matrix is

$$\mathrm{Var}(c_\beta\hat{\beta}) = c_\beta\mathrm{Var}(\hat{\beta})c_\beta'$$

$$= \begin{pmatrix} 1 & 0 & 0 \\ 0 & 0 & 1 \end{pmatrix} \cdot \begin{pmatrix} 0.010982 & 0.001561 & 0.001563 \\ 0.001561 & 0.017227 & 0.001675 \\ 0.001563 & 0.001675 & 0.030597 \end{pmatrix} \cdot \begin{pmatrix} 1 & 0 \\ 0 & 0 \\ 0 & 1 \end{pmatrix}$$

$$= \begin{pmatrix} 0.010982 & 0.001563 \\ 0.001563 & 0.030597 \end{pmatrix}$$

The Wald statistic for testing the null hypothesis that there are no differences among the nonoriental groups is

$$W^2 = (c_\beta \hat{\beta})' \mathrm{Var}(c_\beta \hat{\beta})^{-1} c_\beta \hat{\beta}$$

$$= (-0.30434 \; -0.08651) \cdot \begin{pmatrix} 0.010982 & 0.001563 \\ 0.001563 & 0.030597 \end{pmatrix}^{-1} \cdot \begin{pmatrix} -0.30434 \\ -0.08651 \end{pmatrix}$$

$$= 8.495$$

which is compared to a chi-square distribution with 2 df ($p = .014$), thus leading to a rejection of the null hypothesis.

An analysis based on the $-1\ 0\ 1$ coding yields exactly the same conclusions even though the intermediate results may be different. In this instance, the contrast for the regression parameters would be

$$c_\beta = c_\theta X$$

$$= \begin{pmatrix} -1 & 1 & 0 & 0 \\ -1 & 0 & 0 & 1 \end{pmatrix} \cdot \begin{pmatrix} -1 & -1 & -1 \\ 1 & 0 & 0 \\ 0 & 1 & 0 \\ 0 & 0 & 1 \end{pmatrix} \qquad (7.13)$$

$$= \begin{pmatrix} 2 & 1 & 1 \\ 1 & 1 & 2 \end{pmatrix}$$

However, the estimate of the effect is

$$c_\beta \hat{\beta} = \begin{pmatrix} 2 & 1 & 1 \\ 1 & 1 & 2 \end{pmatrix} \cdot \begin{pmatrix} 0.13973 \\ -0.94138 \\ 0.35757 \end{pmatrix}$$

$$= \begin{pmatrix} -0.30434 \\ -0.08651 \end{pmatrix}$$

with a covariance matrix given by

$$\mathrm{Var}(c_\beta \hat{\beta}) = c_\beta \mathrm{Var}(\hat{\beta}) c_\beta'$$

$$= \begin{pmatrix} 2 & 1 & 1 \\ 1 & 1 & 2 \end{pmatrix} \cdot \begin{pmatrix} 0.008204 & -0.002804 & -0.006147 \\ -0.002804 & 0.011270 & -0.007624 \\ -0.006147 & -0.007624 & 0.017955 \end{pmatrix} \cdot \begin{pmatrix} 2 & 1 \\ 1 & 1 \\ 1 & 2 \end{pmatrix}$$

$$= \begin{pmatrix} 0.010982 & 0.001563 \\ 0.001563 & 0.030597 \end{pmatrix}$$

both of which are identical to the results obtained using a 0 1 coding. Hence, the Wald statistic is still 8.495 with 2 df, thus illustrating once again that choice of codes is unimportant, as long as we are careful when interpreting the parameters.

Likelihood ratio tests for linear hypotheses

Instead of a Wald test for a general linear hypothesis, we might use a likelihood ratio test. This approach directly uses changes in the log-likelihood, a measure of the contribution of data to the statistical inference, without necessarily appealing to a multivariate normal approximation for the estimators. This method requires the careful choice of variables to be included and excluded from the model, so that we can test the particular hypothesis of interest by calculating the change in the scaled deviances: $\Delta G^2 = G^2(\text{restricted model}) - G^2(\text{full model})$.

Returning to the melanoma example discussed earlier, recall that a hypothesis of interest was whether subjects with European ancestry had identical risk. Using a 0 1 coding scheme with a design matrix given in equation 7.6, we are left with the following effects for each country, expressed in terms of the regression parameters:

$$
\begin{array}{ll}
\text{England} & \theta_1 = 0 \\
\text{France} & \theta_2 = \beta_1 \\
\text{Italy} & \theta_3 = \beta_2 \\
\text{China} & \theta_4 = \beta_3 \\
\text{Japan} & \theta_5 = \beta_4
\end{array}
$$

Hence, the null hypothesis, $H_0: \theta_1 = \theta_2 = \theta_3$, is equivalent to the null hypothesis $H_0: \beta_1 = \beta_2 = 0$ for the regression parameters. This can be tested using $\Delta G^2 = G^2(X_3 \ X_4) - G^2(X_1 \ X_2 \ X_3 \ X_4)$, which has 2 df, associated with the two regressor variables that were dropped from the model.

We can construct a likelihood ratio test that corresponds to a Wald test of any general linear hypothesis, although the choice of regressor variables to be used for this purpose is not always obvious. With experience, our intuition in defining appropriate regressor variables will improve, but it is always prudent to check our choice in order to be sure that the restricted hypothesis is making the comparison of interest. When intuition fails, we can always make use of the following algorithm (4) that will provide the variables required for testing a linear hypothesis.

Suppose that there are p parameters in the full model, given by the vector $\boldsymbol{\beta}$, and one wishes to test $H_0: \mathbf{c}_\beta \boldsymbol{\beta} = \mathbf{0}$, where $\mathbf{c}_\beta$ is an $r \times p$ matrix. Let $\mathbf{G}$ be a nonsingular matrix, given by the partitioned matrix

$$
\mathbf{G} = \begin{pmatrix} \mathbf{G}_1 \\ \text{---} \\ \mathbf{G}_2 \end{pmatrix}
$$

where $\mathbf{G}_1 = \mathbf{c}_\beta$, and $\mathbf{G}_2$ is an arbitrarily defined matrix that is linearly independent of the rows of $\mathbf{G}_1$. The product

$$\mathbf{G}\beta = \left(\begin{array}{c} \mathbf{G}_1\beta \\ \hline \mathbf{G}_2\beta \end{array}\right) = \left(\begin{array}{c} \gamma_1 \\ \hline \gamma_2 \end{array}\right)$$

so that the null hypothesis is $H_0: \mathbf{G}_1\beta = \gamma_1 = 0$. To set up a test for this hypothesis, notice that the linear predictor can be represented by

$$\mathbf{X}\beta = \mathbf{X}\mathbf{G}^{-1}\mathbf{G}\beta$$
$$= \mathbf{Z}\gamma$$
$$= (\mathbf{Z}_1 \mid \mathbf{Z}_2) \left(\begin{array}{c} \gamma_1 \\ \gamma_2 \end{array}\right)$$

where $\mathbf{Z} = \mathbf{X}\mathbf{G}^{-1}$. Hence, we can use the likelihood ratio test

$$\Delta G^2(\mathbf{Z}_1 \mid \mathbf{Z}_2) = G^2(\mathbf{Z}_2) - G^2(\mathbf{Z}_1\mathbf{Z}_2) = G^2(\mathbf{Z}_2) - G^2(\mathbf{X})$$

which is compared to a chi-square distribution with r degrees of freedom.

Example 7–1 (Continued)   Returning once again to the association between ethnic group and yield of breast fluid, one can construct a likelihood ratio test of the null hypothesis that there are no differences among the non-Asian groups, or a test that is equivalent to the Wald test computed in the preceding section. In the case of a 0 1 coding, the four ethnic groups can be represented by the variables given in Table 7–2, and the appropriate contrast matrix for the parameters is shown in equation 7.12. Hence, we define

$$\mathbf{G} = \left(\begin{array}{ccc} 1 & 0 & 0 \\ 0 & 0 & 1 \\ \hline 0 & 1 & 0 \end{array}\right)$$

For this particular choice of $\mathbf{G}$, it so happens that $\mathbf{G}^{-1} = \mathbf{G}$, so that

$$\mathbf{Z} = \left(\begin{array}{ccc} 0 & 0 & 0 \\ 1 & 0 & 0 \\ 0 & 1 & 0 \\ 0 & 0 & 1 \end{array}\right) \cdot \left(\begin{array}{ccc} 1 & 0 & 0 \\ 0 & 0 & 1 \\ \hline 0 & 1 & 0 \end{array}\right)$$

$$= \left(\begin{array}{ccc} 0 & 0 \mid & 0 \\ 1 & 0 \mid & 0 \\ 0 & 0 \mid & 1 \\ 0 & 1 \mid & 0 \end{array}\right)$$

$$= (\mathbf{Z}_1 \mid \mathbf{Z}_2)$$

and the likelihood ratio test becomes

$$\Delta G^2(\mathbf{X} \mid \mathbf{Z}_2) = G^2(\mathbf{Z}_2) - G^2(\mathbf{X})$$
$$= 30.061 - 21.611 \qquad (7.14)$$
$$= 8.450$$

which is compared to a chi-square distribution with 2 df ($p = .015$). This statistic is very similar to the value of 8.495 obtained for the Wald test in the preceding section.

When a $-1\ 0\ 1$ coding is used for the four ethnic groups, the contrast for the regression parameters is given in equation 7.13, and we can define

$$\mathbf{G} = \begin{pmatrix} 2 & 1 & 1 \\ 1 & 1 & 2 \\ \hline 0 & 0 & 1 \end{pmatrix}$$

which has an inverse given by

$$\mathbf{G}^{-1} = \begin{pmatrix} 1 & -1 & 1 \\ -1 & 2 & -3 \\ \hline 0 & 0 & 1 \end{pmatrix}$$

The matrix of regressor variables that yields the appropriate constraint is

$$\mathbf{Z} = \begin{pmatrix} 1 & -1 & 1 \\ -1 & 2 & -3 \\ \hline 0 & 0 & 1 \end{pmatrix} \cdot \begin{pmatrix} -1 & -1 & -1 \\ 1 & 0 & 0 \\ 0 & 1 & 0 \\ 0 & 0 & 1 \end{pmatrix}$$

$$= \begin{pmatrix} 0 & -1 & | & 1 \\ 1 & -1 & | & 1 \\ -1 & 2 & | & -3 \\ 0 & 0 & | & 1 \end{pmatrix}$$

$$= (\mathbf{Z}_1 \mid \mathbf{Z}_2)$$

Notice that $\mathbf{Z}_2\gamma_2$ gives the following effects for each of the four ethnic groups:

White	γ_3
Black	γ_3
Chinese	$-3\gamma_3$
Latin American	γ_3

Hence, we see that the model in which $\gamma_1 = \gamma_2 = 0$ satisfies the condition of the hypothesis of interest: equal effects for the non-Asian ethnic groups. The likelihood ratio statistic is identical to that obtained using the 0 1 coding.

Power Transformations of Continuous Regressor Variables

We have already discussed the use of polynomial regression as an approach for relaxing the linearity assumption for a continuous regressor variable. Another approach is to select an alternative way of expressing the actual exposure dose for a particular subject. For example, in studies of workers in the nuclear industry there are often quite detailed records maintained of their occupational history, including measures of radiation exposure obtained from badges worn while on the job. If we decide that a cumulative estimate of radiation exposure is of interest, we still may need to determine whether the actual level should be included in the model or whether we should first transform the dose, perhaps by taking its logarithm. After all, in many studies of the physiological effect of factors it has been found that the dose–response relationship is linear in log dose. In this section, we describe a general approach for selecting an expression or transformation for a regressor variable that will enable us to use generalized linear models for the analysis.

For the regression models we are considering, the exposure–response curve is defined by way of the linear predictor, and we must select a scale on which to express the exposure level, because this can effect the shape of the exposure–response curve. Selecting an appropriate transformation of the exposure can provide a way of representing an appropriate model by using a linear predictor when the relationship is monotone—that is, the risk continues to increase (or decrease) with the level of exposure. The power family of transformations gives us some control over the degree of curvature for the exposure–response function by providing a family of transformations that depend on a single parameter, which can be either specified or estimated, to yield the optimal transformation for a particular set of data.

Suppose that Z is a positive variable and represents the measured level of exposure to a particular agent. The power family of transformations defines the variable to be included in the regression model as

$$X = Z^\rho \qquad \text{when } \rho > 0$$
$$= \log(Z) \qquad \text{when } \rho = 0$$
$$= -Z^\rho \qquad \text{when } \rho < 0$$

where ρ is the power to be used. If $\rho = 1$, then there is no change of scale and the actual value itself is included in the model. The relationship between X and Z for various values of ρ is shown in Figure 7–4. If one chooses values of ρ greater than 1, the concave or hollow side of the curve is facing upward and the bend becomes sharper as ρ increases. Similarly, when

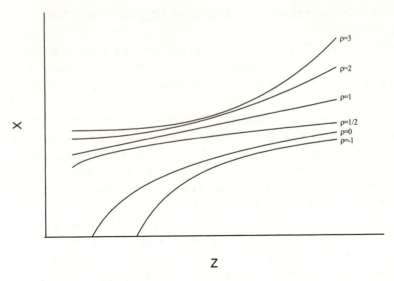

Figure 7-4 Plot of curves from the Box-Cox transformation for various values of ρ.

ρ is less than 1, the concave side is downward and the bend becomes more pronounced as ρ decreases.

Box and Cox (5) described an alternative way of expressing the power transformations:

$$X = (Z^\rho - 1)/\rho \qquad \rho \neq 0$$
$$= \log(Z) \qquad \rho = 0$$

The only difference between the two is that the Z^ρ is divided by ρ, and $1/\rho$ is subtracted from the result. Taking a linear function of a regressor variable does not change the fit of the model, but it does change regression coefficients in a predictable way. For example, if β is the coefficient for the power transformed variable, then $\rho\beta$ would be the coefficient for the corresponding Box-Cox transformation.

When the transformation is expressed in this form, it is easy to see how the log fits in with the power family by considering the limit as $\rho \to 0$. Because the limit for both the numerator and the denominator of this expression is zero, the limit for this ratio is equal to the limit of the ratio of derivatives with respect to ρ:

$$\lim_{\rho \to 0} \left(\frac{Z^\rho - 1}{\rho} \right) = \lim_{\rho \to 0} \left(\frac{Z^\rho \log(Z)}{1} \right)$$
$$= \log(Z)$$

When considering a power transformation for an exposure–response relationship, we can choose to transform either the dose or the response. The four quadrants shown in Figure 7–5 give the fundamental shapes that can occur for curves that are monotone. A simple mnemonic for the selection of ρ is the "bulging rule" (6) which can be simply stated as, "Move along the scale for ρ in the direction of the bulge."

For example, if we wish to straighten a line based on an untransformed exposure–response curve that bends in the direction shown in quadrant IV—that is, from a steep slope to one that is less steep—the bulge is in the direction of an increase in ρ for the response, and a decrease for the dose. If we are interested in transforming the response, we need to look for larger values of ρ. Alternatively, if we choose to transform the dose, we should must explore smaller values of ρ. Hence, starting with an untransformed variable, we might first try the square root ($\rho = \frac{1}{2}$), and if the curve still showed the same general pattern we could move on to the log ($\rho = 0$). Similarly, if at some point we discover that we have gone too far, we can always return to a less severe transformation. While it is possible to transform either the dose or the response in the context of the generalized linear model, if we limit ourselves to logistic regression, say, then we can only transform the dose.

Example 7–3 Let us return to the data on the association between asbestos exposure and the risk of lung cancer presented in Table 6–1 (7). We might first choose to use logistic regression for our analysis, which gives rise to the log odds link function. In Figure 7–6 we see a plot of the estimated log odds for disease against the

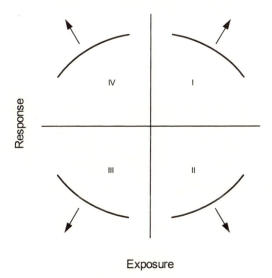

Figure 7–5 Type of curvature for possible application of the Bulging Rule.

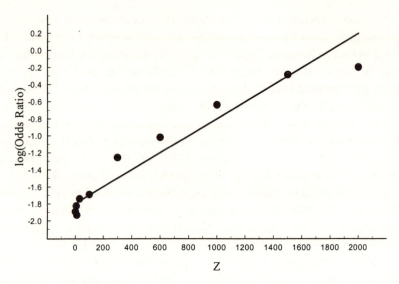

Figure 7–6 Plot of the log odds ratio against the untransformed dose for the data in Table 4–1.

untransformed estimate of asbestos exposure, Z. Because we can see a systematic departure from linear trend, we might try to straighten the curve by using a power transformation. The bulge points in the direction of smaller values with respect to the Z axis, so we would need to try powers less than 1. Suppose we try the log transformation, but the fact that it is undefined for zero dose, requires that we first add a small constant, 1 say, before taking the logarithms. The result is displayed in Figure 7–7, and it is clear that we have gone too far in that the exposure–response

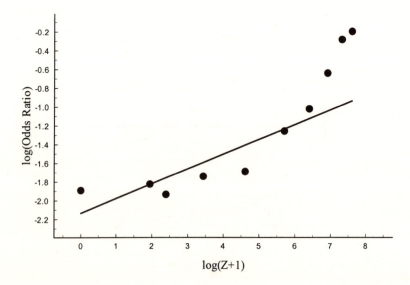

Figure 7–7 Plot of the log odds ratio against log exposure for the data in Table 4–1.

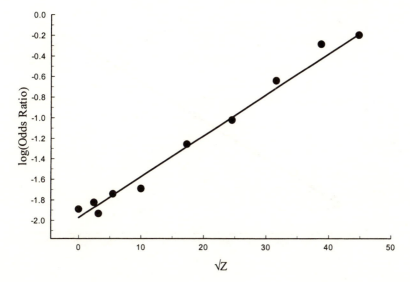

Figure 7–8 Plot of the log odds ratio against the square root of asbestos exposure for the data in Table 4–1.

curve is now bent in the opposite direction. Moving up from the log, we can try a value of ρ between 0 and 1, say $\frac{1}{2}$ or the square root, which is shown in Figure 7–8. This appears to be a good choice, as the relationship is now linear, and thus one that can be well described by the linear logistic model.

An advantage of using generalized linear models is that we are not locked into using one specific link function, but we can in fact reexpress the response, as well as the dose. If we apply the bulging rule to the response axis in Figure 7–6, we should try powers greater than that represented by the logarithm, or $\rho > 0$. Suppose that instead we choose the untransformed odds, $\rho = 1$, with the resulting exposure–response relationship shown in Figure 7–9. Once again, we have succeeded in straightening the curve, and for these data it appears that either choice gives an adequate description of the exposure-response relationship over this range of exposures. Thus, a clear choice of a final model may not emerge, and we may be left with several choices. We can see that by using the square root of the dose we can obtain an excellent model using logistic regression. However, we may not like to explain results based on the square root of exposure to a substantive audience, so we might choose instead to employ the equally valid model that is linear on the odds for disease.

When the range of observed values for the exposure is far from zero, we might see little effect from using a power transformation. In these circumstances, we can magnify the effect of the transformation by first subtracting a constant before taking the power:

$$X = (Z - C)^\rho \qquad \text{when } \rho > 0$$

$$= \log(Z - C) \qquad \text{when } \rho = 0$$

$$= -(Z - C)^\rho \qquad \text{when } \rho < 0$$

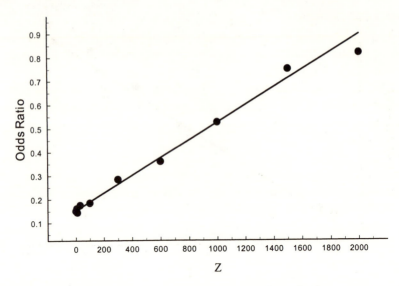

Figure 7–9 Plot of the odds ratio against the untransformed asbestos exposure for the data in Table 4–1.

This is equivalent to adding a negative value before applying the transformation, a technique we employed in the example in order to avoid undefined transformations. The results are usually not sensitive to this added constant when it does not result in a substantial shift toward or away from 0.

While the power family offers an extremely useful set of transformations, it is important to remember that they can only work for monotone relationships. If the exposure–response relationship changes from increasing to decreasing at some point, then we must look elsewhere for a reasonable model for the data. Polynomials is one such approach. However, there are also some useful nonparametric models for the exposure effect, including regression splines, that do not require a restrictive assumption about the form for the relationship.

Summary

The coding of categorical variables can result in very different values for the parameters in a regression model, but when they are correctly understood in term of effects on estimates of risk, they do not affect the overall conclusions. We have considered two commonly used coding schemes that use either 0 1 values only or −1 0 1. The former are generally easier to interpret, especially when the reference level is identified by all zeroes, because the individual regression parameters can then be interpreted as estimates of risk. Significance tests, however, are unaffected by the choice of coding.

Dividing a continuous variable into categories and comparing the resulting trends with that obtained by fitting a particular model offers a simple and somewhat crude method for assessing goodness of fit. The strategy of using flexible approaches to estimating trends for continuous variable are useful in assessing the fit of more specific models. Inevitably we must trade off the minimal assumptions required from the less restrictive nonparametric methods of analysis against the additional power that can be achieved when a highly parametric model is appropriate. Hence, this idea of allowing an exposure–response relationship to emerge from the data is fundamental to data analysis, and we will explore other more powerful techniques in later chapters.

In this chapter, we also explored specially defined variables that allowed us to consider thresholds, as well as questions of whether associations are consistent for all subgroups of the population. We have thus seen that although we are restricting our methods primarily to those that involve effects that are linear after a transformation on the mean, we still have a very rich family of models available to us. By creatively defining our regressor variable, we can still explore an extensive variety of different types of exposure–response relationships.

Another very powerful tool that we can employ in regression analyses is the linear hypothesis. This extends the basic concept of comparing different groups, which is the most common approach to hypothesis testing, by opening up ways to formulate different types of hypotheses that can be generated by scientific questions of interest. We have seen how this fundamental idea can be employed using either the Wald test or the likelihood ratio test.

Finally, we considered an approach for reexpressing either the regressor variable or the response in order to achieve a relationship that can be described by a generalized linear model. The power family, or the Box–Cox transformation, offers one useful set of transformations that can be employed to effectively straighten curves when there is a monotone exposure–response relationship. Another approach for considering curvilinear relationship is by using polynomial regression, as we saw in Example 7.1. While polynomials offer the possibility of fitting curves that are not monotone, we saw also that they had limitations, either by not having sufficient flexibility or by imposing biologically implausible curves, especially for high-degree polynomials. Spline functions and generalized additive models offer alternative formulations that go some way to resolving some of these difficulties, and this remains a fruitful area for further methodological work in statistical aspects of epidemiological research.

Exercises

7.1 In this exercise we return to the clinical trial of adult-onset diabetes. The full trial considered four treatment arms, including a placebo (8, 9). The outcome in this analysis is death from cardiovascular disease (CHD), which we also considered in Chapter 6. Two insulin treatments were also employed: a fixed dose based on characteristics of the patients, and an effort to titrate the dose to achieve a desired level of blood sugar control.

Age	Treatment	*Male* No. patients	*Male* No. CHD deaths	*Female* No. patients	*Female* No. CHD deaths
≤53	Placebo	28	1	85	1
	Oral agent	26	5	71	1
	Insulin 1	28	0	71	1
	Insulin 2	21	1	72	1
>53	Placebo	35	6	58	2
	Oral agent	37	6	70	14
	Insulin 1	29	5	74	7
	Insulin 2	25	1	76	9

a. Use a Wald test to:
   i. Compare the two insulin groups
   ii. Compare the mean of the insulin groups to the oral agent
   iii. Compare the three non-placebo treatments
b. Repeat (a) using likelihood ratio tests.

7.2. The data reported in the table are from the Framingham study (10). Men were followed from September 1948 to August 1951; at the end of that period it was noted whether clinically manifest heart disease (MI or angina pectoris) had occurred. The table shows the number of men broken down by whether they had coronary heart disease (CHD), systolic blood pressure, and serum cholesterol.

CHD	Serum cholesterol (mg/100 cc)	Systolic blood pressure (mm Hg)				
		−127	127–146	147–166	167+	Total
No	−199	2	3	3	4	12
	200–219	3	2	0	3	8
	220–259	8	11	6	6	31
	260+	7	12	11	11	41
	Total	20	28	20	24	92
Yes	−199	117	121	47	22	307
	200–219	85	98	43	20	246
	220–259	119	209	68	43	439
	260+	67	99	46	33	245
	Total	388	527	204	118	1237

a. Fit a linear logistic model to these data, treating blood pressure and cholesterol categories as nominal variables.
b. Give a Wald test and a likelihood ratio test of the effects of blood pressure and cholesterol estimated in (a).
c. Plot the log odds for CHD as a function of blood pressure and cholesterol, using the results in (a).
d. Use the linear logistic model to fit a linear trend to the log odds for disease, using blood pressure and cholesterol as the covariates. Give tests for linear trend, as well as tests for departure from linear trend.
e. Construct a table summarizing the likelihood ratio chi-square statistics from the models you have fitted. For each factor, partition the overall chi-square so that you have a test for linear trend and a test of deviations from linearity.

7.3. Bain et al (11) studied the relationship between the number of moles on limbs and malignant melanoma using 98 cases and 190 controls. The data for arms and legs are tabulated here.

Site	Total no. of moles at site					
	0	1–5	6–15	16–30	31–50	51+
Arm						
Cases	16	20	20	12	13	17
Controls	57	40	45	20	16	12
Leg						
Cases	29	20	27	14	5	3
Controls	101	44	30	8	3	4

    a. Summarize the dose–response relationship between the number of moles on the arms and legs and the risk of malignant melanoma.

    b. Does a model that assumes a linear relationship between the number of moles and the log odds ratio provide an adequate description of these data?

    c. Are the trends similar for arms and legs?

    d. Fit a model that allows the trend to change for individuals with more than 15 moles.

        i. Is there evidence of a significant change in trend at 15 moles for the arm? leg? both?

        ii. Does the trend with number of moles reach a plateau at 15 for the arm? leg? both?

References

1. Petrakis NL, Ernster VL, Sacks ST, King EB, Schweitzer RJ, Hunt TK, King MC. Epidemiology of breast fluid secretion: association with breast cancer risk factors and cerumen type. *Journal of the National Cancer Institute* 1981;67: 277–284.

2. Hills M. *Statistics for Comparative Studies*. London: Chapman and Hall, 1974.

3. Cox DR, Hinkley DV. *Theoretical Statistics*. London: Chapman and Hall, 1974.

4. Graybill FA. *An Introduction to Linear Statistical Models*. New York: McGraw-Hill, 1961.

5. Box GEP, Cox DR. An analysis of transformations (with discussion). *Journal of the Royal Statistical Society, Series B* 1964;26:211–252.

6. Mosteller F, Tukey JW. *Data Analysis and Regression: A Second Course in Statistics*. Reading, MA: Addison-Wesley, 1977.

7. Thomas DC. General relative risk models for survival time and matched case-control analysis. *Biometrics* 1981;37:673–686.

8. University Group Diabetes Program. A study of the effects of hypoglycemic agents on vascular complications in patients with adult onset diabetes: I. Design, methods, and baseline results; II. Mortality results. *Diabetes* 1970;12, Suppl. 2:747–783, 787–830.

9. Committee for the Assessment of Biometric Aspects of Controlled Trials of Hypoglycemic Agents. Report of the Committee for the Assessment of Biometric Aspects of Controlled Trials of Hypoglycemic Agents. *Journal of the American Medical Association* 1975;231:583–608.

10. Bishop YMM, Fienburg SE, Holland PW. *Discrete Multivariate Analysis: Theory and Practice*. Cambridge, Mass.: MIT Press, 1973.

11. Bain C, Colditz GA, Willett WC, Stampfer MJ, Green A, Bronstein BR, Mihm MC, Rosner B, Hennekins CH, Speizer FE. Self-reports of mole counts and cutaneous malignant melanoma in women: methodological issues and risk of disease. *American Journal of Epidemiology* 1988;127:703–712.

8

Parametric Models for Hazard Functions

In this chapter we extend our set of analytic tools for analyzing rates and survival times by introducing regression models that allow us to consider many parameters at the same time. This offers us much more flexibility than we might have had using the techniques discussed in Chapter 4, where we discussed the problem of comparing two groups and testing for trend. While other factors may be controlled in such methods through stratification, we can quickly run into situations in which we run out of data in forming strata, so that there is essentially no information left in the data to actually make an inference about the question at hand. A regression framework allows us to adjust for many more factors than is possible through stratification. Each time we include another variable in the stratification, we not only include a main effect for that factor, but we also implicitly include interactions between that factor and all other covariates in the model. However, this gain from regression is achieved by making restrictive assumptions about the form for the relationship between the hazard function and the regressor variables. It is essential that we be aware of this potential limitation and that we look for violations of the underlying assumptions of the model.

As we discuss regression methods for hazard functions, we also need to keep in mind the alternative approaches for selecting regressor variables described in Chapter 7. These general principles for handling regressor variables hold in any regression problem, and we can still take advantage of these approaches to formulating linear hypotheses and specifying flexible functions that can describe the effect of continuous measures of exposure.

Each of the models described in this chapter corresponds to a specific distribution for the failure times, so that when we use these methods of analysis, we need to be aware of the possibility that our data may not be well described by this distribution. Regression diagnostics offer a way of checking the validity of distributional assumptions, but another alternative is available through the use of nonparametric models, which are described in Chapter 9.

Constant Hazard Model

The simplest regression model for the hazard function is independent of time, and dependent only on the regressor variables, $\mathbf{X} = (X_1, X_2, \ldots, X_p)$, or, $\lambda(\mathbf{X},t) \equiv \lambda(\mathbf{X})$. We have already seen in our discussion of rates in Chapter 4, that a close relationship exists between a rate and a constant hazard function in that each one can be expressed as the ratio of an "expected" frequency over a denominator, $\lambda(\mathbf{X}) = \mu(\mathbf{X})/T$, where $\mu(\mathbf{X})$ is the expected number of failures and T is the denominator. We can make a conceptual distinction for the case in which we are modeling a failure rate and one in which we are dealing with a population-based rate: in the first instance the denominator represents total person-years' experience observed in a group of individuals, while in the second we have an estimated mid-period population size. However, we have already seen that for purposes of carrying out the calculations, they can both be handled in an identical fashion. In the discussion of the theoretical considerations for the methods in Appendix 6, we consider this distinction in some more detail, but the fact that both problems yield the same set of calculations means that we can develop the concepts for fitting these models together.

Log-linear model for rates

The most commonly employed regression model for rates assumes that the log rate is linearly related to the regressor variables,

$$\log \lambda(\mathbf{X}) = \beta_0 + X_1\beta_1 + X_2\beta_2 + \cdots + X_p\beta_p = \mathbf{X}\boldsymbol{\beta} \qquad (8.1)$$

or, alternatively,

$$\lambda(\mathbf{X}) = \exp\{\mathbf{X}\boldsymbol{\beta}\} \qquad (8.2)$$

If X_1 is a 0–1 dummy variable representing two groups, then this model implies that

$$\lambda_2 = \exp\{\beta_0 + \beta_1\} = \exp\{\beta_0\}\exp\{\beta_1\} = \lambda_1\exp\{\beta_1\}$$

That is, there is a multiplicative relationship between the rates. Hence, the log-linear model for the rates is sometimes referred to as a multiplicative model.

By definition, rates cannot be negative, and a strength of the log-linear model is that negative rates are impossible for any value of the regressor variables. This is not the case with some alternatives, in which a fitted rate can take negative values, which is clearly wrong. This can result in a serious problem in model fitting, because inadmissible values for one or more observations may cause the fitting algorithm to fail. Such a failure can arise when an inadmissible value occurs at an intermediate step in the iterative fitting process, even though all values may be admissible for the maximum likelihood estimates. The log-linear hazard model avoids this potential problem by employing a transformation on the rate that forces the possible values into the positive range.

A log-linear model for the rates implies that the "expected" frequency is

$$\mu(\mathbf{X}) = T\exp\{\mathbf{X}\boldsymbol{\beta}\} = \exp\{\mathbf{X}\boldsymbol{\beta} + \log(T)\} \tag{8.3}$$

which is also a log-linear model with the same regressor variables and parameters. The difference is the introduction of a known proportionality constant for the mean, T, or an added constant for the linear component, $\log(T)$. Hence, we can fit a log-linear model to the rates by fitting a model to the "expected" frequencies. We shall explore a method that employs the Poisson distribution for observed frequencies, a distribution that depends only on the expectation.

Generalized linear model

One approach to obtaining a maximum likelihood fit for a log-linear model for rates is to consider a generalized linear model in which the log link function is used to relate the mean to the linear component of the model. As we can see from equation 8.3,

$$\log \mu(\mathbf{X}) = \mathbf{X}\boldsymbol{\beta} + \log T = \eta + \log T$$

where η is the linear predictor and $\log(T)$ is an added constant referred to as the *offset*.

We shall assume that the observed number of failures for a particular combination of regressor variables, Y, has a Poisson distribution:

$$\Pr\{Y = y\} = \frac{\mu^y \exp\{\mu\}}{y!} \propto \mu^y \exp\{\mu\}$$

An important feature of the Poisson distribution is the equality of the mean and variance, or $E[Y] = \text{Var}(Y) = \mu$. We can directly obtain maximum likelihood estimates of the parameters by defining:

1. Response, Y, is the observed number of failures
2. Link is the log
3. Distribution of the response is Poisson
4. Offset is log T

Example 8–1 Let us continue our analysis of the data from the Paris Prospective Study, shown in Table 4–1 (1), which investigated the association between leukocyte count and myocardial infarction (MI) while controlling for cigarette smoking. We now employ a regression approach to the analysis and attempt to develop a model that can be used to provide a quantitative description of the data. First, consider a model in which smoking and leukocyte count are each considered as additive factors in a log-linear model. Such a model does not induce any assumption about the structure for the effect of either factor, but if we do not include an interaction term in our model, then we have not allowed for the possibility that the effect of leukocyte count, say, may be modified by cigarette smoking. Hence, we need to keep such a possibility in mind when assessing the fit of our model.

In Figure 8–1 is a SAS procedure that calls on PROC GENMOD to fit a log-linear model for rates using these data. A variable named "log_t" has been defined as the log person-years of follow-up which is included in the model as an offset. The variables "leuk" and "smoke" are defined as integer variables, indexing the categories identified in Table 4–1. Including these factors in the "class" statement instructs the procedure to establish dummy variables for each level of the factor, and the convention employed by this software uses a 0–1 coding, in which the final category is always 0. The resulting parameters thus yield estimates of adjusted log hazard ratios, using the final category as the reference. If we prefer another reference category, we can accomplish that by recoding the variables so that reference would occur last.

```
data one;   input n t @@;

leuk = mod(_N_-1,3)+1;         /* Codes for leukocyte counts */
smoke = floor((_N_-1)/3)+1;    /* Codes for smoking status   */
log_t = log(t);                /* Calculate the offset       */
cards;

2 4056   4 2892   2 1728   2 4172   3 3467   1 2183   7 4616   6 3835
6 3102   2  888   5 1101   2 1674   6 2456  10 3740  46 7269

proc genmod;   class leuk smoke;
       model n = leuk smoke / dist=p offset=log_t type3;   run;
```

Figure 8–1 SAS procedure for fitting log-linear model for rates to observed frequencies.

The output from the SAS procedure in Figure 8–1 is shown in Figure 8–2. We can first check on the overall fit of the model by noting that the scaled deviance is 9.70 with 8 df, which can be compared to a chi-square distribution ($p = .29$). Thus, the lack of significance for the goodness-of-fit statistic provides little evidence against our model, so we will proceed to use it. Unlike the usual hypothesis test, in which we hope to reject H_0 in order to establish the existence of an effect, the lack of a significance for the goodness-of-fit statistic is desirable because it suggests that the model provides an adequate description of the data. The option "type3" in the "model" statement requests a likelihood ratio statistic, ΔG^2, for each term

---

The GENMOD Procedure

Class Level Information

Class	Levels	Values
LEUK	3	1 2 3
SMOKE	5	1 2 3 4 5

Criteria For Assessing Goodness Of Fit

Criterion	DF	Value	Value/DF
Deviance	8	9.7042	1.2130
Scaled Deviance	8	9.7042	1.2130
Pearson Chi-Square	8	9.6662	1.2083
Scaled Pearson X2	8	9.6662	1.2083
Log Likelihood	.	159.9840	.

Analysis Of Parameter Estimates

Parameter		DF	Estimate	Std Err	ChiSquare	Pr>Chi
INTERCEPT		1	-5.1938	0.1459	1266.5675	0.0001
LEUK	1	1	-0.6470	0.2763	5.4840	0.0192
LEUK	2	1	-0.3581	0.2350	2.3223	0.1275
LEUK	3	0	0.0000	0.0000	.	.
SMOKE	1	1	-1.4049	0.3842	13.3751	0.0003
SMOKE	2	1	-1.8378	0.4335	17.9701	0.0001
SMOKE	3	1	-0.8736	0.2691	10.5415	0.0012
SMOKE	4	1	-0.5844	0.3571	2.6786	0.1017
SMOKE	5	0	0.0000	0.0000	.	.
SCALE		0	1.0000	0.0000	.	.

NOTE: The scale parameter was held fixed.

LR Statistics For Type 3 Analysis

Source	DF	ChiSquare	Pr>Chi
LEUK	2	6.3896	0.0410
SMOKE	4	37.5609	0.0001

Figure 8–2 Output from SAS procedure in Figure 8–1.

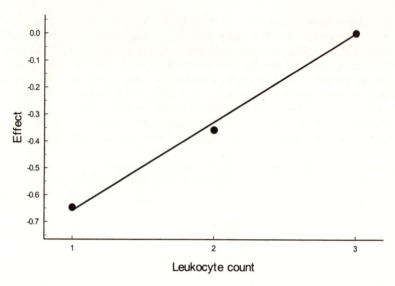

Figure 8–3 Effect of leukocyte count using dummy variables (*dots*) and linear trend (*line*).

in the model, in the presence of the others. Clearly, smoking is highly significant, as expected. In addition, there is fairly strong support for an effect of leukocyte count after adjusting for the effect of smoking ($\Delta G^2 = 6.39$, $\Delta df = 2$, $p = .041$).

To better understand the factors in our model, we can plot the estimated effects, as shown by the plot of the leukocyte effects in Figure 8–3. Notice that each point lies close to a line, the slope of which was estimated by fitting a similar model that did not include the variable "leuk" in the "class" statement. The difference between the scaled deviances for the model with "leuk" in the "class" statement and that without it yields a likelihood ratio test for deviation from linear trends. In Table 8–1 we see a partition of the effect of leukocyte count into the linear and deviations from linear components, and it is clear that the deviations are very small. Hence, the test for linear trend is valid for these data, and we can see that the results are even more conclusive with respect to the effect of leukocyte count.

Table 8–1. Analysis of deviance for effects of leukocyte count and cigarette smoking on MI rates for the Paris prospective study

Source	df	ΔG^2	p
Goodness of fit	8	9.70	.2864
Leukocyte count	2	6.39	.0410
Linear	1	6.37	.0116
Deviations from linear	1	0.02	.8808
Smoking	4	37.56	.0000
Linear	1	34.30	.0000
Deviations from linear	3	3.26	.3527
Nonsmokers	1	2.23	.1355
Deviations among smokers	2	1.04	.5959

A similar analysis of the effect of cigarette smoking is provided by the plot in Figure 8–4, and the partition shown in Table 8–1. Despite the crude nature of these smoking categories that we noted in Chapter 4, there still appears to be a strong dose–response relationship among the smokers. While the overall trend among the smoking categories does seem plausible, there is a suggestion that the first category, the nonsmokers, may in fact not fit in with the overall trend. Possible biologic reasons for such a phenomenon could be that there is a threshold, so that there is little effect for the lowest exposure level among smokers, or the nonsmokers may not smoke because they have lower general health that also influences their risk of MI. We can partition the smoking effect one step further, by introducing a dummy variable to distinguish between smokers and nonsmokers, thus leaving the linear effect to only involve the smoking categories. As we can see in Table 8–1, there was no significant deviation from linear trend in either case, and the effect for nonsmokers in a model that includes linear trend was not significant ($p = .1355$), indicating that these data do not provide strong evidence for such a threshold phenomenon. Actually, the results from this final step could have been foreseen from the previous step in which we obtained a likelihood ratio statistic for deviation from linear trend among all smoking categories, $\Delta G^2 = 3.26$ with $\Delta df = 3$. Even if we could have obtained a model in which all of the deviation was concentrated in 1 df, ΔG^2 could never be greater than 3.26 and thus could not have achieved significance as the nominal 5% level which requires a value of at least 3.84 for a test with 1 df.

An alternative approach to using generalized linear models for the number of events is to directly use the rates. In this case, the log is still the link

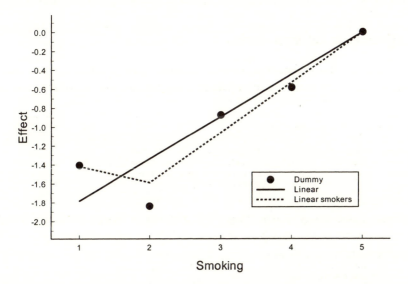

Figure 8–4 Smoking effects using dummy variable (*dots*), linear trend (*solid line*), and linear trend for smokers only (*broken line*).

function under consideration, only now it is not necessary to include an offset, as we can see from equation 8.1. The variance of a rate is

$$\text{Var}\left(\frac{Y}{T}\right) = \frac{\text{Var}(Y)}{T^2} = \frac{\mu}{T^2} = \frac{\lambda}{T}$$

which is clearly proportional to the mean. The reciprocal of the constant of proportionality, T, is the weight given to each observation. Hence, another approach for obtaining a maximum likelihood fit for a log linear model for rates is to define the following:

1. Response, $\hat{\lambda}$, is the observed rate
2. Link is the log
3. Distribution of the response is Poisson
4. Weight for each observation is T

The estimates and all aspects of statistical inference are identical using either approach.

Example 8–1 (continued)   To illustrate this approach to fitting a log-linear model to rates, we return once again to the Paris Prospective Study (1). Figure 8–5 gives a SAS procedure using PROC GENMOD, only this time each observation is weighted by the variable "wght," which is identical to the total follow-up time. Notice that we no longer are required to include an offset in the model, because we are now directly fitting the rates and not the number of failures. The scaled deviance, parameter estimates, and variances are all identical to those given in Figure 8–2.

Alternatives to log-linear models

We have thus far considered a model in which the hazard is a linear function of regressor variables after taking a log transformation of the rate. As

```
data one;  input n t @@;

leuk = mod(_N_-1,3)+1;        /* Codes for leukocyte counts */
smoke = floor((_N_-1)/3)+1;   /* Codes for smoking status   */
rate = n/t;                   /* Calculate observed rate    */
wght = t;                     /* Calculate the weight       */
cards;

2 4056   4 2892   2 1728   2 4172   3 3467   1 2183   7 4616   6 3835
6 3102   2  888   5 1101   2 1674   6 2456  10 3740  46 7269

proc genmod;  class leuk smoke;
        model rate = leuk smoke / dist=p type3;
        scwgt wght;  run;
```

Figure 8–5 SAS procedure for fitting log-linear model rates to observed rates.

we have already seen, this is but one of many such transformations that may be used. For example, we might easily choose instead to employ a power (or Box–Cox) family of transformations, similar to those discussed in Chapter 7 (2). For the power family we have the link

$$\lambda(\mathbf{X})^\rho = \mathbf{X}\boldsymbol{\beta} \qquad \rho \ne 0$$
$$\log \lambda(\mathbf{X}) = \mathbf{X}\boldsymbol{\beta} \qquad \rho = 0$$

(8.4)

or, alternatively, the inverse link

$$\lambda(\mathbf{X}) = (\mathbf{X}\boldsymbol{\beta})^{1/\rho} \qquad \text{if } \rho \ne 0$$
$$= \exp(\mathbf{X}\boldsymbol{\beta}) \qquad \text{if } \rho = 0$$

(8.5)

where ρ is either given in advance or estimated from the data. Not only does this family of models include the log-linear model for rates, but it also includes a linear model for the rates when $\rho = 1$.

As in the previous section, we can fit this model by specifying the observed rate as arising from a Poisson distribution, weighting by the denominator for the rate. Hence, it only remains to specify the link function, which is defined for a given value of ρ.

Example 8–2   The British Doctors' Study (3) was designed to explore the effect of cigarette smoking on health, and some of the data relevant to cardiovascular death are shown in Table 8–2. We consider fitting the power model to these data using only main effects due to age and smoking status. Maximum likelihood estimates of the regression parameters can be found by specifying that the cardiovascular death rate has a Poisson distribution in which the case weights are given by the denominator for the rate. Figure 8–6 shows a plot of the profile scaled deviances for ρ when age is included as a categorical variable, as well as when it is a linear function of the category index.

When age is categorical, the log-linear model does not seem to give a good fit to the data ($G^2 = 12.13$, df = 4, $p = .016$). While the linear rate model ($\rho = 1$)

Table 8–2. Number of cardiovascular deaths and person-years' experience by age and smoking status from the British Doctors's Study (3)

Age	Nonsmoker		Smoker	
	C.V. deaths	Person-years	C.V. deaths	Person-years
35–44	2	18,790	32	52,407
45–54	12	10,673	104	43,248
55–64	28	5,710	206	28,612
65–74	28	2,585	186	12,663
75+	31	1,462	102	5,317

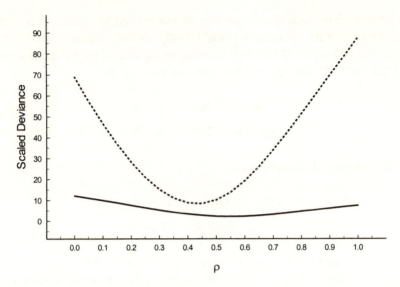

Figure 8–6 Plot of the scaled deviance against ρ for the data in Table 8–3 when age is categorical (*solid line*) and linear (*broken line*).

does not provide strong evidence for lack of fit ($G^2 = 7.43$, df $= 4$, $p = .115$), it is clear from Figure 8–6 that values of ρ that suggest a transformation of the rate that is somewhere between linear and log linear on the ladder of reexpression provides a much better fit. The scaled deviance is minimized for the categorical age model at $\hat\rho = 0.550$, the maximum likelihood estimate, for which the fit is very good indeed ($G^2 = 2.14$, df $= 3$, $p = .544$).

We can see from Figure 8–6 that the profile scaled deviance for the model that is linear in age is much more sharply curved, thus suggesting a much more precise estimate of ρ. In fact, neither the log-linear ($G^2 = 69.18$, df $= 7$, $p < .0001$) nor the linear ($G^2 = 87.64$, df $= 7$, $p < .0001$) model comes close to providing an adequate fit in this instance. The maximum likelihood estimate for the power term is $\hat\rho = 0.433$, which provides a good fit to the data ($G^2 = 8.36$, df $= 6$, $p = .213$). The standard error for $\hat\rho = 0.0598$, which strongly suggests that neither the log-linear nor the linear model for the rate is appropriate for these data. Estimates of the regression parameters are shown in Table 8–3, along with their standard errors. Notice that the crude standard error estimates obtained directly from the generalized linear model do not allow for the fact that we have estimated ρ from the data. If

Table 8–3. Regression parameter estimates for the power model, along with their standard errors, assuming ρ is known and correcting for the fact that it has been estimated for the data in Table 8–2 ($\hat\rho = 0.433$)

Parameter	Coefficient	Crude SE	Corrected SE
Intercept	−0.0195	0.0046	0.0073
Smoking	0.0188	0.0040	0.0065
Age	0.0389	0.0013	0.0077

we obtain the correct covariance matrix, using the method described in Appendix 7, the standard errors are in fact much larger. However, our qualitative conclusions about the statistical significance of smoking and age remain unchanged in this particular example.

Models for standardized ratios

In our motivation for the estimation of standardized mortality ratios (SMRs) in Chapter 4, we considered a proportional hazards model in which the underlying rate was given by population rates. We now extend the problem to the consideration of multiple risk groups identified by covariates, $\mathbf{X}$. The underlying log-linear proportional hazards model for the jth individual is given by $\lambda(t; \mathbf{X_j}) = \lambda_j^*(t) \exp\{\mathbf{X_j} \cdot \boldsymbol{\beta}\}$, where $\lambda_j^*(t)$ are determined by rates from a relevant population as applied to the jth individual. The contribution to the expected number of failures for the jth subject, who enters the study at age t_{Lj} and is last seen at age t_{Uj}, is $\Lambda_j = \int_{t_{Lj}}^{t_{Uj}} \lambda_j^*(u)du$, which is the area under the known hazard function. This is determined by first calculating the number of years the subject was in an age group at a time period when a particular rate applied. We then multiply the rate by the number of years exposed to that rate and sum over all possible combinations, giving the contribution to the *expected* number of failures, Λ_j for the jth subject.

We now consider the analysis of data in which we have tabulated the observed number of failures, along with the corresponding expected number based on the sum of each individual's contribution. For the ith cell of the table we have summary statistics given as d_i, observed failures, and E_i, expected failures. The kernel of the log likelihood under this model—that is, the portion that is available to making inferences—is equivalent to a Poisson distribution with mean $E_i \exp\{-\mathbf{X_i}\boldsymbol{\beta}\}$. This is identical to the model we considered for rates, only now we have an expected number of failures to deal with, rather than the total follow-up time. Otherwise, the model distributions are identical, so we can proceed as before, either by using an offset of $\log(E_i)$ for a model on the number of failures or by using E_i as a weight for a model on the observed ratio, or, the SMR for group i.

Example 8–2 We now return to the study of employees in a Montana smelter (4), which we discussed briefly in Chapter 4. Recall that we saw that these workers were indeed at greater risk of mortality than the general population and that those who were foreign born were at even greater risk than those who were not. We now explore more specific information available on actual levels of exposure to potentially harmful chemicals. Of particular interest were exposures to arsenic trioxide (As_2O_3) and sulfur dioxide (SO_2). Unfortunately, the investigators were not able to make separate assessments of risk from these two factors because the estimates of exposure were very highly correlated. This difficulty often occurs in observational studies such as this one because an unhealthy work environment often exposes subjects to a wide variety of potentially harmful substances, not to just a single agent. Hence, it may not be possible to tease out the separate contribution to risk of a single chemical. In this analysis, we focus on arsenic exposure, although we must keep in mind that this exposure can also be considered as a surrogate for sulfur dioxide exposure so that any effect we see may be caused by the combination of these two chemicals, as well as other factors that were not measured.

Depending on the job, a worker would have different levels of exposure, which were classified as moderate or heavy, and workers could hold several jobs over the history of their employment. In addition, duration of exposure was categorized within each level of exposure. For years of moderate exposure ("MOD"), the categories were: 0, <1, 1–4, 5–14, and ≥15. Likewise, for years of heavy exposure ("HVY") we have 0, 1–4, and ≥5. Finally, we represent place of birth ("FOR") by U.S. born and foreign born. Table 8–4 gives the tabulated data which we will now consider for analysis.

Before fitting a model to these data, it is important to note the substantial number of cells with 0 observed frequencies. This implies that we may well encounter divergence or infinite parameter estimates if we try to fit a model with many interaction terms, so we might be better off trying to fit a model with fewer parameters and then add as few interactions as might be necessary. Table 8–5 presents a summary of the results from analyzing scaled deviances from an initial model that includes just main effects for the three factors, and then adds two-factor interactions one at a time. Notice that the HVY*FOR interaction is highly significant, while neither of the other two interactions come close to significance. As the next step in building a model for these data, we consider a model with this interaction, along with the two main effects that are its lower order relatives and with a main effect for MOD. If we drop MOD, we can evaluate the change in scaled deviance

Table 8–4. Observed and expected numbers of deaths among workers at a Montana smelter by place of birth and years of arsenic exposure

Moderate arsenic exposure (years)	Heavy arsenic exposure (years)					
	0		1–4		≥5	
	Observed	Expected	Observed	Expected	Observed	Expected
U.S.-BORN						
0	28	20.86	5	1.77	6	0.60
<1	7	4.91	3	0.96	2	0.29
1–4	8	3.10	5	0.43	1	0.11
5–15	4	1.58	0	0.20	0	0.01
≥15	4	1.14	1	0.16	0	0.03
FOREIGN-BORN						
0	33	7.34	1	0.50	2	0.28
<1	2	1.31	0	0.12	0	0.05
1–4	4	0.91	0	0.08	0	0.04
5–15	6	1.05	0	0.15	0	0.04
≥15	16	1.60	3	0.30	0	0.01

Table 8–5. Analysis of scaled deviance for models fitted to the data in Table 8–4

Source	df	G^2	p
GOF for HVY, MOD, FOR	22	24.981	.2980
+HVY*MOD	8	10.069	.2602
+HVY*FOR	2	10.825	.0045
+MOD*FOR	4	5.444	.2447
GOF for HVY, MOD, FOR, HVY*FOR	20	14.156	.8225
−MOD	4	16.713	.0022

to determine whether this is a significant factor that should be included in a final model, and, indeed, it is also highly significant. Hence, we have arrived at our final model, which incidentally also shows a goodness-of-fit statistic that is not close to statistical significance.

Regression coefficients for the final model are shown in Table 8–6, along with their standard errors. The effect of years of moderate arsenic exposure suggests a dose–response relationship, although it is not monotone increasing. We could explore this further to determine whether the departure from such a trend is statistically significant. The effects of heavy arsenic exposure and place of birth are more difficult to sort out because of the interaction term in the model. In Table 8–7, we calculate the sum of main effects and interactions as they apply to each of the six combinations for HVY and FOR. It is interesting to note that there is a strong dose–response relationship with years of heavy exposure among the U.S. born, but not the foreign born. We can also see that the excess risk among the foreign born is only seen in those with no heavy exposure, while foreign born with some heavy exposure actually appear to have lower risk than the U.S. born. Clearly, the effect of place of birth is more complex than what we might have thought in our first analysis in Chapter 4, because it now becomes apparent that not all groups are at increased risk, and further work is necessary if we are to understand the reasons for this pattern. Among the possibilities we need to consider is the whether the records on which duration of heavy exposure in foreign born was determined have the same accuracy as those in the U.S. born.

Table 8–6. Parameter estimates for the final model for the data in Table 8–4

Variable	Estimate	SE	Variable	Estimate	SE
Intercept	2.3722	0.7405	FOR		
MOD			1	0.6453	0.7831
1	−0.8922	0.2424	2	Ref	
2	−1.2046	0.3466			
3	−0.4182	0.3198	HVY*FOR		
4	−0.6685	0.3778	11	−1.6497	0.8063
5	Ref		12	Ref	
HVY			21	−0.2362	0.9693
1	−0.0757	0.7202	22	Ref	
2	−0.5860	0.8710	31	Ref	
3	Ref		32	Ref	

Table 8–7. Calculation of relative risk for all combinations of HVY and FOR, and the relative risk for FOR by HVY adjusted for MOD for the data in Table 8–4

	Coefficients			log(RR)		
	FOR	1	2			
HVY	Main	0.6453	0.0000	1	2	RR(FOR)
1	−0.0757	−1.6497	0.0000	−1.0801	−0.0757	2.73
2	−0.5860	−0.2362	0.0000	−0.1769	−0.5860	0.66
3	0.0000	0.0000	0.0000	0.6453	0.0000	0.52

FOR, foreign born; HVY, years of heavy; MOD, years of moderate exposure.

Weibull Hazard Model

An alternative to the constant hazard model is the Weibull hazard, in which the form for the way in which time enters the model is represented by $\lambda_0(t) = \alpha \cdot \lambda \cdot t^{\alpha-1}$, where α is a shape parameter that allows the hazard to either remain constant ($\alpha = 1$), increase ($\alpha > 1$), or decrease ($0 < \alpha < 1$) with time. If the parameter, λ, is a log-linear function of covariates, we have a parametric version of a proportional hazards models in which $\lambda(\mathbf{X};t) = \alpha \cdot \lambda_0 \cdot t^{\alpha-1} \cdot \exp\{\mathbf{X}\boldsymbol{\beta}\}$. The cumulative hazard from 0 to t_i, which is the area under the hazard curve, yields the corresponding "expected" value for δ_i,

$$\Lambda(\mathbf{X_i};t_i) = \int_0^{t_i} \lambda(\mathbf{X_i};u)\,du$$

$$= \lambda_0 \, t_i^{\alpha} \, \exp\{\mathbf{X_i}\boldsymbol{\beta}\}$$

$$= \exp\{\beta_0 + \mathbf{X_i}\boldsymbol{\beta} + \alpha \log t_i\}$$

where $\beta_0 = \log(\lambda_0)$. If we know the shape parameter, α, we can conceptualize the Weibull model in terms of a power transformation of the time scale, in that if we consider $Y = t^{\alpha}$ as the response, then Y has an exponential distribution that arises from a constant hazard model. Moreover, the hazard associated with this distribution is the log-linear model given in equation 8.1. Hence, if we know α, the problem reduces to the one we have just considered for Poisson regression. The difference is that, in general, α needs to be estimated from the data. In Appendix 6 we show how this analysis can be conducted by using software for fitting a generalized linear model in which the response for the ith individual is represented by $\delta_i = 1$ for a complete or uncensored observation and is 0 otherwise. For purposes of finding the maximum likelihood estimates, we can assume that the response has a Poisson distribution. The offset, in this instance, is given by $\alpha \cdot \log(t)$.

Yet another formulation that is used in regression for a response that has a Weibull distribution is derived from considering the transformed response, $Y = t^{\alpha}$, directly. When t has a Weibull distribution with shape α, and covariates enter in a manner described by the proportional hazards model, it turns out that Y has an exponential distribution with hazard $\lambda(\mathbf{X})$. Using the fact that the mean for an exponential random variable is the reciprocal of the hazard implies that

$$E[t^{\alpha}] = \frac{1}{\lambda(\mathbf{X})} = \exp\{-\mathbf{X}\boldsymbol{\beta}\}$$

for the log-linear model. Notice that this formulation involves using the power transformation on time. Thus, as a final step, we can take the inverse power in order to return to the original units of time, or:

$$E[t^{\alpha}]^{1/\alpha} = \exp\{-\mathbf{X}\boldsymbol{\beta}/\alpha\}$$

It is important to realize that under either formulation, the same set of βs are used to describe the effect of the regressor variables on the response. However, for a model describing the effect on the mean length of time to the event, the regression parameters change sign, because an increase (decrease) in the hazard results in a decrease (increase) in the mean time to the event. Notice that there is also a scale change for the slope, and this change is sometimes indicated by the inclusion of an estimate of $1/\alpha$. Therefore, we can translate regression parameter estimates from an analysis of time to the event, β^{*}, to estimates of parameters for the proportional hazards model through division by this scale factor, or $\beta = -\beta^{*}/(1/\alpha)$.

Example 8–3 Let us return to the data on the effect of treatment on remission times for leukemia shown in Table 5–1, fitting a model that assumes they are described by a Weibull distribution. This was accomplished using PROC LIFEREG in SAS, and the corresponding output is displayed in Figure 8–7. The effect of treatment achieves a high level of statistical significance, but if we wish to express the magnitude of the effect in terms of the a log rate ratio, we must change sign and divide by the "Scale" estimate, $-1.26733/0.73219 = -1.731$. Thus, the estimate of the rate ratio is $\exp\{-1.731\} = 0.177$.

The estimate of the scale is somewhat interesting in its own right, because the exponential distribution corresponds to the case in which it takes the value of 1. A test of the null hypothesis that the scale is 1 actually allows us to formally test whether the distribution is exponential, compared to the alternative hypothesis of a Weibull distribution. In this instance, we can obtain an approximate test by cal-

```
                          Analysis of Parameter Estimates

                                   Standard
             Variable   DF   Estimate    Error  Chi-Square  Pr > ChiSq  Label

             Intercept   1   0.98102   0.42976    5.2108     0.0224  Intercept
             treat       1   1.26733   0.31064   16.6444    <.0001
             Scale       1   0.73219   0.10785                       Extreme value scale
```

Figure 8–7 Output from fitting a Weibull model to the data in Table 5–1 using PROC
LIFEREG (SAS).

culating $z = (1 - 0.73219)/0.10785 = 2.48$, which can be compared to a standard
normal distribution ($p = .013$). This suggests that the Weibull distribution offers a
significant improvement in fit to these data.

Other Parametric Models

We have discussed the analysis of data that arise from a hazard that is constant over time; this analysis gives rise to failure times that have an exponential distribution. In addition, we have considered the Weibull distribution for failure times. However, these are by no means the only possibilities
that might be considered. In this section we briefly describe some other
failure-time models that can be employed.

Gamma failure times

The gamma distribution offers another way of generalizing the exponential distribution, and the form for the density function is given by

$$f(t) = \frac{\lambda \cdot (\lambda t)^{k-1} \cdot \exp\{-\lambda T\}}{\Gamma(k)}$$

where t, k, and λ are all positive numbers, and $\Gamma(\ )$ is the gamma function. The parameter of primary interest is λ, and if we were to introduce
covariates into the model, it would be most natural to express λ as a function of $\mathbf{X}$. The shape parameter is given by k, which affects the shape of
the probability density, as well as the hazard function. A special case in
which $\lambda = 1$ yields the density function,

$$f(t) = \frac{t^{k-1} \cdot \exp\{-t\}}{\Gamma(k)}$$

which is closely related to the chi-square distribution. When $2k$ is an integer representing the degrees of freedom for a chi-square random variable,

Y, then $Y/2$ has a gamma distribution with $\lambda = 1$ and shape parameter k. Figure 8–8 shows the hazard for the gamma distribution for several values of the shape parameter, and we can see that it can be either decreasing $(k < 1)$, constant $(k = 1)$, or increasing $(k > 1)$.

One way in which we can motivate the use of a gamma model is if we think that the failure time arises by taking the sum of independent and identically distributed exponential random variables. The resulting distribution has a shape parameter equal to the number of variables in the sum. It is not possible to give a closed form expression for either the survival or the hazard functions for the gamma distribution, so we would need to use numerical algorithms to find these values in practice. This makes it more awkward to set up a gamma model for the analysis of failure-time data, but the ready availability of relevant numerical algorithms has made it possible to develop the necessary software for fitting this model.

Log-normal failure time

The normal distribution generally does not lend itself to fitting failure-time data because the response can take any value, including negative values. However, the log of positive numbers can take the full range from $-\infty$ to $+\infty$, which suggests that we might consider a model in which log time has a normal distribution—the log-normal distribution. This distribution has some of the same disadvantages of not having a closed form for the sur-

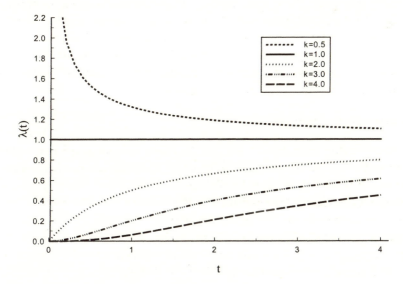

Figure 8–8 Plot of the hazard function for the gamma distribution when $\lambda = 1$ and $k = 0.5, 1.0, 2.0, 3.0,$ and 4.0.

vival or hazard function as does the gamma, but it does not negate the use of numerical methods for evaluating these functions.

While the normal distribution may not be particularly relevant for failure time, there are other instances in which this type of regression can be useful in the analysis of epidemiologic data. This is sometimes referred to as Tobit regression (5), and it was originally proposed for regression in the economics setting in which the response is cost, which cannot be negative. A similar problem can arise in epidemiologic studies when one has measured the level of a biomarker, but the method of analysis has a specified quantitation limit, so that the lowest possible value for the exposure really indicates that the level is less than the quantitation limit. Conceptually, the measured level of exposure, X, might arise from a true level of exposure, Z. If Z is greater than the quantitation limit, then $X = Z$; otherwise, the only information we have is that X is less than the quantitation limit. Tobit regression can be used to fit a model in which the level of exposure is X. From the standpoint of statistical inference, knowledge that the response is less than a specified value means that it is censored on the left, so it should not be surprising that this is very similar to the right-censored models considered in this chapter. See O'Conner et al. (6) for an example of the use of Tobit regression in the analysis of factors associated with passive exposure to cigarette smoke.

Gompertz–Makeham model

The Gompertz–Makeham form for the hazard function is $\lambda(t) = \xi + \exp\{\alpha + \gamma t\}$, where the special case, $\xi = 0$, is referred to as the Gompertz model. For the Gompertz model, the hazard is a log-linear function of time, as compared to the Weibull model, which was log linear with log time. Once again, we have the exponential as a special case, $\xi = \gamma = 0$, and the family allows for hazards that are either increasing or decreasing with time, depending on whether γ is positive or negative.

Extreme-value distribution

Another conceptualization of the way in which failures occur is to think of an individual as being made up of many different components, and if any one of these fails, then the individual as a whole fails. Hence, the distribution of interest is the minimum or the extreme value for the distribution of all components. The probability density function for the extreme-value or Gumbel distribution is given by $f(t) = \alpha^{-1} \exp\{(t - \gamma)/\alpha\} \exp\{-\exp[(t - \gamma)/\alpha]\}$. This distribution is closely related to the Weibull, in that if Z has a Weibull distribution then $T = \log(Z)$ has an extreme value distribution.

Extra Poisson Variation

One of the important characteristics of the Poisson distribution is the equality of the mean and the variance, which plays a critical role in the formulae used for obtaining variance estimates. However, it is not uncommon for count data to violate this assumption by exhibiting a variance that is greater than the mean. One way in which this might occur is when the population identified as belonging to a particular risk group actually consists of a mixture of individuals, some of whom are more prone to the illness than others. It is not hard to imagine this happening because of the potential existence of an unknown, or unmeasured, risk factor, and the effect that this has on the distribution of the observed number of cases usually results in a variance that is larger than the mean. The effect that this violation of the Poisson assumption can have on our inference is generally most profound for the estimated standard errors of the parameter estimates, which will also be smaller than they really are. This will lead to confidence intervals that are narrower than they should be, as well as concluding too often, on average, that results are statistically significant.

The form of overdispersion that is analytically most convenient to deal with occurs when the variance is proportional to the mean $\text{Var}(Y) = \phi\mu$, where ϕ is an unknown scale parameter. Of course, in the case of the Poisson distribution, this scale parameter is assumed to be 1, but in other instances we would need to estimate it. An estimate that works well in many instances is the ratio of the Pearson chi-square goodness-of-fit statistic to its degrees of freedom:

$$\tilde{\phi} = \frac{\chi^2}{(n-p)}$$

where χ^2 is the Pearson chi-square statistic, n is the number of observations included in the analysis, and p is the number of model parameters, including the intercept (7). This is reminiscent of the estimate of the error variance in ordinary least squares regression, and, indeed, the same distributional assumptions would be used when making inferences based on a model in which the scale parameter was estimated. For example, confidence limits and tests for individual parameters would make use of the t_{n-p} distribution, instead of the normal, z. The likelihood ratio tests would also be modified, using

$$F_{\Delta df, \, (n-p)} = \frac{\Delta G^2 / \Delta df}{\tilde{\phi}}$$

where Δdf is the number of regressor variables dropped from a nested set of models, which is compared to an F distribution.

Of course, a variance that is in proportion to the mean is just one of many possible candidate models for the relationship between the mean and the variance. Other models of potential interest are discussed by Mc-Cullagh and Nelder (7). In fact, the development of models for the variance can become a critical preparatory step in an analysis, especially in situations that involved longitudinal observations on the individuals under study. Fortunately, the inferences on parameters associated with the means are not overly sensitive to getting the model for the variance exactly right, so that we can often be satisfied with an analysis that provides a rough approximation of the form for the relationship.

Summary

In this chapter, we have considered several approaches to using regression models when a mathematical expression that describes the way in which the hazard varies with time is known. The simplest of these is the constant hazard model, which does not vary with time. If this assumption is correct, then we can directly analyze failure rates, and the approaches available to us extend to count data that are widely available from disease and vital statistics registries. It is particularly convenient to make use of Poisson regression models in these instances. While the log-linear model has particularly nice statistical properties, we saw that, within the class of generalized linear models, we could also consider alternative transformations that led to the linear component of our regression model. In particular, we were able to illustrate this by using the power family of transformations.

Another application of the Poisson regression model arose from the analysis of indirect adjusted rates—that is, the standardized morbidity/mortality ratio. In this case, the ratio of observed to expected numbers of cases is the outcome of interest, and these analyses allow us to compare these effects among many subgroups.

While the constant hazard case is the simplest model for the effect of time, we are by no means limited to such a restrictive assumption. The Weibull distribution is one class of distributions that has been found to provide very useful generalizations to the constant hazard assumption, and we looked at this model in some detail. However, there are also others that are used in practice, including: gamma, log-normal, Gompertz–Makeham, and extreme-value distributions. Very often, the actual form for the distribution is only of peripheral interest, the main purpose of most studies being the estimation of estimates of risk. But if we do not get the distribution right in a parameteric model for the effect of time, our estimates of relative risks and their standard errors can be invalid. In Chapter 9 we consider approaches to the analysis that are nonparametric with respect to time, only focusing on the association between exposure and disease.

The final generalization that we considered for the Poisson regression model addressed the situation in which the variance was greater than that predicted by the Poisson distribution. We considered in some detail the particular instance in which the variance was proportional to the mean, which is the simplest case to handle numerically. The problem is to arrive at an appropriate model that describes the relationship between the mean and the variance. In practice, the effect of this adjustment can be quite large for the standard errors and all statistical inferences that flow from them, but not on the regression parameters themselves.

Exercises

8.1. Return to the data in exercise 4.2 to answer the following questions.

    a. Conduct a Wald test for comparing the effect of adrenalectomy with hypophysectomy, adjusting for age and type of mastectomy, that is formally equivalent to the test in exercise 4.2 (b).

    b. Repeat (a) using a likelihood ratio test.

    c. Find the best-fitting log-linear model for rate using these data.

    d. What do you now conclude about the appropriateness of the analysis in (a) and (b)?

8.2. The following table reports the results of a study of the effect of physical activity on the risk of heart attack (HA) in a group of 16,936 Harvard male alumni.

| | | Physical activity | | | |
| | | <2000 kcal/week | | ≥2000 kcal/week | |
Cigarette smoker	History of hypertension	Person-years	No. HA	Person-years	No. HA
Yes	Yes	1,712	42	1,020	9
Yes	No	18,319	100	11,809	49
No	Yes	2,618	38	1,434	9
No	No	26,684	89	18,648	45

    a. Is there a statistically significant association between level of physical activity and risk of heart attack, adjusting for smoking and history of hypertension?

    b. Each of these three factors is thought to be a risk factor for heart disease. Create a new variable, number of risk factors, and investigate its relationship with heart attack.

    c. The analysis in (b) assumes that each of these factors has the same effect on risk of heart disease. Give an overall comparison of the adjusted relative risks for these three factors using

       i. Wald test

       ii. Likelihood ratio test

8.3. Using the data from exercise 4.3, answer the following:

    a. Fit a constant hazards model to these data, including the effects of sex, age, nephrectomy, and treatment. Summarize your conclusions.

    b. Repeat (a) using a Weibull model. Does the Weibull offer a significant improvement in fit? Are the results changed?

References

1. Zalokar JB, Richard JL, Claude JR. Leukocyte count, smoking, and myocardial infarction. *New England Journal of Medicine* 1981;304:465–468.
2. Aranda-Ordaz FJ. An extension of the proportional hazards model for grouped data. *Biometrics* 1983;39:109–117.
3. Doll R, Hill AB. Mortality in relation to smoking: ten years observations of British doctors. *British Medical Journal* 1964;1:1399–1410.
4. Breslow NE, Lubin JH, Marek P, Langholz B. Multiplicative models and cohort analysis. *Journal of the American Statistical Association* 1983;78:1–12.
5. Tobin J. Estimation of relationships for limited dependent variables. *Econometrica* 1958;26:24–36.
6. O'Connor TZ, Holford TR, Leaderer BP, Hammond SK, Bracken MB. Measurement of exposure to environmental tobacco smoke in pregnant women. *American Journal of Epidemiology* 1995;142:1315–1321.
7. McCullagh P, Nelder JA. *Generalized Linear Models*. London: Chapman and Hall, 1989.

9

Proportional Hazards Regression

In Chapter 8, we considered regression models in which the time component was represented in the model as a fully specified function. We began by assuming that the hazard was a constant, independent of time, and then considered more flexible models in which the hazard might vary with time, such as the Weibull model. However, each of these approaches to data analysis relies on a fully parametric representation of the way in which time affects risk of disease. We now consider some useful methods that relax this assumption to the point where time enters the model as an unparameterized variable, while at the same time the remaining covariates are fully parameterized. These semiparametric models offer extremely powerful methods for analyzing associations between exposure and well-defined events that occur in time, like disease and death.

It should be understood that these methods of analysis are not fully nonparametric, in that we still need to be concerned about the choice of variables used to represent exposure to putative risk factors. In that sense, the methods retain all of the strengths and the limitations of standard regression methods. We should realize, however, that representing time as a parameter-free factor is a two-edged sword. On the one hand, we have eliminated the possibility that incorrectly parameterized time might bias our regression parameter estimates by allowing the function to be completely arbitrary. On the other hand, if we really do wish to make statements involving the way in which time affects the hazard, our power is severely limited when nothing is assumed about the form of that relationship. Predictions about the absolute level of risk near the end of the observed period of data collection are especially affected by an unspecified time component.

The methods of analysis discussed here flow from a seminal paper in which Cox (1) proposed the proportional hazards model that is now often referred to as the Cox model. A formal representation of this regression model gives the hazard as

$$\lambda(\mathbf{X}, t) = \lambda_0(t) \, h(\mathbf{X}) \tag{9.1}$$

Thus, the hazard separates time, t, and the regressor variables, $\mathbf{X}$, into two functions that are multiplied together. While the regressor function, $h(\cdot)$, is specified in this model, the time function, $\lambda_0(\cdot)$, is not. In that sense, it bears some similarity to the relationship between the failure rate approach to analyzing failure time data and the estimation of survival curves. The former approach is reasonable under the highly parametric constant hazard, while the latter enjoys the survival curve's generality of a completely unspecified time effect.

In this chapter, we follow an outline similar to the one used in Chapter 5, by first dividing the follow-up time into a series of intervals and then assuming that the hazard function is a step function of time. We shall see that this piecewise exponential model can give rise to an arbitrarily flexible hazard function by letting the interval widths go to zero as the number of intervals becomes large. Passing to the limit, we arrive at the method proposed by Cox, in which the hazard function is completely arbitrary.

Piecewise Constant Hazards Model

We now consider an approach for approximating a hazard function that varies with time by introducing a step function. We divide the follow-up time into a series of intervals, identified by cutpoints: $\tau_0 = 0, \tau_1, \tau_2, \ldots, \tau_{\mathcal{J}}$. In this section we consider models in which the hazard is constant with respect to time during an interval, but it may vary from interval to interval; so:

$$\lambda(\mathbf{X},t) = \lambda_j(\mathbf{X}) \qquad \tau_j < t \leq \tau_{j+1} \tag{9.2}$$

In most cases, the hazard is likely to be a smooth function, rather than one that makes discrete jumps at a priori cutpoints, However, we should remember that this is only a means of approximating an arbitrary function and such an approximation can become arbitrarily close to the true function by specifying many narrow intervals. In the next section, we shall adopt such a process by passing to the limit, but let us first consider the piecewise exponential model.

Proportional piecewise constant hazards

We begin to specify the model for our analysis by considering proportional hazards, in which we represent the hazard for the jth interval by

$$\lambda(\mathbf{X},t) = \lambda_j \, h(\mathbf{X}) \qquad \tau_j < t \leq \tau_{j+1} \tag{9.3}$$

As we saw in Chapter 2, such a model results in a hazard ratio that is independent of time, in that a comparison of a risk group represented by regressor variables $\mathbf{X_1}$ compared to the reference group $\mathbf{X_0}$ reduces to

$$R(\mathbf{X_1},\mathbf{X_0}) = \frac{\lambda_k\, h(\mathbf{X_1})}{\lambda_k\, h(\mathbf{X_0})} = \frac{h(\mathbf{X_1})}{h(\mathbf{X_0})}$$

Proceeding a step further, we will specify the covariate component as a log-linear model, so that

$$\lambda(\mathbf{X},t) = \lambda_j \exp(\mathbf{X}\boldsymbol{\beta})$$
$$= \exp\{\mu + \alpha_j + \mathbf{X}\boldsymbol{\beta}\} \tag{9.4}$$

where μ is an intercept, α_j is the interval effect which includes a constraint such as $\alpha_1 = 0$, and $\lambda_j = \exp\{\mu + \alpha_i\}$. An interesting feature of this model is that it looks very much like the constant hazards model that we considered in Chapter 8, only now we have introduced a time interval effect into the model, α_j. We can take advantage of this, because this relationship actually carries through to the point where there is the equivalence to the Poisson likelihood, as shown in Appendix 7.

In setting up the problem for analysis, we consider a set of regressor variables for the ith group, which we represent by $\mathbf{X}_i$. Similar to the approach used to formulate the piecewise exponential model estimate of the survival function in Chapter 5, we must determine the total length of follow-up by group i in the jth interval, T_{ij}. Finally, we specify the number of failures by group i in interval j by d_{ij}. These are the raw summary data required for fitting our model, and from these we can fully represent the log likelihood and conduct statistical inference. We have presented the model in terms of groups, but this does not preclude the possibility that each individual forms a group of one, so that the times, T_{ij}, correspond to the length of time the ith subject was followed during interval j, and $d_{i+} = 1$ if the subject ultimately fails and $d_{i+} = 0$ otherwise. If we do not have the raw data on individual subjects, but only the summary statistics used in the calculation of an actuarial life table, then we can approximate the observed time for the ith group in the jth interval by $T_{ij} \approx 1_{ij} - \frac{1}{2}(W_{ij} + d_{ij})$.

As before, the model is formulated in terms of the "expected" number of failures by group i in interval j:

$$\mu_j(\mathbf{X_i}) = T_{ij} \exp\{\mu + \alpha_j + \mathbf{X_i}\boldsymbol{\beta}\}$$
$$= \exp\{\mu + \alpha_j + \mathbf{X_i}\boldsymbol{\beta} + \log(T_{ij})\}$$

The kernel of the log likelihood is equivalent to that of a Poisson distribution (2–4), and we can employ software for fitting a log-linear Poisson regression model by specifying the following:

1. d_{ij} is the response that has a Poisson distribution
2. $\log(T_{ij})$ is an offset
3. Interval is introduced as a categorical factor, and the corresponding model parameter to be estimated is α_j

Example 9–1   Boyle (5) studied the effects that stage at diagnosis and tumor histology had on survival from lung cancer. The data were obtained from cases reported to the Connecticut Tumor Registry in 1973. Stage was categorized into three levels (local, regional, and remote), as was histology (1, epidermoid; 2, glandular origin; 3, undifferentiated and anaplastic). Table 9–1 presents a summary of the essential statistics for these data that can be used in fitting a log-linear hazards model.

It is well known that stage at diagnosis is strongly related to prognosis, so the primary interest here is in the effect of tumor histology. Notice that the stage distribution of total follow-up times within each histology shown at the bottom of Table 9–1 suggests that while the distributions for epidermoid and glandular are quite similar, undifferentiated has relatively much more follow-up among those with remote stage at diagnosis. Hence, it would appear to be important that we control for stage in the analysis.

Figure 9–1 gives a SAS program for fitting a log-linear proportional hazards model to these data, and the results are shown in Figure 9–2. Not shown is a preliminary analysis that checked for an interaction between stage and histology, but this was not significant ($\Delta G^2 = 2.89$, $\Delta df = 4$, $p = .576$). The Type 3 likelihood ratio statistics shown in the output indicate that stage is highly significant ($\Delta G^2 = 112.07$, $\Delta df = 2$, $p < .0001$), which was expected. However, histology adjusted for the effect of stage is not ($\Delta G^2 = 1.89$, $\Delta df = 2$, $p = .388$). By way of contrast, a test for the effect of histology not adjusting for stage yields $\Delta G^2 = 8.85$ ($\Delta df = 2$, $p = .012$), which provides fairly strong evidence of a histology difference in prognosis, but we can see that this can readily be accounted for by differences in the stage distribution.

Testing for constant hazards

The constant hazards model is a special case of the more general piecewise exponential model in which the hazard is shown in equation 9.2; in fact, it can be obtained by constraining the interval parameters to be zero. Hence, we can regard a test of H_0: $\alpha_j = 0$ for all j as a test of goodness of fit for the exponential survival model. If there are many intervals, however, the test suffers from being too broad; this is because the many parameters associated with the dummy variables needed to represent the intervals can

Table 9–1. Summary data on lung cancer survival by cell type and stage at diagnosis (5)

Mon.	Epidermoid			Glandular			Undifferentiated		
	Local	Reg.	Rem.	Local	Reg.	Rem.	Local	Reg.	Rem.
NO. OF DEATHS									
0–1	9	12	42	5	4	28	1	1	19
2–3	2	7	26	2	3	19	1	1	11
4–5	9	5	12	3	5	10	1	3	7
6–7	10	10	10	2	4	5	1	1	6
8–9	1	4	5	2	2	0	0	0	3
10–11	3	3	4	2	1	3	1	0	3
12–13	1	4	1	2	4	2	0	2	3
14–15	3	3	3	1	2	0	0	1	1
16–17	2	3	3	0	1	1	2	0	1
18–19	2	1	1	0	0	0	0	0	0
20–21	1	0	2	1	3	0	0	0	0
22–23	1	1	0	0	0	0	0	0	0
24–25	0	0	1	1	0	0	0	0	0
26–27	0	0	1	0	0	0	0	0	0
28–29	0	0	0	0	0	0	0	0	0
Total	44	53	111	22	29	68	7	9	54
TOTAL FOLLOW-UP TIME									
0–1	157	134	212	77	71	130	21	22	101
2–3	139	110	136	68	63	72	17	18	63
4–5	126	96	90	63	58	42	14	14	43
6–7	102	86	64	55	42	21	12	10	32
8–9	88	66	47	50	35	14	10	8	21
10–11	82	59	39	45	32	13	8	8	14
12–13	76	51	29	42	28	7	6	6	10
14–15	71	38	28	34	19	4	6	4	3
16–17	62	21	19	30	14	4	5	2	2
18–19	49	16	13	28	11	2	2	2	0
20–21	42	12	9	25	9	2	2	2	0
22–23	34	10	6	19	4	2	2	2	0
24–25	19	4	4	15	2	1	0	0	0
26–27	5	2	1	11	2	0	0	0	0
28–29	4	4	0	8	4	0	0	0	0
Total	1056	709	697	570	394	314	105	98	289
	43%	29%	28%	45%	31%	25%	21%	20%	59%

Reg. = Regional; Rem. = Remote

reduce the power if a relatively simple function can represent the pattern. Therefore, it is important to supplement this test with a graphical exploration of the interval parameters to determine whether there is an underlying pattern that might suggest that the constant hazard model was inappropriate for the data.

```
options nocenter;
data deaths;  infile 'filename';
input deaths @@;

data times;  infile 'filename';
input time @@;

stage = mod(_N_-1,3)+1;
histol = mod(floor((_N_-1)/3),3)+1;
flup = floor((_N_-1)/9)+1;
log_time = log(time);

data all;  merge deaths times;

proc genmod data=all;  classes stage histol flup;
      model deaths = stage histol flup / dist=p offset=log_time type3;  run;
```

Figure 9–1 SAS procedure for fitting a log-linear model to the data in Table 9–1.

Criteria For Assessing Goodness Of Fit

Criterion	DF	Value	Value/DF
Deviance	101	82.3870	0.8157
Scaled Deviance	101	82.3870	0.8157
Pearson Chi-Square	101	86.5366	0.8568
Scaled Pearson X2	101	86.5366	0.8568
Log Likelihood	.	406.7036	.

Analysis Of Parameter Estimates

Parameter	DF	Estimate	Std Err	ChiSquare	Pr>Chi
INTERCEPT	1	-1.8310	1.0124	3.2709	0.0705
STAGE 1	1	-1.3546	0.1411	92.1723	0.0001
STAGE 2	1	-0.8053	0.1276	39.8319	0.0001
STAGE 3	0	0.0000	0.0000	.	.
HISTOL 1	1	-0.1470	0.1413	1.0821	0.2982
HISTOL 2	1	-0.0122	0.1542	0.0062	0.9371
HISTOL 3	0	0.0000	0.0000	.	.
FLUP 1	1	0.2893	1.0074	0.0825	0.7740
FLUP 2	1	0.1609	1.0097	0.0254	0.8734
FLUP 3	1	0.2077	1.0114	0.0422	0.8373
FLUP 4	1	0.4045	1.0123	0.1597	0.6894
FLUP 5	1	-0.3781	1.0308	0.1346	0.7137
FLUP 6	1	-0.0620	1.0263	0.0036	0.9518
FLUP 7	1	0.1133	1.0273	0.0122	0.9122
FLUP 8	1	0.0634	1.0365	0.0037	0.9512
FLUP 9	1	0.2969	1.0390	0.0817	0.7751
FLUP 10	1	-0.5599	1.1190	0.2504	0.6168
FLUP 11	1	0.2077	1.0699	0.0377	0.8461
FLUP 12	1	-0.7571	1.2256	0.3816	0.5368
FLUP 13	1	-0.1789	1.2258	0.0213	0.8840
FLUP 14	1	-0.0309	1.4146	0.0005	0.9826
FLUP 15	0	0.0000	0.0000	.	.
SCALE	0	1.0000	0.0000	.	.

NOTE: The scale parameter was held fixed.

LR Statistics For Type 3 Analysis

Source	DF	ChiSquare	Pr>Chi
STAGE	2	112.0680	0.0001
HISTOL	2	1.8940	0.3879
FLUP	14	17.0813	0.2519

Figure 9–2 Output from the SAS procedure shown in Figure 9–1.

Example 9–1 (continued) In the previous section, we fitted a log-linear model for the lung cancer data in Table 9–1, including the main effects for stage and histology, along with effects for follow-up intervals. The overall test for the follow-up effects is not statistically significant ($\Delta G^2 = 17.08$, $\Delta df = 14$, $p = .252$), but a plot of the estimated effects against the number of months of follow-up reveals an overall negative trend, as seen in Figure 9–3. We can test for the significance of this slope by including follow-up interval in the model, but not placing it in the "CLASSES" statement, thus forcing the effect to be linear. In this case, the effect of follow-up is significant ($\Delta G^2 = 4.27$, $\Delta df = 1$, $p = .0388$), due in part to a more focused alternative hypothesis compared to the overall test.

Alternatives to proportional hazards

We have seen that a fundamental assumption that underlies the proportional hazards model is the implication that the effect of exposure does not vary with time. In the short term, such a concept may be quite feasible to comprehend, but over the long term it becomes increasingly problematic. This is especially true of exposures that may change over time. Consider the effect of cigarette smoking among those who have quit, for instance. In studies of heart disease, the excess risk among smokers tends to return quite quickly to the lower risk levels of nonsmokers. A similar phenomenon has also been observed for lung cancer, a disease in which the relative effect of cigarette smoking is even greater. While the risk never returns to the low levels of a nonsmoker, it is nevertheless considerably better than for a smoker, thus providing a strong rationale for smoking cessation programs.

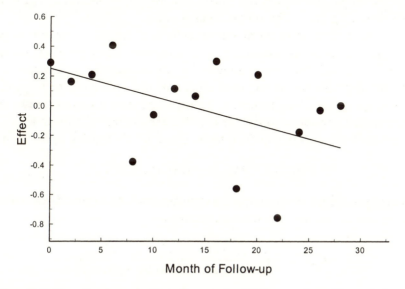

Figure 9–3 Plot of estimated effects for month of follow-up from Figure 9–2.

It is also not uncommon to observe a wash-out of an initially strong effect, especially when individuals are followed over a long period of time. In an unpublished study of survival among colorectal cancer patients reported to the Connecticut Tumor Registry, surgical treatment was found to be highly associated with survival. While some of this effect was undoubtedly due to beneficial therapeutic effects of surgery, there was also a strong component of self-selection in these population-based data. The treatment decision for a patient diagnosed with very advanced disease may be to simply not treat because of poor prognosis, choosing instead to relieve symptoms and pain. A wash-out in the effect of surgery was apparent in these data, 10 to 15 years after diagnosis, while those treated surgically experienced a much better prognosis in the years immediately after diagnosis. The implication is that if somehow a patient survived 15 years without surgical treatment, then their future prognosis was essentially the same as those who had been treated. Of course, not many untreated patients were fortunate enough to live that long.

Effects that vary with time have also been observed in clinical trials that cover shorter time periods. In the Veterans Administration Coronary Artery Bypass Surgery Study, patients were randomized to receive either surgical or medical treatment regimens (6). Immediately after treatment, surgically treated patients had lower survival, partly because of the complications of the surgery itself. Later, however, the surgically treated patients showed a better prognosis than did the medically treated patients. Such crossover effects often pose difficult treatment decisions in that, by exposing a patient to some initial excess risk, it is possible to eventually achieve a long-term benefit among those who survive long enough.

In our discussion of specifying variables in Chapter 7, we saw how interaction terms can be introduced to investigate whether the effect of one factor varies with the level of another. We can employ the same idea when investigating effects that vary with time, only now the interactions involve follow-up as one of the factors. If the exposure level is represented by X, then we can consider a model for the jth interval that includes an interaction between exposure and the interval index, jX, thus giving us the model

$$\lambda(\mathbf{X(j)},t) = \exp\{\mu + \alpha_j + X\beta_x + jX\boldsymbol{\beta}_{jX}\}$$

Hence, the hazard ratio, comparing exposure level X_1 to the reference level X_0 in the jth interval of follow-up, becomes

$$R(X_1,X_0;t) = \frac{\exp\{\mu + \alpha_j + X_1\beta_X + jX_1\beta_{jX}\}}{\exp\{\mu + \alpha_j + X_0\beta_X + jX_0\beta_{jX}\}}$$

$$= \exp\{(X_1 - X_0)(\beta_X + j\beta_{jX})\}$$

in which the log hazard ratio is proportional to a linear function of the interval index.

In principle, we can include interactions with all dummy variables representing follow-up intervals, but this would present us with a vague alternative hypothesis that would tend to have little power relative to a linear trend when the latter represents the true situation. Hence, it is preferable to reduce the number of parameters by investigating interactions with linear components of follow-up interval (perhaps after a transformation), low-order polynomials, categorical splits, or other flexible models with relatively few parameters.

Example 9–1 (continued) In fitting the proportional hazards model, we introduced histology as a classification variable by listing it in the "CLASSES" statement. This is equivalent to introducing two dummy variables for histology:

$$X_1 = 1 \quad \text{if histology} = 1$$
$$= 0 \quad \text{otherwise}$$
$$X_2 = 1 \quad \text{if histology} = 2$$
$$= 0 \quad \text{otherwise}$$

If we wish to fit a model in which the effect of histology changes linearly with follow-up interval, we include a product between each histology variable and the interval index:

$$X_3 = j \quad \text{if histology} = 1$$
$$= 0 \quad \text{otherwise}$$
$$X_4 = j \quad \text{if histology} = 2$$
$$= 0 \quad \text{otherwise}$$

Thus, the log hazard ratio for level 1 of histology compared to level 3 becomes $\beta_1 + j\beta_3$, as shown in Figure 9–4. Similar models can be considered for the effect of stage of disease. In these data, there was no strong evidence for effects that varied over time, as the histology interaction that controlled for the stage interaction (along with the other factors) was not significant ($\Delta G^2 = 4.15$, $\Delta df = 2$, $p = .126$), nor was the corresponding stage interaction with follow-up interval ($\Delta G^2 = 2.37$, $\Delta df = 2$, $p = .306$).

Nonparametric Proportional Hazards

As we saw in our discussion of survival curve estimates in Chapter 5, a completely nonparametric model with respect to the time component could be realized by passing to the limit as the width of each interval goes to zero

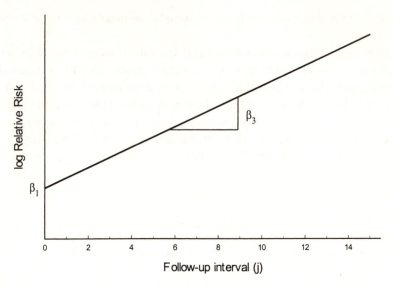

Figure 9–4 Trend in log relative risk for a model with an interaction with follow-up interval.

and the number of intervals to infinity. Our objective now is to establish a method for estimating the association between exposure and the hazard function, which is represented by equation 9.1. For a small interval, most individuals who enter survive for the entire interval, except for those who fail or are censored. If we adopt the same rule for the censored as we did to motivate the product limit estimate of the survival curve—that is, move each censored observation to the end of the interval—then these subjects are also followed for the entire interval. All that remains is the failure, and if we adopt a similar convention of regarding these as being followed for the entire width of the small interval, then the total follow-up experience for the ith group during the interval that includes jth failure is ΔR_{ij}, where Δ is the width of the interval and R_{ij} is the number of subjects in exposure group i at the jth follow-up interval. The expected number of failures in the interval is

$$\mu(\mathbf{X_i},j) = R_{ij}\,\Delta\,\exp\{\mathbf{X_{ij}}\,\beta\}$$
$$= R_{ij}\,\exp\{\alpha_0(t_j) + \mathbf{X_{ij}}\,\beta\}$$

where $\alpha_0(t_j) = \log[\Delta\,\lambda_0(t_j)]$. We could proceed to find maximum likelihood estimates of the parameters by substituting this formulation into the method we already employed for the piecewise exponential model, except for the awkwardness that arises from the fact that there are a great many uninteresting nuisance parameters, $\alpha_0(t_j)$, to be estimated (2–4). A somewhat simpler representation of the analysis method results from only considering the parameters of interest, β. Intervals that do not include failures contribute no information about the parameters that associate the regressor variables with risk of failure, β, and the only relevant information is provided by intervals that include failure times. This results in the approach used by software specifically designed to fit proportional hazards models, as is discussed in further detail in Appendix 7.

Example 9–2 The Veteran's Administration conducted a clinical trial of lung cancer therapy (7) in which the current standard was compared to a new test therapy. We have information on the following covariates:

1. Length of follow-up in days
2. Survival status (0, alive; 1, dead)
3. Performance status (scale from 0 to 100 that measures degree of illness)
4. Months from diagnosis
5. Age in years
6. Prior therapy (0, no; 10, yes)
7. Treatment (1, standard; 2, test)
8. Cell type (1, squamous; 2, small; 3, adeno; 4, large)

Let us consider a model in which all of these factors are included, some continuous (performance status, months from diagnosis, age) and some categorical (prior therapy, treatment, cell type). Previous therapy and treatment are both binary, which we will code as 1 for yes and 0 otherwise. As there are four cell types, we require three dummy variables, and we will arbitrarily use squamous as the reference level, thus introducing the variables:

Cell type	X_{H2}	X_{H3}	X_{H4}
Squamous	0	0	0
Small	1	0	0
Adeno	0	1	0
Large	0	0	1

Figure 9–5 shows a SAS program used for fitting these data, and the resulting output is given in Figure 9–6.

One of the primary interests in these data is the potential efficacy of treatment, but there is little evidence to suggest a treatment difference ($W^2 = 2.09$, df $= 1$, $p = .148$). In fact, the hazard ratio of death for treatment controlling for these other factors is $\exp\{0.303\} = 1.35$, so that our best estimate points in the direction of a harmful effect for the new treatment. Among the other covariates with 1 df, only performance status shows a very strong association with survival, and none of the others is statistically significant. Finally, we consider histology, which by our coding scheme compares each group to squamous. Taking the difference in -2(log likelihood) we obtain a likelihood ratio test, $\Delta G^2 = 951.882 - 932.170 = 19.712$, with Δdf $= 3$ ($p = .0002$), which is highly significant. The hazard ratio for large

```
data one; infile 'filename';
input t status perform dx_mon age p_trt trt hist;
*                        ;
* DEFINE DUMMY VARIABLES ;
*                        ;
trt = trt-1;
p_trt = p_trt/10;
h2 = (hist = 2);
h3 = (hist = 3);
h4 = (hist = 4);
*                             ;
* FIT MODEL WITH ALL COVARIATES ;
*                             ;
proc phreg data=one;
    model t*status(0) = perform dx_mon age p_trt trt h2 h3 h4;  run;
*                             ;
* FIT MODEL DROPPING HISTOLOGY  ;
*                             ;
proc phreg data=one;
    model t*status(0) = perform dx_mon age p_trt trt;  run;
```

Figure 9–5 SAS procedure for fitting a proportional hazards model to the VA lung cancer trial.

```
                          The PHREG Procedure

                  Testing Global Null Hypothesis: BETA=0

                      Without       With
          Criterion   Covariates    Covariates   Model Chi-Square

          -2 LOG L     995.773        932.170      63.603 with 8 DF  (p=0.0001)
          Score           .              .         68.063 with 8 DF  (p=0.0001)
          Wald            .              .         63.587 with 8 DF  (p=0.0001)

                  Analysis of Maximum Likelihood Estimates

                     Parameter    Standard     Wald        Pr >        Risk
       Variable  DF   Estimate     Error     Chi-Square  Chi-Square    Ratio

       PERFORM    1   -0.033827    0.00555    37.15500    0.0001       0.967
       DX_MON     1   -0.003282    0.00975     0.11331    0.7364       0.997
       AGE        1   -0.009674    0.00934     1.07372    0.3001       0.990
       P_TRT      1    0.096207    0.23601     0.16617    0.6835       1.101
       TRT        1    0.303168    0.20952     2.09372    0.1479       1.354
       H2         1    0.927447    0.28226    10.79656    0.0010       2.528
       H3         1    1.238946    0.30670    16.31864    0.0001       3.452
       H4         1    0.475165    0.28830     2.71647    0.0993       1.608

                          The PHREG Procedure

                  Testing Global Null Hypothesis: BETA=0

                      Without       With
          Criterion   Covariates    Covariates   Model Chi-Square

          -2 LOG L     995.773        951.882      43.891 with 5 DF  (p=0.0001)
          Score           .              .         47.974 with 5 DF  (p=0.0001)
          Wald            .              .         45.413 with 5 DF  (p=0.0001)

                  Analysis of Maximum Likelihood Estimates

                     Parameter    Standard     Wald        Pr >        Risk
       Variable  DF   Estimate     Error     Chi-Square  Chi-Square    Ratio

       PERFORM    1   -0.034801    0.00540    41.53666    0.0001       0.966
       DX_MON     1   -0.001000    0.00960     0.01084    0.9171       0.999
       AGE        1   -0.004371    0.00930     0.22095    0.6383       0.996
       P_TRT      1   -0.068918    0.22477     0.09402    0.7591       0.933
       TRT        1    0.182624    0.18795     0.94415    0.3312       1.200
```

Figure 9–6 Output from the SAS procedure shown in Figure 9–5.

compared to squamous is only 1.61, but small and adeno patients clearly have much worse prognosis with hazard ratios of 2.53 and 3.45, respectively.

Evaluating the Fit of a Proportional Hazards Model

An extension to the basic proportional hazards model (7) introduces stratification, which gives even more flexibility to the model and offers a way of validating the underlying proportionality assumption. In this case, we form strata based on the level of one of our factors, and for the kth stratum, the log-linear hazard is given by $\lambda(\mathbf{X};t,k) = \lambda_{0k}(t) \exp\{\mathbf{X\beta}\}$. We have already seen that variables that are categorical in nature can be included in the proportional hazards model by using dummy variables. However, the time component of these models was assumed to be the same for all strata, $\lambda_0(t)$. Now we are considering a model with a fundamental difference, in that the time component can vary among strata; that is, for the kth stratum, time enters as $\lambda_{0k}(t)$. One approach to validating the proportional hazards model is to obtain summaries that characterize the stratum-specific time component and check to see whether they in fact behave in the way we would expect if proportional hazards are applied to the stratified variable.

One such summary is the adjusted survival curve, which depends on the best estimates of the model parameters, and the covariates are fixed so that we are comparing each stratum at the same level of risk with respect to the other factors, $\mathbf{X_0}$. This is most easily accomplished by setting $\mathbf{X_0} = \mathbf{0}$, and so that we estimate

$$\hat{\mathscr{F}}_k(\mathbf{X} = \mathbf{0};\mathbf{t}) = \exp\{-\int_0^t \hat{\lambda}_{0k}(u)\, du\}$$

If proportional hazards applies to the k strata, then we expect that a plot of $\log[-\log \hat{\mathscr{F}}_k(\mathbf{X} = \mathbf{0};\mathbf{t})]$ would result in a series of parallel lines, and a lack of parallelism would suggest that, in fact, proportional hazards did not apply.

Example 9–2 (continued) Returning to the data from the lung cancer clinical trial, let us graphically consider the question of whether the proportional hazards assumption applies to these data. Instead of including the dummy variable for histology, we now stratify by histology to obtain an adjusted survival curve based on arbitrarily setting the other covariates to 0. Figure 9–7 shows a plot of the log-log adjusted survival curve estimates plotted against time on a log scale. The most striking feature of this graph is that squamous cell cancers are not parallel to adeno or large. Small, on the other hand, is less clear cut, in that before 30, small appears to be more nearly parallel to large and adeno, but after 30 it appears to be paral-

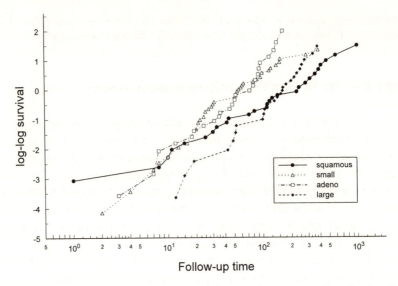

Figure 9–7 Plot of log-log survival adjusted for covariates against time for data from the VA lung cancer clinical trial.

lel with squamous. We see that the effect of histology on lung cancer survival may be more complex than can be adequately represented by the basic proportional hazards model. This means that single estimates of the hazard ratio that apply over the entire period of follow-up simply do not apply, and to more precisely describe what is happening, we must present time-dependent estimates of the association. It is also interesting to note that early in the follow-up, squamous had an experience similar to small and adeno and worse than large. However, ultimately, those patients with squamous cell tumors had the best prognosis. In the following section, we consider a more formal exploration of this phenomenon by introducing effects that vary with time.

Time-Dependent Covariates

The proportional hazards model provides us with a very rich framework for studying associations between exposure and disease risk; it also allows us to consider covariates that may themselves change over the course of follow-up. We actually encountered one example of the way in which this can arise in the section "Alternatives to Proportional Hazards," by including in our model interactions with interval of follow-up, thus allowing the effect of one factor to vary over time. However, interactions with time are just one type of regressor variable that can broadly be referred to as a time-dependent covariate, which we shall represent as $\mathbf{Z}(t)$, and the general representation of the model is

$$\lambda(\mathbf{X},\mathbf{Z}(t);t) = \lambda_0(t) \exp\{\mathbf{X}\beta_{\mathbf{X}} + \mathbf{Z(t)}\beta_{\mathbf{Z}}\} \qquad (9.5)$$

in which β_X are the parameters associated with variables that remain the same over time and β_Z are those associated with the time-dependent covariates. This extension allows us to fit models in which the effect of exposure is not limited to the same multiplicative value over time, so that it is no longer just a proportional effect, as is implied by the proportional hazards model.

The added flexibility that time-dependent covariates provide allows us to also consider exposures that may vary over the course of follow-up. In addition, it allows us to begin to consider models for disease progression, in which we analyze factors associated with the development of different stages in the overall illness process. Followed to the next logical step, we might also consider an analysis of various events in time, some of which are intermediate stages in the development of a disease, which is referred to as event time analysis (8).

Effects that vary with time

In our discussion of covariates in Chapter 7, we explored the use of interactions to characterize risk associated with exposure to two or more factors when the effect of one depended on the level of another. When we considered interactions with follow-up interval in the preceding section on alternatives, the idea followed easily from any other type of interaction, in part due to the fact that we set up the analysis as a table of rates. The follow-up interval was simply another dimension of the table, so it seemed natural to treat it as just another regressor variable in our analysis. We now consider an approach for setting up the analysis in the context of the usual representation of a typical proportional hazards model.

Let us now consider a model in which exposure is represented by X, and we also wish to consider interactions with time, which we represent by the regressor variable $Z(t) = Xt$. If there are no other variables in the model, then

$$\lambda(X, Z(t); t) = \lambda_0(t) \exp\{X\beta_X + Xt\beta_Z\}$$

The hazard ratio implied by this model, letting X_0 represent the reference level, is given by

$$R(X, X_0) = \frac{\lambda(X, Z(t); t)}{\lambda(X_0, Z(t); t)}$$

$$= \frac{\lambda_0(t) \exp\{X\beta_X + Xt\beta_Z\}}{\lambda_0(t) \exp\{X_0\beta_X + X_0t\beta_Z\}}$$

$$= \exp\{(X - X_0)\beta_X + (X - X_0)t\beta_Z\}$$

Hence, the log hazard ratio is a linear function of t, in which $(X - X_0)\beta_X$ represents the intercept, or the log hazard ratio when $t = 0$, and $(X - X_0)\beta_Z$ is the amount by which the log hazard ratio changes for a unit change in time, t.

For time interactions, we can include products of exposure and any function of time, $Xf(t)$. Thus we might consider including a transformation of the time scale, such as log time, rather than the original scale. In addition, we can consider more complex models that can involve multiple parameters, such as polynomials. A model in which the log hazard ratio behaves as a quadratic function of time can be represented by including not only the exposure variable but also the time-dependent covariates, Xt and Xt^2. Thus the log hazard ratio becomes

$$\log R(X,X_0) = (X - X_0)\beta_X + (X - X_0)t\beta_{Z_1} + (X - X_0)t^2\beta_{Z_2}$$

A general rule of thumb when including higher order interactions in a model is to also include the lower order relatives. With respect to time interactions, this would imply that parameters associated with the main effects for $f(t)$ should also be included, but it is not immediately clear that we have abided by that rule because nowhere do we see such a function in our model specification. However, we need to remember that the main effect for time—the element that does not depend on exposure—was represented by the arbitrary function $\lambda_0(t)$, which becomes the similarly arbitrary function $\log \lambda_0(t)$ when we bring it into the exponent of our log-linear hazard model. The fact that this function of time is completely arbitrary means that it would also include $f(t)$ as a special case. Thus, we have actually accounted for the main effect for time, even though we have not explicitly entered it into our model. In fact, any attempt to do so would result in an error because it would be completely redundant.

Example 9–2 (continued)   In our analysis of the VA lung cancer trial in which we stratified on histology, we noticed that the adjusted log-log survival curves appeared to be linear in log time, but the lines were not parallel. We can represent this situation by adding products of log time and the dummy histologies to our model:

Cell type	Z_{H2}	Z_{H3}	Z_{H4}
Squamous	0	0	0
Small	$\log t$	0	0
Adeno	0	$\log t$	0
Large	0	0	$\log t$

```
data one; infile 'filename';
input t status perform dx_mon age p_trt trt hist;
*                                      ;
* DEFINE DUMMY VARIABLES ;
*                                      ;
trt = trt-1;
p_trt = p_trt/10;
h2 = (hist = 2);
h3 = (hist = 3);
h4 = (hist = 4);
*                                                      ;
* PROPORTINAL HAZARDREGRESSION WITH TIME-DEPENDENT COVARIATES;
*                                                      ;
proc phreg data=one;
    h2t = h2*log(t);
    h3t = h3*log(t);
    h4t = h4*log(t);
    model t*status(0) = perform dx_mon age p_trt trt h2 h3 h4 h2t h3t h4t;
    run;
```

Figure 9-8 SAS procedure for fitting a log-linear model with time-dependent covariates to the VA clinical trial data.

A SAS procedure for such a model is shown in Figure 9–8. Notice that the time-
dependent covariates are defined in statements that are part of PROC PHREG, and
not in the "DATA" step in which variable transformations are defined. If we had
included the statement in the "DATA" step then the same level of the covariate,
calculated at the observed length of follow-up, would have been considered at each
failure time, and we would not have a function that could change with time, as envisioned by this representation. In fact, the inclusion of some function of the observed length of follow-up would be like including a function of the response as
one of the covariates, which would make no sense. The results of this analysis are
shown in Figure 9–9, and the likelihood ratio statistic resulting from the inclusion
of these time interactions is found by comparing these results to those in the model
without the time-dependent covariate in Figure 9–6, $\Delta G^2 = 932.170 - 916.692 =
15.478$ (Δdf $= 9 - 6 = 3$, $p = .0015$), providing strong evidence that the effect of
histology varies with time. Our choice of dummy variables makes squamous the
convenient referent group, and the parameters imply the relationship among the
hazard ratios that is shown in Figure 9–10.

One of the preliminary suggestions from our graphical analysis of the histology
strata was that the trends for large and adeno were parallel, and small may be parallel with squamous or perhaps large and adeno. If there is a lack of parallelism
just between two groups, we can indicate that by introducing just a single time-
dependent variable:

$$Z(t) = \log t \quad \text{if group 2}$$

$$= 0 \quad \text{otherwise}$$

When we partition the time-dependent effect by grouping small with squamous
and comparing with the rest, we have strong evidence of a difference between the
groups ($\Delta G^2 = 13.344$, Δdf $= 1$, $p = .0003$), and the parameters within groups are
not at all significant ($\Delta G^2 = 0.570$, Δdf $= 2$, $p = .752$). Alternatively, when we compare squamous with the remaining three histologies, we have the suggestion

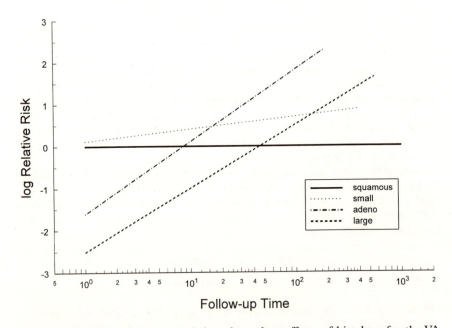

```
                        The PHREG Procedure

                  Testing Global Null Hypothesis: BETA=0

                     Without       With
          Criterion   Covariates   Covariates   Model Chi-Square

          -2 LOG L     995.773       916.692     79.081 with 11 DF (p=0.0001)
          Score          .             .         81.470 with 11 DF (p=0.0001)
          Wald           .             .         74.352 with 11 DF (p=0.0001)

                  Analysis of Maximum Likelihood Estimates

                        Parameter    Standard      Wald        Pr >        Risk
        Variable   DF   Estimate     Error      Chi-Square   Chi-Square   Ratio

        PERFORM    1    -0.037023    0.00575    41.44877      0.0001      0.964
        DX_MON     1    -0.006560    0.00960     0.46724      0.4943      0.993
        AGE        1    -0.012056    0.00968     1.55168      0.2129      0.988
        P_TRT      1     0.187848    0.23738     0.62620      0.4288      1.207
        TRT        1     0.375917    0.21341     3.10273      0.0782      1.456
        H2         1     0.018789    0.72689     0.0006681     0.9794      1.019
        H3         1    -1.852691    1.09308     2.87277      0.0901      0.157
        H4         1    -2.771218    1.20194     5.31587      0.0211      0.063
        H2T        1     0.198625    0.18004     1.21712      0.2699      1.220
        H3T        1     0.812122    0.28045     8.38582      0.0038      2.253
        H4T        1     0.739165    0.25738     8.24789      0.0041      2.094
```

Figure 9–9 Output from the SAS procedure shown in Figure 9–8.

Figure 9–10 Plot of the estimated time-dependent effects of histology for the VA lung cancer clinical trial.

of some heterogeneity among small, large, and adeno ($\Delta G^2 = 9.416$, $\Delta df = 2$, $p = .0090$). This suggests that the trend in the effect for small is more nearly like squamous and that the lack of parallelism can be adequately defined by just considering two groups of histologies.

Exposures that vary with time

A second type of time-dependent covariate arises when the exposure itself changes over the course of follow-up. For example, in a study of occupational exposures at a plant, an individual may change jobs several times during the course of employment and thus be exposed to different levels of risk over time. Hence, the time-dependent covariate, $Z(t)$, represents the exposure level at time t. The following example is a classic illustration of such a change in an exposure over time.

Example 9–3 The Stanford heart transplant study (7, 9) was conducted to assess the efficacy of heart transplants in a qualified group of patients with severe heart disease. Unlike a standard clinical trial like the VA trial we considered in the previous section, treatment was not necessarily immediately available because it required a satisfactory donor heart. There could be weeks of waiting for a donor heart, so patients would often die while waiting for treatment. Evaluating survival from the time of transplant was considered, but the investigators recognized that to receive surgery, the patient must live long enough for a donor heart to be identified. Inevitably, the healthier patients would be better able to survive long enough to receive a transplant, so there would not be a valid comparison if we were to only consider those who received this new form of treatment and compared it to the group who did not.

It would also be impossible to randomize patients into a group that could receive a transplant and another who could not, and compare the two groups' survival from the time of enrollment into the study. A study that simply randomized patients into a group in which the intended treatment was transplant and control group that received only standard available treatment would perhaps get at the effect of a particular treatment strategy, but it would dilute the estimated effect of the treatment. Because of the difficulty in finding donor hearts, many patients in the intend-to-transplant group might not receive the treatment because they had died before a donor was found, thus diluting any potential benefit. This strategy would also not make the best use of the limited number of qualified patients and donors, because undoubtedly there would be some in a control group for whom a donor was more readily available, so this was not the best use of very limited resources.

An alternative form of analysis measured time from the point at which a subject was enrolled in the study. Thus, in a nonparametric analysis the hazard could, for example, be very high initially, as the most severely ill patients died shortly after enrollment, and then decline over time as the stronger patients remained under active follow-up. Treatment was considered as a time-dependent dummy variable that changed at the follow-up time when the patient received the transplant,

$$Z(t) = 1 \quad \text{if (time of transplant)} \leq t$$
$$\quad\quad = 0 \quad \text{otherwise}$$

In this model, we are comparing the hazard for a patient who has received a transplant at t with one who has not, thus the hazard ratio is represented by

$$R(1,0) = \frac{\lambda(1;t)}{\lambda(0;t)} = \frac{\lambda_0(t) \cdot \exp\{1\beta_Z\}}{\lambda_0(t) \cdot \exp\{0\beta_Z\}} = \exp\{\beta_Z\}$$

The risk set that determines the contribution at each failure time considers a patient's treatment status at that particular point in time. Hence, patients would remain in the untreated group until they received a transplant, and thereafter they would be counted among the treated patients.

The data from this study are coded as follows:

1. Patient identification number
2. Survival time in days
3. Survival status: 0, censored; 1 or 2, dead
4. Waiting time to transplant in days
5. Age at transplant
6. Tissue mismatch score (a measure of donor compatibility)

We first define the time-dependent variable that will yield the estimated effect of transplant. If we represent the waiting time to a transplant by w, and t is the survival time, then treatment can be represented by

$$Z_1(t) = 1 \qquad \text{if } w \leq t$$

$$= 0 \qquad \text{otherwise}$$

Two other factors related to the transplant are also of interest, as they may suggest a transplant effect that was modified by one of them. The first factor we consider is age at transplant, in order to explore whether the transplants are equally effective in old and young patients. A potentially serious complication in transplant surgery is rejection of the donor organ, so a second factor related to the treatment was the tissue mismatch score, which was an attempt to measure the compatibility between the donated heart and the patient. Let X represent the putative treatment modifier, or, age at surgery or mismatch score, and the corresponding time-dependent covariate is defined by

$$Z_2(t) = X \qquad \text{if } w \leq t$$

$$= 0 \qquad \text{otherwise}$$

Hence, the log hazard ratio for transplant with related covariates at time t is given by

$$\log R[(Z_1(t),Z_2(t)),(0,0);t] = \log \left[\frac{\lambda_0(t)\exp\{Z_1(T)\,\beta_{Z_1} + Z_2(T)\,\beta_{Z_2}\}}{\lambda_0(t)\exp\{0\,\beta_{Z_1} + 0\,\beta_{Z_2}\}} \right]$$

$$= \beta_{Z_1} + X\beta_{Z_2} \qquad \text{if transplant received}$$

$$= 0 \qquad \text{otherwise}$$

where β_{Z_1} represents the treatment effect when $X = 0$, and β_{Z_2} the change in treatment effect per unit change in X.

```
data;   infile 'stanhrt.dat' missover;
input id 3.  survtime 5.  stat 3.  waittime 5.  op_age 3.  mismatch 5.2;
if (waittime = .) then waittime=99999;
*                            ;
* Model for transplant ;
*                            ;
proc phreg;
    if (survtime >= waittime) then tr_plant = 1;  else tr_plant=0;
    model survtime*stat(0) = tr_plant;
run;
*                                          ;
* Model for the effect of age on transplant ;
*                                          ;
proc phreg;
    if (survtime >= waittime) then tr_plant = 1;  else tr_plant=0;
    if (survtime >= waittime) then trp_age = op_age;  else trp_age=0;
    model survtime*stat(0) = tr_plant trp_age;
run;
```

Figure 9–11 SAS procedure for fitting a log-linear model to the Stanford heart transplant data.

Figure 9–11 shows a SAS procedure set up to first fit a model with only the treatment effect and then, with the putative modifier, age at transplant. The resulting output is shown in Figure 9–12. While the estimate of the treatment effect by itself is in the direction of a beneficial effect, the tiny value for the corresponding Wald statistic, $W^2 = 0.006$, suggests that there is essentially no evidence of a treatment effect in these data. However, in the second model that also includes the age at transplant variable, there is quite strong evidence that these two factors together are important ($\Delta G^2 = 7.320$, $\Delta df = 2$, $p = .0257$). While the Wald tests for the individual parameters indicate that both variables are statistically significant, we should remember that in this case the transplant parameter estimates the efficacy of transplant at age 0, which is an obviously silly extrapolation. Figure 9–13 plots the estimated effect of treatment within the observed range of ages at transplant. We can see that the line centers about a log hazard ratio of zero, hence the absence of any treatment effect when we consider treatment alone. However, it is now clear that the surgery was far more successful in the younger patients, while those who were older appear to actually suffer a worse prognosis.

Summary

In this chapter, we relaxed the parametrically restrictive parameterization for time that we had considered in the previous chapter, adopting instead a nonparametric set of models in which the exact form for the effect of time was left as an arbitrary function. This proportional hazards (or Cox) model provides a very rich framework for data analysis, enabling us not only to consider factors that were measured at the beginning of follow-up but also to update the risk status over time.

```
                         The PHREG Procedure

                 Testing Global Null Hypothesis: BETA=0

                     Without        With
         Criterion   Covariates    Covariates    Model Chi-Square

         -2 LOG L     561.646       561.640      0.006 with 1 DF (p=0.9362)
         Score           .             .         0.006 with 1 DF (p=0.9362)
         Wald            .             .         0.006 with 1 DF (p=0.9362)

                  Analysis of Maximum Likelihood Estimates

                     Parameter    Standard     Wald        Pr >        Risk
       Variable  DF  Estimate     Error     Chi-Square   Chi-Square    Ratio

       TR_PLANT   1  -0.024219    0.30256    0.00641      0.9362       0.976


                         The PHREG Procedure

                 Testing Global Null Hypothesis: BETA=0

                     Without        With
         Criterion   Covariates    Covariates    Model Chi-Square

         -2 LOG L     561.646       554.327      7.320 with 2 DF (p=0.0257)
         Score           .             .         6.346 with 2 DF (p=0.0419)
         Wald            .             .         6.456 with 2 DF (p=0.0396)

                  Analysis of Maximum Likelihood Estimates

                     Parameter    Standard     Wald        Pr >        Risk
       Variable  DF  Estimate     Error     Chi-Square   Chi-Square    Ratio

       TR_PLANT   1  -2.703591    1.13742    5.64986      0.0175       0.067
       TRP_AGE    1   0.056694    0.02241    6.39920      0.0114       1.058
```

Figure 9–12 Output from the SAS procedure shown in Figure 9–11.

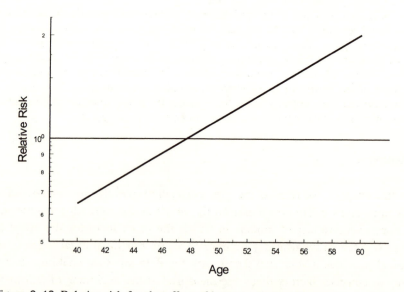

Figure 9–13 Relative risk for the effect of heart transplant by age.

We began this discussion by considering the piecewise constant hazards model, which directly generalized the approach used for the analysis of failure rates. This not only allowed us to relax our assumptions about the form for the time effect, but also it provided a direct method of testing for the adequacy of the proportional hazards assumption. In addition, it enabled us to consider whether the effects of the covariates of interest in the analysis varied over time.

The flexibility of the piecewise constant hazards approach can be improved by letting the interval widths become small while the number of intervals becomes large. This provides a justification for the methods used in fitting the proportional hazards model, although there are other approaches that provide deeper insights into the inferential subtleties involved. The types of variables that can be included in these regression models are those that are constant over time, as well as those that may vary over time. We saw that time-varying covariates may involve interactions with time, but they may also include exposures that change during the course of follow-up. Hence, we have a set of data analytic tools that allow us to study the processes involved in developing a disease, including the identification of intermediate steps that are critical to the ultimate outcome.

Exercises

9.1. For this exercise we return to the data first discussed in exercise 4.3, and then continued in exercise 8.3.

 a. To evaluate the effect of nephrectomy on mortality, fit a proportional hazards model to the data.
  i. Test for significance of the effect of nephrectomy using a Wald test and a likelihood ratio test.
  ii. Estimate the hazard ratio.
  iii. Give confidence limits for the hazard ratio.
 b. Repeat (a), adjusting for the effects of sex, age, and treatment.
 c. Present a graphical display that demonstrates whether the effect of nephrectomy, adjusting for the effects of sex, age, and treatment, behave in the way described by a proportional hazards model.
 d. Test whether the effect of nephrectomy varies over time in the study, adjusting for sex, age, and treatment.

References

1. Cox DR. Regression models and life-tables (with discussion). *Journal of the Royal Statistical Society, Series B* 1972;34:187–220.
2. Holford TR. Life tables with concomitant information. *Biometrics* 1976;32: 587–597.

3. Holford TR. The analysis of rates and survivorship using log-linear models. *Biometrics* 1980;36:299–305.
4. Laird N, Olivier D. Covariance analysis of censored survival data using log-linear analysis techniques. *Journal of the American Statistical Association* 1981;76: 231–240.
5. Boyle CM. *Some Aspects on Utilization of Connecticut Tumor Registry Data in the Estimation of Survival from Lung Cancer: Epidemiology and Public Health.* New Haven, CT: Yale University, 1976.
6. Veterans Administration Coronary Artery Bypass Surgery Study Group. Eleven-year survival in the Veterans Administration randomized trial of coronary artery bypass surgery for stable angina. *New England Journal of Medicine* 1984;311: 1333–1339.
7. Kalbfleisch JD, Prentice RL. *The Statistical Analysis of Failure Time Data.* New York: Wiley, 1980.
8. Vermunt JK. *Log-Linear Models for Event Histories.* Thousand Oaks, CA: Sage, 1997.
9. Crowley J, Hu M. Covariance analysis of heart transplant survival data. *Journal of the American Statistical Association* 1977;72:27–36.

IV

STUDY DESIGN AND NEW DIRECTIONS

10

Analysis of Matched Studies

The methods of analysis that we have discussed thus far have sought to control for differences in the distribution of covariates among subjects in the risk groups of interest by either stratifying or including those variables in a regression model. An alternative strategy would be to put more effort into designing a study in which the risk groups were fully comparable in the first place, so that the analysis would be completely straightforward and only the factor that defined the risk groups of interest would vary. In practice, it is not possible to control for everything so during the analysis phase of a study inevitably we will wish to control certain factors that were not balanced when the study was designed. In addition, the effect of a factor of interest may vary with the level of a factor controlled by design, which we will wish to describe in our analysis. In this chapter we discuss methods of analysis that incorporate the matching aspect of the study design into the analysis.

In some instances the matches arise naturally, such as studies that enroll siblings or twins, in which one is controlling not only factors like socioeconomic status that might be measurable but also a host of potential factors that cannot easily be determined. In the case of monozygotic twins, this would include the fact that they were raised in essentially the same environment and that they also share an identical set of genes, thus allowing us to introduce even more control than is possible with an unmatched design. In other instances, easily determined variables that are strong potential confounders are employed in the matched design to achieve balance among the groups of particular interest in the study.

Matching offers an especially useful design strategy in nested case-control studies in which banks of tissue or serum samples have been preserved in a population that is followed prospectively (1, 2). For example, one might recruit subjects from a large health plan, in which part of the initial enrollment might include a brief questionnaire that obtained demographic information along with some fundamental baseline data. In addition, blood samples might be obtained and stored for later analysis. When a sufficient number of cases of a particular disease of interest has occurred, one or more controls can be selected for each case from among the individuals who were disease free at the time the case was diagnosed. The baseline questionnaire provides a convenient way of balancing potential confounders by matching them to the levels observed for the case. If the aim of the project is to learn about the association between the level of a biomarker at baseline and disease risk, the necessary lab analyses can be conducted using the stored samples. This approach enables investigators to conserve research funds by only conducting expensive laboratory analyses of biomarkers on a subset of subjects, and this design is highly efficient for studying the associations of interest. In addition, such a strategy can avoid the difficulty of having the study become dated, as scientific theories about specific biomarkers that may have been in vogue when the study was launched can later be replaced by others that appear to be more promising. This might include the use of assays for compounds or genetic polymorphisms that were developed well after the inception of the study.

Designing Matched Studies

The rationale for matching resembles that of blocking in statistical design, in that each stratum formed by the matching strategy is essentially the same with respect to the factors being controlled. However, there are many variations on this underlying theme, and we now explore some of these approaches.

Matched pairs

Study designs that employ matched pairs or one-to-one matching are often approached by methods that assume a certain uniqueness of each member of the pair. Twin studies, in which one twin is compared to the other, offers one of the best examples of such a study, in that each twin pair is indeed unique with respect to their genes and their shared environment. In other instances, readily determined factors like age, gender, and ethnicity are used to ensure that each member of a particular stratum is identical in these respects. A much weaker matching strategy would be one in which the "matched pair" is selected through a method that is convenient to implement. For example, one might select a control for each individual in a study by recruiting a neighbor in the first house on the right. This could offer some control for things like the similar socioeconomic status of a neighborhood, but residual differences would remain. In these cases the benefits of matching over a design that controlled for factors at the end in a regression analysis are likely to be small (3, 4).

Many-to-one matching

Instead of selecting just a single control subject for the analysis, additional controls are sometimes used to increase the power of a study. Such a strategy is especially useful when one is dealing with a small group of cases that cannot be readily increased. Herbst et al. (5) studied the occurrence of adenocarcinoma of the vagina in young women to estimate the risk associated with exposures experienced by their mothers during pregnancy. As the disease is extremely rare in women in their late teens and early twenties, the investigators decided to select four controls for each case enrolled in the study, thus increasing the information provided by each case. Some of the results from this study are presented in Table 10–1.

This strategy of selecting multiple controls for each case can improve the power of a study when there are a limited number of cases. However, there are diminishing returns on such an approach: a study's precision will ultimately be limited by the size of the case group, so the precision of a study can only be improved to a point by obtaining further information on the controls. Breslow et al. (2) suggest that there is little benefit to using more than six controls for each case in a matched case-control study.

Table 10–1. Summary of the results from a case-control study of DES with 4-to-1 matching (5)

| | Case | | Controls | | | | | | | |
| | | | 1 | | 2 | | 3 | | 4 | |
Match	Est.	Loss.	Est.	Loss.	Est.	Loss.	Est.	Loss.	Est.	Loss.
1	Y	Y	N	Y	N	N	N	N	N	N
2	Y	Y	N	Y	N	N	N	N	N	N
3	Y	N	N	Y	N	N	N	N	N	N
4	Y	Y	N	N	N	N	N	N	N	N
5	N	N	N	Y	N	N	N	N	N	N
6	Y	Y	N	N	N	N	N	N	N	N
7	Y	Y	N	Y	N	N	N	N	N	N
8	Y	Y	N	N	N	N	N	N	N	N

Est. = Used DES

Loss. = History of pregnancy loss

Y = Yes

N = No

While a study design might call for M-to-one matching, it is sometimes impossible to obtain the appropriate number of controls in each instance, or it may be found later that some controls are ineligible for the study. In these situations the number in the matched sets varies from stratum to stratum, so that we might better refer to this case as M_i-to-one matching.

Frequency matching

In frequency matching, an investigator attempts to balance the frequency distribution for one or more factors among the various comparison groups. One way of accomplishing this is by forming broad categories based on potential confounding variables and then selecting the same number of individuals from the comparison groups for each category. Under this scenario, the categories are essentially strata, or blocks. For a two-group comparison, we might refer to these as M_i-to-N_i matching. In this chapter, we discuss conditional methods of analysis, and fundamental questions that need to be asked when deciding whether this is necessary are (1) Would the number of possible strata remain fixed if we were to conduct a larger study? and (2) How large are the strata? If we are matching on age by balancing the number of cases and controls within 10-year intervals, then by doubling the size of the study, the number of strata remains the same, which might suggest that the conditional analysis is unnecessary. In this case, we can adjust for our selected design by including a dummy variable for the age strata. A fundamentally different situation would arise from a study that selected siblings for study; by doubling the number of subjects we would necessary be selecting twice as many families, thus generating twice as many levels of the family factor. In this situation, we can make use of the conditional methods discussed later in this chapter.

Caliper matching

Each of the matching strategies we have discussed thus far can be most directly applied to variables that are categorical because they assume that each member of the set is identical with respect to the factor. For continuous variables, it becomes almost impossible to find matches that are identical, so one option is to use an approach we have already suggested—that is, divide a continuous variable into categories. When a case is identified for a match case-control design, we would select a control from among those falling into the same category identified by specified interval cutpoints. For example, one approach to age-matching would be to divide ages into 10-year intervals: 20–29, 30–39, and so on. If a 31-year-old case is recruited, then the corresponding control(s) would be 30–39 years of age.

Caliper matching offers an alternative strategy for finding controls with nearly the same age by setting an interval about the case's age, which is found by adding and subtracting the amount specified by the caliper setting. In the age example, we might specify a 5-year caliper, so that the appropriate controls for a 31-year-old case would be aged 26–36. Hence, there is never more than 5 years difference between the ages of cases and controls, even though there is a 10-year interval formed by the caliper. By contrast, with interval matching, the difference between two subjects in a matched set can be as large as the length of the interval. Bradley (6) discusses the efficiency for various strategies of selecting matched subjects for study.

Strategies for analysis

A rationale for establishing a method of analysis for case-control studies is to regard the matched sets themselves as units of observation. Each set consists of individuals with an observed mixture of covariates that are putatively associated with the risk of disease. The method we shall rely on is conditional: it is based on the probability of the observed assignment of covariates to cases and controls, given the mix of covariates in the set. These probabilities give the contribution of each set to the conditional likelihood, and it offers an important way of incorporating the matched design into the analysis. To illustrate, let us consider the relatively simple case in which each matched set has just one case. We can think of this as essentially a pooled set of individuals, and X_0 are the regressor variables observed in the case. In addition, there are J controls in the pool, and these have regressor variables $X_1, X_2, \ldots X_J$. The conditional likelihood contribution is the probability that X_0 occurs for the case given that we have a set with a given mix of covariates, $X_0, X_1, X_2, \ldots, X_J$. For the types of models we are considering, this strategy results in a likelihood that no longer depends on set-specific parameters but on the covariates only, thus achieving our goal of providing a method of analysis that appropriately allows for our study design.

While it would be possible to prepare software to directly use the overall conditional likelihood, it turns out that for many of the common matched designs, we can express the contribution of each matched set within the framework of one of the methods of analysis we have already considered. To understand the details that justify the methods of setting up the analysis, we need to work through the theoretical discussion provided in Appendix 8. However, in the following sections we shall describe and illustrate rules for setting up a conditional analysis using software for fitting either standard linear logistic or proportional hazards models. At times the rules may seem arbitrary or inconsistent with other rules of thumb for regression, but we must keep in mind that these have been carefully developed to achieve equivalence with the contributions shown by the theoretical development.

Conditional inference is not the only way of incorporating the matched design in the analysis. Baysean methods, for example, offer an alternative that in some circumstances can be very effective. However, the conditional inference approach has proved to be quite successful in appropriately allowing for this study design in the analysis, by providing estimates of risk that are consistent and significance tests that are valid. In addition, widely available software can be adopted to perform the calculations, making it an extremely practical approach as well, which is the reason it will be the primary focus of our discussion.

Case-Control Studies with Matched Pairs

In this section, we first consider an approach that is reminiscent of the techniques we discussed in Part II that did not require formal model fitting. We shall then discuss two approaches for using standard logistic regression software to perform conditional inference on more than one factor at a time. As we will see, matched-pair designs also give rise to goodness-of-fit statistics that are do not arise in a study with all observations independent of each other, and the second method of analysis provides a way to calculate these statistics.

McNemar's test and its extensions

A typical layout for data from a matched-pair case-control study with two levels of exposure is shown in Table 10–2. The frequencies show the number of pairs exhibiting the four possible combinations of exposure status:

Table 10–2. Layout of results from a typical case-control study with a binary exposure variable

	Case		
Control	Not exposed $(X_0 = 0)$	Exposed $(X_0 = 1)$	Total
Not exposed $(X_1 = 0)$	a $(X_0 - X_1 = 0)$	b $(X_0 - X_1 = 1)$	$a + b$
Exposed $(X_1 = 1)$	c $(X_0 - X_1 = -1)$	d $(X_0 - X_1 = 0)$	$c + d$
Total	$a + c$	$b + d$	N

a, b, c, d = Frequencies

the first row and column gives the number of pairs in which neither the case nor the control was exposed. Cells along the diagonal in this table (frequencies a and d) represent the concordant pairs in which the exposure status is identical for cases and control. Marginal totals provide the frequencies in a corresponding summary of the number of cases and controls falling into each exposure category, which gives rise to a tabular summary that we are already familiar with from the analysis of independent observations. Notice that the difference in the proportion exposed for cases and controls is

$$\frac{c+d}{N} - \frac{b+d}{N} = \frac{c-b}{N}$$

which does not involve the concordant frequency, d. Hence, it should not be surprising that these concordant pairs do not contribute information about the difference in the proportion exposed.

Matched pairs can effectively be regarded as strata in which there is just one case and one control, but the response to a query about exposure is random. The four possible 2×2 tables that can summarize the results from such a stratified design are shown in Table 10–3. If we apply the Mantel–Haenszel statistic (7) to these data, we have the total observed cases who are exposed:

$$O = 0 \cdot a + 1 \cdot b + 0 \cdot c + 1 \cdot d = b + d$$

Table 10–3. Possible 2×2 tables from the strata of a match case-control study

Disease	Exposure No	Yes	Total	Frequency	Expected	Variance	R	S
No	1	0	1					
Yes	1	0	1	a	0.0	0.00	0	0
Total	2	0	2					
No	1	0	1					
Yes	0	1	1	b	0.5	0.25	.5	0
Total	1	1	2					
No	0	1	1					
Yes	1	0	1	c	0.5	0.25	0	0.5
Total	1	1	2					
No	0	1	1					
Yes	0	1	1	d	1.0	0.00	0	0
Total	0	2	2					

with the corresponding total expected,

$$E = 0.0{\cdot}a + 0.5{\cdot}b + 0.5{\cdot}c + 1{\cdot}d = 0.5(b + c) + d$$

The sum of the variance contributions over the entire dataset is

$$Var = 0.00{\cdot}a + 0.25{\cdot}b + 0.25{\cdot}c + 0.00{\cdot}d = 0.25(b + c)$$

Hence, the resulting score statistic reduces to

$$S^2 = \frac{(O - E)^2}{Var} = \frac{(b - c)^2}{(b + c)} \tag{10.1}$$

which is compared to a chi-square distribution with 1 df. This is identical to the test proposed by McNemar (8) for comparing the difference in the proportion exposed for such as matched design.

The Mantel–Haenszel estimators for the overall odds ratio is found by taking the ratio of the sums for the contributions to R and S from equation 3.31,

$$\tilde{\Omega} = \frac{0.5{\cdot}b}{0.5{\cdot}c} = \frac{b}{c} \tag{10.2}$$

and the variance of its logarithm is

$$Var(\log \tilde{\Omega}) = \frac{1}{b} + \frac{1}{c} \tag{10.3}$$

Example 10–1 Kelsey and Hardy (9) report the results of a matched case-control study of factors that are associated with low back pain or acute herniated lumbar discs. One of the factors considered in their analysis was whether a subject lived in the suburbs, and the results are shown in Table 10–4. A score test for such an association is provided by applying equation 10.1:

$$S^2 = \frac{(57 - 37)^2}{(57 + 37)} = 4.255$$

which is compared to a chi-square distribution with 1 df ($p = .039$), suggesting that there is indeed an association. An estimate of the relative risk is provided by applying equation 10.2:

$$\tilde{\Omega} = \frac{57}{37} = 1.541$$

Table 10–4. Results from a case-control study of acute herniated lumbar discs (9); in this analysis the factor of interest is whether the subject was a suburban resident

	Case suburban resident		
Control suburban resident	No	Yes	Total
No	53	57	110
Yes	37	70	107
Total	90	127	217

with a standard error of its logarithm, equation (10.3) given by

$$SE(\log \tilde{\Omega}) = \sqrt{\frac{1}{37} + \frac{1}{57}} = 0.211$$

We can now construct a 95% confidence interval for the relative risk,

$$1.541 \cdot \exp\{\pm(1.96)\,(0.211)\} = (1.019, 2.330)$$

suggesting a slightly increased risk of low back pain associated with suburban residence.

McNemar (8) proposed the test in equation 10.1 as a way of testing the null hypothesis of equality of two correlated proportions. If we have an exposure with three or more levels, we can set up a table similar to Table 10–5, in which we enumerate the frequency of pairs with each possible combination of exposure levels. Equality of the distribution of exposures between cases and controls involves a comparison of the distribution of the row totals with the column totals. The null hypothesis of an equal distribution of these totals is called the hypothesis of *marginal homogeneity*. The

Table 10–5. Tabular summary of the results from a matched-pairs case-control study with three levels of exposure

	Case $(X_{01}, X_{02})^*$			
	Exposure 1	Exposure 2	Exposure 3	
Control (X_{11}, X_{12})	(0,0)	(1,0)	(0,1)	Total
Exposure 1	a	b	c	$a+b+c$
(0,0)	(0,0)	(1,0)	(0,1)	
Exposure 2	d	e	f	$d+e+f$
(1,0)	(−1,0)	(0,0)	(−1,1)	
Exposure 3	g	h	i	$g+h+i$
(0,1)	(0,−1)	(1,−1)	(0,0)	
Total	$a+d+g$	$b+e+h$	$c+f+i$	N

* Numbers in parentheses are the differences between the covariates for the case and the control.

Stuart–Maxwell statistic (10–13) provides a test of this hypothesis, but a preferable test is described next, because it incorporates all of the features implied by the models we are considering.

Logistic regression method I

Two variations to the approach for setting up data for analysis will allow us to use standard logistic regression software for conducting a conditional logistic analysis. The first follows from the recognition that the contribution of each matched pair to the conditional likelihood had the same mathematical form as an observation for logistic regression, if the data are set up as follows:

1. The intercept is dropped from the model.
2. The covariates for each pair are the differences between values for the case and the control.
3. The response is 1 for each pair.

These rules are somewhat counterintuitive; for example, dropping the intercept from a model is generally bad advice. However, if one cares to follow the theoretical details in Appendix 8, it becomes clear that the method works; in fact, the derivation did indeed start with an intercept, so in effect we have allowed for such a term in the analysis. We are essentially using logistic regression software for something other than its original purpose, so we must follow the rules exactly as stated; otherwise, the results will be incorrect.

The parameters, standard errors, and the resulting covariance matrix can be used in the same way as those from a linear logistic model to obtain estimates of relative risk adjusted for the study design, as well as other factors in the model. In addition, we can use the covariance matrix to construct Wald tests of linear hypotheses that have been defined by a particular set of contrasts. Finally, by adding variables to a model and calculating the change in scaled deviance, we have a likelihood ratio test of the added parameters in the presence of other factors already in the model.

Example 10–1 (continued)   Continuing our analysis of the data on acute herniated lumbar discs, in which we had previously found a significant association with suburban residence, it is important to also note from the overall summary in Table 10–6 that another factor strongly associated with herniated discs is driving a car. The fact that suburban residents must, out of necessity, drive cars presents the possibility of confounding between these two factors. Therefore, we are interested in also considering an analysis in which we evaluate the effect of suburban residence adjusted for driving. This also raises the possibility for an interaction between these two factors, as the effect of driving may be modified by suburban residence, or vice versa.

Table 10–6. The data tabulated below are frequencies and covariates (differences in the body of the table) from a case-control study of acute herniated lumbar discs (9). In this analysis the two factors of interest are whether the subject drove a car and suburban residence.

Control drove a car	Control suburban residence	Case drove a car			
		No		Yes	
		Case suburban resident			
		No (0,0,0)*	Yes (1,0,0)	No (0,1,0)	Yes (1,1,1)
No	No (0, 0, 0)*	9 (0, 0, 0)†	2 (1, 0, 0)	14 (0, 1, 0)	22 (1, 1, 1)
No	Yes (1,0,0)	0 (−1, 0, 0)	2 (0, 0, 0)	1 (−1, 1, 0)	4 (0, 1, 1)
Yes	No (0,1,0)	10 (0, −1, 0)	1 (1, −1, 0)	20 (0, 0, 0)	32 (1, 0, 1)
Yes	Yes (1, 1, 1)	7 (−1, −1, −1)	1 (0, −1, −1)	29 (−1, 0, −1)	63 (0, 0, 0)

* Numbers in parentheses for row and column tables are the exposure covariates: X_1 = suburban residence; X_2 = driver; and $X_3 = X_1 X_2$.

† Numbers in parentheses for body of table are covariates for inclusion in logistic regression, obtained by taking the difference between case and control.

To conduct our analysis, we introduce 0–1 dummy variables for nonsuburban and suburban residents, respectively, and similarly for nondrivers and drivers. The next step is to create the variables for the pair by taking the difference between the variables for the case and the control. In addition, we will consider an interaction between these two variables, remembering that to create such a variable for the pair, we must first calculate the product of the dummy variables for suburb and driving for cases and controls, and then construct the pair variable by taking the difference between these products. It is important to note that this is not the same as taking the product of the main effect variables we have already created for the pair. Figure 10–1 shows a SAS program for setting up the data for a conditional analysis using PROC GENMOD to fit a linear logistic model. Notice that we can no

```
data;  infile 'filename';
input drv1 sub1 drv2 sub2;
sub = sub1-sub2;                      *Create suburb difference
drv = drv1-drv2;                      *Create driver difference;
int = (sub1*drv1)-(sub2*drv2);        *Create interaction difference;
one = 1;                              *Response and number of subjects;
*;
* Model with interaction and main effects;
*;
proc genmod;
        model one/one = drv sub int / dist=binomial noint;  run;
*;
* Model with main effects only;
*;
proc genmod;
        model one/one = drv sub / dist=binomial noint type3;  run;
```

Figure 10–1 SAS procedure for the analysis of the acute herniated lumbar disc data using Method I logistic regression.

longer use the "CLASSES" statement to automatically establish a set of dummy variables for our categories, but must construct them ourselves.

The output from running this program is shown in Figure 10–2. As is the case when logistic regression is used on single (as opposed to tabulated) observations, the scaled deviance by itself has little meaning. However, we can use the change in scaled deviance to conduct a likelihood ratio test of parameters dropped from the model. For example, comparing the models with and without the interaction term results in a likelihood ratio test of the null hypothesis of no interaction, $\Delta G^2 = 291.2803 - 291.2049 = 0.0754$, $\Delta df = 1$, which is clearly not statistically significant. From the second model we have an estimate of the relative risk for suburban residence adjusting for driving, $\exp(0.2555) = 1.291$, with 95% confidence interval, $1.291 \cdot \exp\{\pm1.96 \times 0.2258\} = (0.829, 2.010)$. The "type 3 analysis" provides tests of each main effect in the presence of the others, thus indicating that "DRV" is statistically significant in the presence of "SUB," while "SUB" is not in the pres-

```
Model with interaction--

              Criteria For Assessing Goodness Of Fit

         Criterion          DF       Value      Value/DF
         Scaled Deviance     214     291.2049     1.3608
         Pearson Chi-Square   214     216.8391     1.0133
         Log Likelihood       .      -145.6024      .

                Analysis Of Parameter Estimates

     Parameter   DF   Estimate   Std Err   ChiSquare  Pr>Chi
     INTERCEPT    0    0.0000     0.0000       .          .
     DRV          1    0.6913     0.3189     4.6984    0.0302
     SUB          1    0.4438     0.7203     0.3797    0.5378
     INT          1   -0.2058     0.7476     0.0758    0.7831
     SCALE        0    1.0000     0.0000       .          .
NOTE:  The scale parameter was held fixed.

Model with main effects only--

              Criteria For Assessing Goodness Of Fit

         Criterion          DF       Value      Value/DF
         Scaled Deviance     215     291.2803     1.3548
         Pearson Chi-Square   215     216.7748     1.0083
         Log Likelihood       .      -145.6402      .

                Analysis Of Parameter Estimates

     Parameter   DF   Estimate   Std Err   ChiSquare  Pr>Chi
     INTERCEPT    0    0.0000     0.0000       .          .
     DRV          1    0.6579     0.2940     5.0079    0.0252
     SUB          1    0.2555     0.2258     1.2796    0.2580
     SCALE        0    1.0000     0.0000       .          .
NOTE:  The scale parameter was held fixed.

              LR Statistics For Type 3 Analysis

          Source     DF   ChiSquare  Pr>Chi
          DRV         1     5.2575    0.0219
          SUB         1     1.2877    0.2565
```

Figure 10–2 Output resulting from fitting a model to the herniated lumbar disc data using the SAS procedure in Figure 10–1.

ence of "DRV." Therefore, it appears that by adjusting for driving, we have accounted for all of the effect of suburban residence.

Some common mistakes in setting up a conditional analysis for matched-pairs using standard logistic regression software are as follow:

1. Including an intercept. This always results in divergence because all of the responses have been set to 1, thus resulting in an intercept estimate that is heading toward infinity in magnitude, and the other parameters would likewise diverge.
2. Including the product of differences as interactions in the model, instead of the correct approach, which was illustrated in the example.
3. Including the square and higher powers when interested in polynomial models, instead of the correct approach, which is to take the power of the covariate for the case and for the control and then to include the difference between these powers as covariates in the model.

Logistic regression method II

In the preceding section on McNemar's test and its extensions, we discussed an analysis of matched pairs with two levels of the covariate of interest. We now consider an analysis for similar tabular summaries of matched pairs when there are more than two levels of exposure. The fact that the number of possible levels for cases and controls is identical results in an equal number of rows and columns—a square table. The analysis of such tables provides new insights that cannot be gleaned from Method I, and in this section we develop these further.

In Table 10–5 we see a typical display of the results of a study in which there are three levels of exposure. If we ignore the results for exposure 3, the tabular summary effectively reduces to a 2×2 table, like that shown in Table 10–2, and the resulting estimate of relative risk for exposure 2 compared to exposure 1 is

$$RR(2,1) = \frac{b}{d}$$

the ratio of the frequencies for cells that are symmetric about the diagonal. Similarly,

$$RR(3,1) = \frac{c}{g} \quad \text{and} \quad RR(3,2) = \frac{f}{h}$$

The null hypothesis, H_0: $RR(2,1) = RR(3,1) = RR(3,2) = 1$, is realized when the frequencies for cells that are symmetric about the diagonal are equal, and it is referred to as the test for *complete symmetry*.

However, another symmetry arises from the relationship among relative risks when there are more than two exposure groups. From the definition of the relative risk, we have

$$RR(3,2) = \frac{\lambda(\mathbf{X}_3,t)}{\lambda(\mathbf{X}_2,t)}$$

Dividing both the numerator and the denominator by $\lambda(\mathbf{X}_1,t)$ yields

$$RR(3,2) = \frac{\lambda(\mathbf{X}_3,t)/\lambda(\mathbf{X}_1,t)}{\lambda(\mathbf{X}_2,t)/\lambda(\mathbf{X}_1,t)} = \frac{RR(3,1)}{RR(2,1)}$$

thus showing a theoretical consistency relationship among the three relative risks (14). This consistency relationship results in a relationship among the expected cell frequencies that is sometimes call *quasi symmetry* (15), and its effect is to introduce an additional constraint onto the parameters being estimated. Such a model is equivalent to the Bradley–Terry model for square tables (16). Therefore, instead of the three relative risks being tested under the hypotheses of complete symmetry, there are only $2 = (3 - 1)$ unique relative risks once we impose the condition of quasi symmetry.

Another way to conceptualize what has happened here is to recall what we would have had if the study had not been matched. In an unmatched study, the three levels of risk would be identified by just two dummy variables—that is, only 2 df for the three levels of exposure—and as we have already seen, relative risks for all possible comparisons among these three categories can be derived explicitly from the regression parameters associated with those two variables.

To set up a regression model that will take advantage of the features of a square table, we must first take note of a pattern that arises in the relevant covariates used in the analysis of a matched-pairs design. In Table 10–5, we can see that the differences between the case and the control covariates are identical in cells that are symmetric about the diagonal cells, except for the fact that they have the opposite sign. Also, for cells on the diagonal, the differences are always zero, so they do not contribute to the conditional analysis because they do not depend on the model parameters.

Let us represent the cell frequencies above the diagonal by n_{ij} ($i = 1$, ..., I and $j = i + 1$, ..., $\mathcal{J} = I$), where the ith row represents the exposure level for the case and the jth column for the control. The case-control differences in the covariates are $(\mathbf{X}_i - \mathbf{X}_j)$, and the contribution to the conditional likelihood is

$$\Pr\{\text{above} \mid i,j\} = \frac{\exp\{(\mathbf{X}_i - \mathbf{X}_j\}}{1 + \exp\{(\mathbf{X}_i - \mathbf{X}_j\}}$$

The corresponding cell that is symmetric about the diagonal can be represented in this notation as the cell in which the row and column indices are reversed, n_{ji}, with covariate differences, $(\mathbf{X_j} - \mathbf{X_i})$

$$\Pr\{\text{below} \mid i,j\} = \frac{\exp\{(\mathbf{X_j} - \mathbf{X_i}\}}{1 + \exp\{(\mathbf{X_j} - \mathbf{X_i}\}}$$

$$= \frac{1}{1 + \exp\{(\mathbf{X_i} - \mathbf{X_j}\}}$$

$$= 1 - \Pr\{\text{above} \mid ij\}$$

As we can see, the symmetric cells about the diagonal can be regarded as a binary outcome, so by linking them, and arbitrarily calling the cell above a "success" and the cell below a "failure," gives rise to a second approach to setting up a standard logistic regression program for a conditional logistic analysis.

Steps for Method II for fitting a conditional logistic model to tabulated data using a standard logistic regression program are as follows:

1. Pairs of cells that are symmetric about the diagonal are established, in which the cell above the diagonal is arbitrarily identified as a success, $Y_{ij} = 1$.
2. The response is the proportion of pairs in the cell above the diagonal, $n_{ij}/(n_{ij} + n_{ji})$.
3. The covariates for each pair are the differences between values for the case and the control variable for the above diagonal cell.
4. The intercept is dropped from the model.

The scaled deviance or goodness-of-fit statistic for this model indicates the adequacy of the null hypothesis that the consistency relationship applies to these data, or a test for quasi symmetry. In addition, the scaled deviance for a model that excludes all of these covariates results in a test of complete symmetry.

Example 10–1 (continued) We now return once again to the analysis of the data on acute herniated lumbar discs. From Table 10–6, we can verify the fact that the case-control differences in the covariates are indeed symmetric about the diagonal, except for the change in sign. Figure 10–3 gives a SAS program for conducting this analysis, and we shall pick out the six cells above the diagonal, along with their covariates for inclusion in the analysis. The frequency of the complementary outcome will be determined for each cell by taking the value tabulated in the cell that is symmetric about the diagonal. Hence, we see the first observation in the data is derived from the (1,2) cell, with frequency 2 and covariate differences (1,0,0). The frequency of the complementary outcome is obtained from the (2,1) cell, or 0. The rest of the observations are obtained in a similar manner.

```
data;  input sub drv int abv bel;      *Read data;
num = abv+bel;                         *Create variable with total pairs in off-diagonal cells;
cards;
  1  0  0  2  0
  0  1  0 14 10
  1  1  1 22  7
 -1  1  0  1  1
  0  1  1  4  1
  1  0  1 32 29
*;
* Model with interaction and main effects;
*;
proc genmod;  model abv/num = sub drv int / dist=b noint;  run;
*;
* Model with main effects only;
*;
proc genmod;  model abv/num = sub drv / dist=b noint type3;  run;
*;
* Null model with no parameters;
*;
proc genmod;  model abv/num =  /dist=b noint;  run;
```

Figure 10–3 SAS procedure for the analysis of the acute herniated lumbar disc using Method II logistic regression.

The output from this approach to conducting the analysis is shown in Figure 10–4. The scaled deviance is $\Delta G^2 = 4.0444$, $\Delta df = 3$ ($p = .2567$), thus providing little evidence of a lack of fit or lack of consistency for the odds ratio. In this case the model is saturated with respect to the four levels of exposure, so the goodness-of-fit statistic corresponds to a test of quasi symmetry or conformity to the consistency relationship among the relative risks. If we were to study the fitted cell frequencies for this model, they would indeed satisfy this relationship.

Notice that the other parameters and their standard errors are identical to those obtained using Method I. Hence, there is no difference in the interpretation of the effect of the variables included in the analysis.

The final model fitted in the program given in Figure 10–3 excludes all parameters, which corresponds to complete symmetry, in which subjects are equally likely to be assigned to a cell above or below the diagonal. This test has 6 df because of the 6 pairs of cells involved in the test, and $\Delta G^2 = 13.6654$ ($p = .0336$), which is marginally significant. An alternative test of any effect among the four exposure categories arises from a comparison of the complete symmetry model with the first model that implied quasi symmetry. This test of complete symmetry in the presence of quasi symmetry yields $\Delta G^2 = 13.6654 - 4.0444 = 9.6210$, $\Delta df = 3$ ($p = .0221$), which strongly suggests that DRV and/or SUB are associated with risk of an acute herniated lumbar disk.

Case-Control Studies with More Than One Control per Case

For more complicated matched case-control studies in which more than one control is used in each matched set, it is possible to employ a particular form for the log linear model (17). This is actually an extension to the

```
Model with interaction--
                      Criteria For Assessing Goodness Of Fit

                    Criterion           DF       Value    Value/DF
                    Scaled Deviance      3      4.0444      1.3481
                    Pearson Chi-Square   3      3.2955      1.0985
                    Log Likelihood       .    -80.4466          .

                      Analysis Of Parameter Estimates

             Parameter   DF   Estimate   Std Err   ChiSquare  Pr>Chi
             INTERCEPT    0     0.0000    0.0000          .         .
             SUB          1     0.4439    0.7203     0.3797    0.5378
             DRV          1     0.6913    0.3189     4.6984    0.0302
             INT          1    -0.2058    0.7476     0.0758    0.7831
             SCALE        0     1.0000    0.0000          .         .
NOTE:  The scale parameter was held fixed.


Model with main effects only--
                      Criteria For Assessing Goodness Of Fit

                    Criterion           DF       Value    Value/DF
                    Scaled Deviance      4      4.1198      1.0300
                    Pearson Chi-Square   4      3.3450      0.8363
                    Log Likelihood       .    -80.4843          .

                      Analysis Of Parameter Estimates

             Parameter   DF   Estimate   Std Err   ChiSquare  Pr>Chi
             INTERCEPT    0     0.0000    0.0000          .         .
             SUB          1     0.2555    0.2258     1.2796    0.2580
             DRV          1     0.6579    0.2940     5.0079    0.0252
             SCALE        0     1.0000    0.0000          .         .
NOTE:  The scale parameter was held fixed.

                      LR Statistics For Type 3 Analysis

                     Source    DF   ChiSquare  Pr>Chi
                     SUB        1     1.2877    0.2565
                     DRV        1     5.2575    0.0219


Model with no parametere--
                      Criteria For Assessing Goodness Of Fit

                    Criterion           DF       Value    Value/DF
                    Scaled Deviance      6     13.6654      2.2776
                    Pearson Chi-Square   6     12.3728      2.0621
                    Log Likelihood       .    -85.2571          .
```

Figure 10–4 Output resulting from fitting a model to the herniated lumbar disc data using the SAS procedure in Figure 10–3.

linear logistic model, so in a theoretical sense it flows naturally from the ideas in the previous section. However, there is also an equivalence with a particular way of setting up the analysis of a stratified proportional hazards model that provides yet another convenient way of using existing software for this particular study design (18).

We may regard each matched set as essentially a stratum, and we should treat it as such in our analysis. What distinguishes our case-control study from a typical cohort study is that we have only observed the stratum at a snapshot in time. Only one member of the set has developed the disease, and the eventual fate of the controls is unknown. Hence, the contribution of the matched set is that of an observation over a small interval of time in which disease has occurred in the case member of the set, but for the controls the event may occur at an unobserved time in the future. To capture this, we must order the data so that the case event is recognized as having occurred first and that the control observations are subsequently censored.

To summarize, the information that needs to be conveyed to software used to fit a stratified proportional hazards model include (1) the variable that identifies the stratum, (2) the disease status variable, and (3) the time variable, because order of occurrence and not the actual time is all that matters for inference in a proportional hazards model, this variable can be arbitrarily defined so long as the value for the controls is greater than the value for the case.

Example 10–2 We return to Table 10–1, which gives data from a study of the association between adenocarcinoma of the vagina and the use of stilbesterol therapy during mothers' pregnancies (5). At the time it was used, stilbesterol was assumed to be an effective treatment for protection against spontaneous abortion, although subsequent research showed that it was actually an ineffective drug for this purpose. As we have already noted, four controls were selected from among the mothers in the same service (ward or private) who had given birth within 5 days of the corresponding case.

The main factor of interest, stilbesterol use during pregnancy, showed that the mothers of all but one of the cases had been so treated, while none of the controls had been treated. Hence, the point estimate of the relative risk is undetermined or infinite. However, a score test of the null hypothesis of no association is feasible. The second model in the SAS program shown in Figure 10–5 provides the appropriate setup for this test, and the output in Figure 10–6 reveals the results, $S^2 = 28.00$ (df = 1, $p < .001$). Because of the small number of pairs, eight, we should be concerned that the number of observations may not be sufficiently large for the large sample approximation for the score test to hold. One matched set is concordant, so it does not contribute to the inference. Of the remaining, one member is positive in each instance. The probability that the one positive member is the case is $\exp\{\beta\}/(4 + \exp\{\beta\})$, which becomes 1/5 under the null hypothesis, H_0: $\beta = 0$. The probability that all seven discordant sets exhibit this result is $(1/5)^7 = 1.2 \times 10^{-5}$, a result that is highly significant and thus concurs with the score test.

As already noted, an indication for prescribing stilbesterol in pregnancy is a history of pregnancy loss, so we might wonder whether the unadjusted result partially reflects an artifact due to an increased risk of vaginal cancer in women born to mothers with such a pregnancy history. Figure 10–5 shows a SAS procedure that will evaluate the effect of pregnancy loss, and the results are displayed in Figure 10–6. The score test yields $S^2 = 9.500$ (df = 1, $p = .0021$), and the estimate of the odds ratio is $\exp\{2.174333\} = 8.80$, a strong association, albeit less than the esti-

```
data; input id case pr_loss estrogen;
time = 2-case;
loss_adj = 2.174333*pr_loss;
cards;
1 1 1 1
1 0 1 0
1 0 0 0
1 0 0 0
1 0 0 0
2 1 1 1

{rest of dataa}

run;

title 'Loss of previous pregnancy';
proc phreg;
model time*case(0) = pr_loss / ties=discrete;
strata id;  run;

title 'Stilbesterol use';
proc phreg;
model time*case(0) = estrogen / ties=discrete nofit;
strata id;  run;

title 'Stilbesterol use adjusted for loss of previous pregnancy';
proc phreg;
model time*case(0) = estrogen / ties=discrete offset=loss_adj nofit;
strata id;  run;
```

Figure 10–5 SAS procedure for fitting a conditional logistic to the data shown in Table 10–1.

mated effect of stilbesterol. One might wonder whether the significance of the stilbesterol effect remains after adjusting for the effect of pregnancy loss history.

To obtain a score test for the effect of stilbesterol adjusted for pregnancy loss, we use the point estimate of the pregnacy loss effect as an offset in our model. This can be accomplished by estimating the effect of pregnancy loss for each subject, calculated by the "loss_adj" variable shown in Figure 10–5. What is now a fixed contribution for each subject is included in the model as an offset, and the corresponding score test for stilbesterol use is calculated. The resulting score test is $S^2 = 8.8252$ (df = 1, $p = .0030$), which is not as far out in the tail as before but is nevertheless a strong result. Hence, we would conclude that the effect of stilbesterol use is not due to a history of pregnancy loss.

We have already noted the fact that a point estimate for stilbesterol use cannot be determined, but as a final step, let us estimate the lower bound using the likelihood ratio criterion. While the parameter estimates for stilbesterol and pregnancy loss are diverging to infinity in absolute magnitude, the value for $-2 \times$ (log likelihood) approaches 2.773. Hence, the lower 95% confidence limit would be the value of the estrogen parameter that results in a minimum value of $-2 \times$ (log likelihood) equal to $2.773 + 3.841 = 6.614$. We can find this by a search that sets a value for the estrogen parameter and finds the resulting contribution for each subject, which is included as an offset. To allow for pregnancy loss, this variable is included in the model, and the resulting output includes the minimum of $-2 \times$ (log likelihood). Figure 10–7 shows a plot of $-2 \times$ (log likelihood) against the value of the estro-

```
                         Loss of previous pregnancy
                              The PHREG Procedure

              Dependent Variable: TIME
              Censoring Variable: CASE
              Ties Handling: DISCRETE

                        Testing Global Null Hypothesis: BETA=0

                          Without        With
              Criterion   Covariates   Covariates   Model Chi-Square

              -2 LOG L      25.751        17.549     8.202 with 1 DF (p=0.0042)
              Score           .             .        9.500 with 1 DF (p=0.0021)
              Wald            .             .        6.845 with 1 DF (p=0.0089)

                      Analysis of Maximum Likelihood Estimates

                        Parameter    Standard      Wald        Pr >        Risk
         Variable   DF   Estimate      Error    Chi-Square  Chi-Square     Ratio

         PR_LOSS     1   2.174333     0.83110    6.84464      0.0089       8.796


                              Stilbesterol use
                             The PHREG Procedure

              Global Score Chi-Square = 28.0000 with 1 DF (p=0.0001)


              Stilbesterol use adjusted for loss of previous pregnancy
                             The PHREG Procedure

              Global Score Chi-Square = 8.8252 with 1 DF (p=0.0030)
```

Figure 10–6 Partial output for the data in Table 10–1, using the SAS procedure in Figure 10–5.

gen parameter. The critical value for 95% confidence criterion is achieved when the estrogen parameters is 2.328. Hence, the 95% likelihood-based confidence interval for the effect of stilbesterol adjusted for pregnancy loss is obtained by taking the antilog, $(10.3, \infty)$.

Cohort Studies with Matched Pairs

We now consider the analysis of a matched-pairs cohort design with a binary outcome. In these designs the matching is employed to achieve balance among the exposure categories for some potential confounding variables, in contrast to matching in a case-control design which seeks to achieve balance among the disease categories. One analytic approach that we might employ would be to directly use the method we have already described for case-control studies, except that it is important to keep in mind the objectives of our analysis. In a case-control study, subjects are recruited based on their disease status, so that exposure and the covariates are in ef-

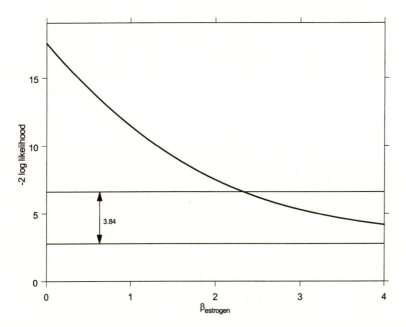

Figure 10–7 Plot of the minimum $-2 \times$ log likelihood against a specified value for the estrogen parameter.

fect random. In a cohort study, however, exposure and covariates are fixed and the disease outcome is random. While the disease–exposure association remains the same in either analysis, there would be a substantive difference in using a case-control analysis with respect to the covariate parameters, in that they would provide estimates of association with exposure and not disease. In general, we are more interested in their association with disease, which can be determined using the methods we shall describe in this section.

Let $i(=1, \ldots, I)$ be an index that can represent the matched pairs, and $j = 1$ for the unexposed, and $j = 2$ for the exposed member of the pair. We shall use a linear logistic model for this discussion:

$$\Pr\{Y_{ij} = 1 \mid i, j, \mathbf{X}_{ij}\} = \frac{\exp\{\alpha_i + E_{ij}\delta + \mathbf{X}_{ij}\boldsymbol{\beta}\}}{1 + \exp\{\alpha_i + E_{ij}\delta + \mathbf{X}_{ij}\boldsymbol{\beta}\}}$$

where α_i is a parameter for the ith matched pair, E_{ij} is a 0–1 dummy variable indicating the exposure status for the jth individual in the ith matched pair, δ is the association between exposure and disease, $\mathbf{X}_{ij}$ is a vector of covariates, and $\boldsymbol{\beta}$ is a vector of corresponding regression parameters that specify the covariate–disease association. The practical problem we would run into if we were to directly use this model arises once again from the many matched pair parameters, α_i, that are estimated with only the two observations in the pair. Once again, a conditional approach can be used to obtain valid estimates for the parameters of primary interest, δ and $\boldsymbol{\beta}$. Details on the more formal aspects of how these are derived will be described in Appendix 8, section "Conditional Likelihood for Cohort Studies," but the result is that the essential unit of analysis is once again the matched pair. The likelihood is based on the probability of the observed pattern of disease outcomes out of all possible patterns that could have occurred, fixing the observed number of diseased individuals occurring in the pair.

A particular matched pair is represented by the index $i = 1, \ldots, I$. One member of a pair is in the control, which is unexposed to the factor of interest, $E_{i1} = 0$, and the other is exposed, $E_{i2} = 1$. In addition, we have a set of covariates, not controlled by matching, that we wish to include in the analysis, $\mathbf{X}_{ij}$ for $j = 1, 2$. The observed disease response is given by Y_{ij} $(= 0, 1)$ for $j = 1, 2$. The first step in our analysis is to exclude the concordant pairs in which the response is the same for both members, $Y_{i+} = 0$ or 2, because they contribute no information on the parameters of interest. The remaining discordant pairs $(Y_{i+} = 1)$, can occur in just two ways, $Y_{i1} = 0$ and $Y_{i2} = 1$, or $Y_{i1} = 1$ and $Y_{i2} = 0$. It is enough to distinguish these two possibilities by only considering Y_{i2}, which will represent our binary outcome for this conditional analysis. As derived in Appendix 8,

$$\Pr\{Y_{i2} = 1 \mid E_{ij}, \mathbf{X}_{ij}, j = 1, 2\} = \frac{\exp\{\delta + (\mathbf{X}_{i2} - \mathbf{X}_{i1})\boldsymbol{\beta}\}}{1 + \exp\{\delta + (\mathbf{X}_{i2} - \mathbf{X}_{i1})\boldsymbol{\beta}\}} \quad (10.4)$$

where δ represents the association between exposure and the disease response. The covariates are included as differences between the levels for the exposed and the control. To make use of conventional software for unconditional fitting of the linear logistic model, we employ the following steps:

1. Drop concordant pairs from the analysis.
2. Set the response to Y_{i2} for the discordant pairs.
3. Adjust for covariates in the discordant pairs by including differences between the levels for the exposed and the unexposed, $(X_{i2} - X_{i1})$.

Notice that the intercept term in this analysis is the effect of exposure.

Example 10–3   Eskenazi et al (19) report the results of a cohort study of the association between exposure to organic solvents during pregnancy and a diagnosis of preeclampsia, and a subset of these data are given by Holford et al. (20). A summary of the data for discordant pairs is shown in Table 10–7, which also provides the gestational age of the fetus, the covariate of interest. Figure 10–8 shows a SAS

Table 10-7. Summary of the results from a matched-pair cohort study of the effect of exposure to organic solvents during pregnancy and risk of preeclampsia (20)

| Unexposed | | Exposed | | |
Response (Y_{i1})	Gestational age* (X_{i1})	Response (Y_{i2})	Gestational age* (X_{i2})	Difference $(X_{i2} - X_{i1})$
0	277	1	307	30
0	302	1	279	−23
0	277	1	286	9
0	313	1	274	−39
1	292	0	293	−19
0	279	1	284	5

* Gestational age is measured in days from first day of last missed period.

program to setup the data and fit the conditional logistic model to these data, and Figure 10-9 gives the corresponding output.

A Wald test for the effect of exposure can be conducted by dividing the parameter estimate by its standard error. For the effect of exposure to solvents adjusted for gestational age, we have $W^2 = (1.9918/1.4726)^2 = 1.83$ ($p = .176$), as shown in the output. The corresponding likelihood ratio test is not given as part of the type 3 analyses, so we need to fit a model without the intercept (not shown) and calculate the difference from the scaled deviance with the model that includes the intercept, which is the exposure effect. For these data we have $\Delta G^2 = 8.3175 -$

```
data analysis (keep=one disease ga_diff);   input pair disease exposed ga;
retain ga0;
one = 1;
*                                              ;
* CREATE PAIR AS UNIT OF OBSERVATION AND COVARIATE DIFFERENCE;
*                                              ;
if (exposed=1) then do;
ga_diff = ga-ga0;
output;
end;

ga0 = ga;
cards;
1 0 0 277
1 1 1 307
2 0 0 302
2 1 1 279
3 0 0 277
3 1 1 286
4 0 0 313
4 1 1 274
5 1 0 292
5 0 1 273
6 0 0 279
6 1 1 284
proc print;   run;
proc genmod data=analysis;
model disease/one = ga_diff / dist=b type3;   run;
```

Figure 10-8 SAS procedure for the analysis of the preeclampsia data shown in Table 10-7.

```
                OBS     DISEASE     ONE     GA_DIFF

                 1         1         1         30
                 2         1         1        -23
                 3         1         1          9
                 4         1         1        -39
                 5         0         1        -19
                 6         1         1          5


                   The GENMOD Procedure

                   Model Information
            Description                    Value

            Distribution                   BINOMIAL
            Link Function                  LOGIT
            Dependent Variable             DISEASE
            Dependent Variable             ONE

              Criteria For Assessing Goodness Of Fit

          Criterion           DF      Value      Value/DF

          Scaled Deviance      4      5.0103       1.2526
          Scaled Pearson X2    4      4.9839       1.2460
          Log Likelihood       .     -2.5051        .

                Analysis Of Parameter Estimates
        Parameter     DF   Estimate   Std Err   ChiSquare  Pr>Chi

        INTERCEPT      1    1.9918     1.4726     1.8295    0.1762
        GA_DIFF        1    0.0327     0.0561     0.3395    0.5601
        SCALE          0    1.0000     0.0000       .         .
NOTE:  The scale parameter was held fixed.


             LR Statistics For Type 3 Analysis
          Source        DF   ChiSquare  Pr>Chi

          GA_DIFF        1    0.3964    0.5289
```

Figure 10–9 Output resulting from fitting a model to the preeclampsia data using the procedure in Figure 10–8.

$5.0103 = 3.31$ ($p = .069$) for the effect of solvent exposure. In this instance, the p value is quite different from that obtained using the Wald test, although it still does not achieve the nominal significance level of .05. The reason for this sizable difference is the small sample size, only six discordant pairs, and of these only one exhibited the disease in the unexposed group. An exact method of analysis (21) would be of use here because it would help establish a p value that did not depend on a large sample approximation.

Summary

In this chapter, we discussed methods of analysis for studies that employed matching in order to adjust for potential confounding of the disease–

exposure association of interest. We have made a distinction between a general strategy of stratification to achieve balance for an important covariate, which can subsequently be included in the analysis, and rigorous matching in which one or two unique controls are identified for a study subject. The methods discussed in this chapter are appropriate for the latter. Whether rigorous matching is in fact the most efficient way of controlling for confounding should be carefully considered at the design phase of a study. Often, it is not, and it has probably been overused by epidemiologists in a mistaken belief that it is increasing precision in the study results. However, regardless of whether it was a good idea to use matching in a study design, once the data have been collected using this approach, the analysis should reflect that fact.

All of the methods considered here employ the general statistical inference strategy of conditioning. The first methods we considered made use of score statistics, which are similar in philosophy to the methods discussed in the Part I of this book. In fact, as we have seen, they are equivalent to the Mantel–Haenszel methods for stratified data analysis. We then extended these methods to model fitting, which can be accomplished using either logistic regression or proportional hazards software that we have already discussed in other chapters. The only real difference in the practical use of these techniques is in the setup, because the subsequent interpretation of the parameters and the use of the likelihood ratio statistic are identical to the methods we have used all along.

Exercises

10.1 The data in the following table are from a study of the effect of exogenous estrogens on the risk of endometrial cancer. The investigators identified 63 cases of endometrial cancer, and a matched control was found for each case. For four controls, the dose level of conjugated estrogen was unknown.

Average dose	Average dose for the case			
for control	0.0	0.1–0.2	0.3–0.5	0.6+
0.0	6	9	9	12
0.1–0.2	2	4	3	2
0.3–0.5	3	2	3	2
0.6+	1	1	1	1

    a. Estimate the relative risk for each level of dose, using 0 as the reference.
    b. Test for the consistency of the odds ratios.

    c. Fit a model for linear trend in the log relative risk with dose.
    d. Test for departure from linear trend.
    e. Summarize your conclusions.

10.2. Tabulated here are results from a pair-matched case-control study. The factor of interest in this analysis is whether the woman ever had a live birth, and in this instance, cases were classified according to whether estrogen receptors (ER) were found in the tumor.

ER	Control	Case No	Case Yes
−	No	32	28
	Yes	20	41
+	No	27	6
	Yes	15	38

    a. Estimate the association between ever had a live birth and risk of ER − breast cancer and ER + breast cancer. Give 95% confidence intervals for your estimates.
    b. Compute a significance test for whether the risk is the same for both types of breast cancer, and summarize your conclusions.

10.3. A matched case-control study of a particular type of cancer was conducted to explore the association between disease and how close the individual's home was to a toxic waste site. Proximity to a toxic site was divided into four categories: town site is <0.5 miles from home, town site is 0.5–2.0 miles from home, town site is >2.0 miles from home, no toxic dump site in this town.

    a. Define contrasts that can be used to test the following hypotheses:
        i. Living in a town with a toxic dump affects disease risk.
        ii. There is a trend in risk with proximity to the dump site.
        iii. Repeat (ii), limiting the comparison to towns with a dump site.
    b. Define a set of regressor variables and describe how they might be used in a regression model to test the hypotheses in (a) using likelihood ratio tests.
    c. A matched-pairs design has been used and the data have been summarized in a 4 × 4 table as shown below:

Control exposure	Case exposure <0.5 miles	0.5–2.0 miles	>2.0 miles	None
<0.5 miles	a	b	c	d
0.5–2.0 miles	e	f	g	h
>2.0 miles	i	j	k	l
None	m	n	o	p

d. In a table, show the regressor variables and the response variable that could be included in a linear logistic model to address c. Describe any additional options necessary for using this procedure to find maximum conditional likelihood estimates of the parameters.

References

1. Mantel N. Synthetic retrospective studies and related topics. *Biometrics* 1973; 29:479–486.
2. Breslow NE, Lubin JH, Marek P, Langholz B. Multiplicative models and cohort analysis. *Journal of the American Statistical Association* 1983;78:1–12.
3. McKinlay SM. The design and analysis of the observational study—a review. *Journal of the American Statistical Association* 1975;70:503–520.
4. McKinlay SM. Pair-matching—a reappraisal of a popular technique. *Biometrics* 1977;33:725–735.
5. Herbst AL, Ulfelder H, Poskanzer DC. Adenocarcinoma of the vagina. *New England Journal of Medicine* 1971;284:878–881.
6. Bradley RA. Science, statistics, and paired comparisons. *Biometrics* 1976;32: 213–239.
7. Mantel N, Haenszel W. Statistical aspects of the analysis of data from retrospective studies of disease. *Journal of the National Cancer Institute* 1959;22:719–748.
8. McNemar Q. Note on the sampling error of the difference between correlated proportions on percentages. *Psychometrika* 1947;12:153–157.
9. Kelsey JL, Hardy RJ. Driving of motor vehicles as a risk factor for acute herniated lumber intvuerteral disc. *American Journal of Epidemiology* 1975;102: 63–73.
10. Stuart A. The comparison of frequencies in matched samples. *British Journal of Statistical Psychology* 1957;10:29–32.
11. Maxwell AE. Comparing the classification of subjects by two independent judges. *British Journal of Psychiatry* 1970;116:651–655.
12. Fleiss JL, Everitt BS. Comparing the marginal totals of square contingency tables. *British Journal of Mathematical and Statistical Psychology* 1971;24:117–123.
13. Fleiss JL. *Statistical Methods for Rates and Proportions.* New York: Wiley, 1981.
14. Pike MC, Casagrande J, Smith PG. Statistical analysis of individually matched case-control studies in epidemiology: Factor under study a discrete variable taking multiple values. *British Journal of Social and Preventive Medicine* 1975; 29:196–201.
15. Bishop YMM, Fienburg SE, Holland PW. *Discrete Multivariate Analysis: Theory and Practice.* Cambridge, MA: MIT Press, 1973.
16. Bradley RA. Some statistical methods in tests testing and quality evaluation. *Biometrics* 1953;9:22–38.
17. Holford TR. Covariance analysis for case-control studies with small blocks. *Biometrics* 1982;38:673–683.
18. Gail MH, Lubin JH, Rubinstein LV. Likelihood calculations for matched case-control studies and survival studies with tied death times. *Biometrika* 1981; 68:703–707.

19. Eskenzai B, Bracken MB, Holford TR, Grady J. Exposure to organic solvents and pregnancy complications. *American Journal of Epidemiology* 1988;14:177–188.

20. Holford TR, Bracken MB, Eskenazi B. Log-linear models for the analysis of matched cohort studies. *American Journal of Epidemiology* 1989;130:1247–1253.

21. Mehta C, Patel N. *StatXact 3 for Windows*. Cambridge, MA: CYTEL Software, 1996.

11

Power and Sample
Size Requirements

An important issue at the planning phase of a study is the question of whether it has enough observations to provide a reasonable opportunity to address the scientific questions being posed. We bring this up near the end of this book, at a point when we have already seen the breadth of approaches to data analysis that can be employed in epidemiologic studies. In practice, however, these calculations would take place at the very beginning, to determine the feasibility of achieving the goals of the work. To estimate a particular parameter we need to consider the precision or the standard error that would be meaningful, or we can express the precision in terms of the width of the confidence interval. To test a hypothesis, by contrast, we must identify the magnitude of the effect that we wish to detect, the strength of evidence given by the significance level needed, and the power or the chance of finding an effect of the specified magnitude.

In still other instances, we may have a limited number of subjects that are available for study. For example, to study the consequences of an industrial accident that resulted in the exposure of employees to toxic chemicals, we are limited to just the workers who were present at the time of the accident. In this instance the appropriate question to ask is whether the power is actually available before extending the effort to conduct a study of this specified size. If there is not sufficient power for effects that are of a size to be scientifically interesting, then there may be little point in wasting valuable resources on the project.

We now address questions of sample size and power for the three primary types of outcomes considered in epidemiologic research—namely, proportions, rates, and time to failure.

Estimation

The standard error, and hence the confidence interval that is typically derived from it, is directly proportional to the reciprocal of the square root of the sample size. Hence, our overall strategy is based on a calculation that finds an expression for the standard error in terms of the variance of a single observation, σ, i.e., $SE = \sigma/\sqrt{n}$. To identify the sample size required to obtain a specified standard error, we simply rearrange this expression by calculating

$$n = (\sigma/SE)^2 \tag{11.1}$$

Confidence intervals based on a normal approximation are related to the standard error by adding and subtracting the boundary factor, $B = z_{1-\alpha/2} \cdot SE$. Thus, the sample size required to obtain a specified boundary factor would be found, once again, by expressing the standard error in terms of σ, and solving for n:

$$n = (z_{1-\alpha/2}\, \sigma/B)^2 \tag{11.2}$$

Finally, the width of the confidence interval, or the difference between the lower and upper bounds, will be twice the boundary factor,

$$W = 2B = 2z_{1-\alpha/2}\, SE \tag{11.3}$$

and the sample size required to obtain a confidence interval of a specified width would be

$$n = (2z_{1-\alpha/2}\, \sigma/W)^2$$

Proportions

We turn now to proportions and the corresponding measures of association that are based on proportions. The outcome of interest is binary, diseased and healthy, so the distribution of the number diseased is governed by the binomial distribution, which has a standard deviation for a single observation of $\sqrt{p(1-p)}$. Table 11–1 provides the standard deviation for a number of common situations for convenient reference.

Example 11–1 A particular gene polymorphism has been identified as a factor that places those with the factor at especially high risk of cancer. For the purpose of public health planning, we would like to know the proportion of the population who have this particular expression of the gene to within 5%. In the context of the terminology just discussed, we can interpret our goal as achieving a 95% boundary of the confidence interval of $B = 0.05$. A preliminary guess suggests that the

Table 11–1. Standard deviations, representing the contribution of a single observation to an estimate that depends on a proportion or a rate ($r = n_2/n_1$)

Parameter	Estimate	Standard error for 1 observation
PROPORTIONS		(Standard error) $\cdot \sqrt{}$ No. subjects in group 1
Proportion	p	$\sqrt{p(1 - p)}$
Log(relative risk)	$\log\left(\dfrac{p_1}{p_2}\right)$	$\sqrt{\dfrac{1 - p_1}{p_1} + \dfrac{1 - p_2}{rp_2}}$
Log(odds ratio)	$\log\left(\dfrac{p_1(1 - p_2)}{(1 - p_1)p_2}\right)$	$\sqrt{\dfrac{1}{p_1(1 - p_1)} + \dfrac{1}{rp_2(1 - p_2)}}$
RATES		(Standard error) $\cdot \sqrt{}$ No. failures in group 1
Failure rate	λ	λ
Log(failure rate)	$\log \lambda$	1
Log(rate ratio)	$\log\left(\dfrac{\lambda_1}{\lambda_2}\right)$	$\sqrt{\dfrac{1}{m_1} + \dfrac{1}{m_2}} = \sqrt{\dfrac{1}{\varphi(\lambda_1)} + \dfrac{1}{r\varphi(\lambda_2)}}$
CORRECTION FOR INCOMPLETE DATA		
Truncation at T_1		$\varphi(\lambda) = 1 - \exp\{-\lambda \cdot T_1\}$
Recruitment to T_0 and truncation at T_1		$\varphi(\lambda) = 1 - \dfrac{\exp\{-\lambda(T_1 - T_0)\} - \exp\{-\lambda T_1\}}{\lambda T_0}$

actual value for the proportion is around 0.2, hence, the sample size required to achieve the goals of this project can be found by using equation 11.2:

$$n = \frac{(1.96)^2 (0.2) (1 - 0.2)}{(0.05)^2} = 245.9$$

In practice, we always round up when selecting a sample size in order to err on the side of increasing our precision; that is, we would select at least 246 subjects for study.

Notice that an accurate calculation of the sample size requires that we know the true proportion, which is the answer we are seeking from the study. Hence, there is a certain irony underlying the process of calculating sample size in that to achieve the best estimate, we must know the results of the study. In practice, we might protect ourselves by calculating the sample size for several plausible values, perhaps selecting the largest n to be certain of obtaining a boundary that is no greater than the proposed design condition. In the case of proportions, the standard deviation is greatest when $p = .5$, which we can use to obtain a conservative estimate of the required sample size. The result of using this value in our calculations suggests a sample size of 385.

Rates

As we saw in Chapter 4, rates can actually be motivated either by considering count data, in which the response has a Poisson distribution, or by considering time to a well-defined endpoint, in which we would calculate the failure rate. In either case, the denominator for the variance is the number of failures, as seen in equation 4.2. When designing a study, there are actually two ways of increasing the number of failures and, hence, the precision: increasing the number of subjects under study, or increasing the period of time they are under observation. As shown in Table 11–1, the contribution to the standard deviation of a single failure is the rate itself, λ, when we are making the calculation on the rate, but it is simply 1, if we are dealing with the log rate. The latter would be of particular interest if we wished to deal with the relative error, and an interesting feature of this approach is that it only depends on the number of failures.

When dealing with failure rates, subjects are weighted depending on the probability the subject is observed until failure. Three strategies that are often employed in follow-up studies with the following resultant weights:

> *Follow until all subjects have failed.* Each subject counts as a complete observation, which can be represented by giving them a weight of $\varphi(\lambda) = 1$. This approach is often impractical, especially if the rate is relatively low because it can require follow-up to continue for many years.
>
> *Truncate the follow-up after time* T_1: Observations for some subjects are now incomplete, so in effect we weight each observation by the expected probability of failure during the period of observation, $\varphi(\lambda) = (1 - \exp\{-\lambda T_1\})$.
>
> *Recruit subjects for time* T_0 *and continue follow-up to time* $T_1 (>T_0)$. If we assume that recruitment occurs at a uniform rate between 0 and T_0, then the effective weight for each observation is $\varphi(\lambda) = [1 - (\exp\{-\lambda(T_1 - T_0)\} - \exp\{-\lambda T_1\})/\lambda T_0]$.

Example 11–2   We are interested in estimating the incidence rate for a complication of a new type of therapy, and the boundary of the 90% confidence interval ($z_{\alpha/2} = 1.645$) should be within 10% of the rate. Subjects will be recruited for 2 years, with 2 additional years of follow-up after the recruitment period ends, so that $T_0 = 2$ and $T_1 = 4$. It is thought that the rate will be around 0.1 per year, so the weight of each observation is

$$1 - \frac{\exp\{-0.1(4 - 2)\} - \exp\{-0.1 \cdot 4\}}{(0.1)(2)} = 0.2579$$

If the boundary of the relative error is to be within 10%, the boundary for the log rate should be $\log(1.1) = 0.09531$. Hence, the required expected number of cases will be

$$n = \left[\frac{(1.645)(1)}{(0.09531)} \right]^2 = 297.88$$

which can be obtained by recruiting $297.88/0.2579 = 1154.8$, or about 1,155 subjects.

Association measure

For estimates arising from responses that have a binomial distribution, the standard deviation can be expressed as a function of the proportion responding, p. Table 11–1 gives the standard deviation for an estimate of the proportion responding, as well as the expressions for the log odds ratio and the log relative risk. As noted in Chapter 3, it is often preferable to use the log transformed values for the odds ratio and the relative risk when using an approximate method for setting confidence limits.

Example 11–3   Suppose that we are planning a cohort study of the risk of giving birth to a low birthweight baby, and we wish to estimate the relative risk in an exposed group of mothers to within 10% error. We shall interpret this to mean that the confidence interval endpoints are within 10% of the point estimate of the relative risk, RR, or $RR \cdot (1.1)^{\pm 1} = \exp\{\log RR \pm \log 1.1\}$. So the $\log(1.1)$ is the boundary factor for the log relative risk. We shall use a 95% confidence level, and we shall assume that the proportion with low birthweight in the controls is 10%, $p_1 = 0.1$, and the relative risk is 2, or, $p_2 = 0.2$. It turns out that it is easier to recruit exposed subjects than controls, so we are planning to enroll half as many controls, $r = 0.5$. Therefore the standard deviation expressed in terms of a single exposed subject is

$$\sigma = \sqrt{\frac{1 - 0.1}{0.1} + \frac{1 - 0.2}{(0.5)(0.2)}} = \sqrt{17} = 4.123$$

Hence, the required sample size for the exposed is

$$n = \left[\frac{(1.96)(4.123)}{\log 1.1} \right]^2 = (84.789)^2 = 7189.2$$

with half as many unexposed, 3,594.6. In general, we would round up in order to be sure that enough subjects were recruited—that is, 7,190 exposed and 3,595 controls.

Clearly, this is a very large study, the size of which is driven largely by the precision requirements. Often, we are only interested in whether exposure increases risk, which implies that the log relative risk is greater than zero. This study will result in a standard error for the relative risk of $\log 1.1/1.96 = 0.0486$, so the null value of 0 is more than 14 standard errors away from the expected value for the log relative risk, which is $\log(2) = 0.693$. In the following section we consider the question of sample size from the standpoint of testing the significance of the null hypothesis.

A similar approach may be applied to the estimation of the rate ratio, a measure of association applied to rates. The following example illustrates the calculation.

Example 11–4   Suppose that we wish to estimate the rate ratio so that the boundary for the 95% confidence limit is within 20% of the actual rate—that is, for the log rate ratio we have $B = \log(1.2) = 0.1823$. Preliminarily, we think that the individual rates are 0.3 and 0.2, so that the first group would be expected to contribute about 50% more failures than the second and thus be more precise. We might achieve some overall efficiency by selecting 50% more subjects in the second group, $r = 1.5$. As in Example 11–2, we will recruit subjects for 2 years, $T_0 = 2$, and the maximum follow-up is 4 years, $T_1 = 4$. The contribution of a single observation in group 1 to the variance of the log rate ratio is given by

$$\mathrm{Var}[\log(\lambda_1/\lambda_2)] = \varphi^{-1}[\lambda_1] + r^{-1}\,\varphi^{-1}[\lambda_2]$$
$$= [1 - (\exp\{-\lambda_1(T_1 - T_0)\} - \exp\{-\lambda_1 T_1\})/\lambda_1 T_0]^{-1}$$
$$+r^{-1}\,[1 - (\exp\{-\lambda_2(T_1 - T_0)\} - \exp\{-\lambda_2 T_1\})/\lambda_2 T_0]^{-1}$$

Substituting in the preliminary values of the parameters, we have the variance contribution of a single observation in the first group of 3.1924. Using equation 11.2, we have the required number in the first group,

$$n = \frac{(1.96)^2\,(3.1924)}{(0.1823)^2} = 368.94$$

or 369, with 554 in the second group.

Two-Group Hypothesis Tests

As we know from the fundamentals of hypothesis testing, there are two types of error that must be considered, and both come into play when designing a study that will address a particular null hypothesis. For the significance test itself, we evaluate the distribution of our test statistic derived under the condition that the null hypothesis is true. In effect, this is a strategy for convincing a skeptic who truly believes that there is no effect of the factor of interest on the response, so we play along by adopting the stance of no effect. If we can show that the observed data are very unlikely to have occurred by chance under this null distribution, then we can reject that point of view, adopting instead the alternative hypothesis, which is the state of affairs we are trying to establish. We do this by setting up a behavior rule, even before we have made any calculations, that results in the identification of a rejection region that will convince us that the null hypothesis is false, a region that occurs with small probability, α.

Suppose that we wish to establish that there is a 10% difference between exposed and unexposed in the proportion of people who develop disease in a specified period of time, and that past history suggests that 10% of the unexposed develop the disease. Hence, we wish to establish that the exposure results in at least 20% disease to be compared to the 10% expected for the controls. If our study is such that equal numbers are recruited to each exposure category, then we expect an average of 15% diseased if there is no effect of exposure. Figure 11–1 shows a two-tailed rejection region under the null hypothesis, where the significance level, or Type I error rate, is 5%, or, 2.5% in each tail. In this instance we are considering a study in which there are an equal number of subjects in each group, and n represents the number in one group. Notice that as the sample size increases, the tails shorten because of the greater precision that has been achieved.

Type II error results from accepting the null hypothesis when the alternative is in fact the truth. Because we are trying to establish that the null hypothesis is false, this would in effect be a failed attempt, assuming that we are right in setting up our conjecture in the form of the alternative hypothesis. The probability of a Type II error is represented by β. Often, this phenomenon is expressed as the power, $1 - \beta$, which is the converse of making a Type II error, or the probability that we successfully establish the alternative hypothesis. Figure 11–1 shows the distribution of the difference in the proportions under our alternative hypothesis, and the shaded area corresponds to a power of 80%, or $\beta = 0.20$. Notice that when the sample size in each group is 150, the region that achieves the desired

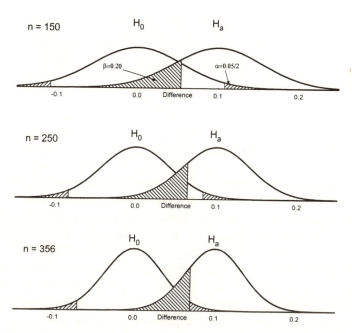

Figure 11–1 Approximate distribution of the difference in proportions under the null ($p_1 = p_2 = 0.15$) and alternative ($p_1 = 0.1, p_2 = 0.2$) hypotheses by sample size.

power is well within the acceptance region for the null hypothesis. As the sample size increases to 250, the cutpoint for the upper tail under H_0 approaches the cutpoint for the desired power under H_a. In fact, an appropriate study design would have a sample size in which the boundaries for α and β coincide, which occurs when the sample size is 356.

In situations in which the normal gives a good approximation to the distribution of the test statistic, the sample size needed to obtain the appropriate Type I and II error rates is given by

$$n = \frac{[z_{\alpha/2}\sigma_0 + z_\beta\sigma_a]^2}{[\theta_a]^2} \tag{11.4}$$

where θ_a is the magnitude of the effect under the alternative hypothesis, and σ_0 and σ_a are the contributions of a single observation to the standard error of an estimate of the effect, θ, under the null and alternative hypotheses, respectively. Power, on the other hand, can be found by rearranging equation 11.4 to obtain an expression for the standard normal deviate for the Type II error rate:

$$z_\beta = \frac{\theta_a\sqrt{n} - z_{\alpha/2}\sigma_0}{\sigma_a} \tag{11.5}$$

The inverse of the normal of z_β yields β, and hence, the power is $(1 - \beta)$.

Proportion comparisons

An expression for directly finding the sample size needed for demonstrating that the difference in two proportions is something other than zero, using α as the specified significance level for a two-tailed test, and with power $(1 - \beta)$ is given by Fleiss (p. 42) (1). If p_1 and p_2 are the proportions in the two groups, then the effect of interest is the difference in these proportions, $\theta = p_1 - p_2$. If $q_i = 1 - p_i$, then the contribution to the variance of a single observation in group 1 is $p_1 q_1$. Let the number of observations in group 2 for each one in group 1 be represented by $r = n_2/n_1$, so that the relative contribution to the variance by those in group 2 for a single subject in group 1 is $r^{-1}p_2 q_2$. Thus the overall contribution of one observation in group 1 to the variance of an estimate of the effect is $\sigma_a = \sqrt{p_1 q_1 + r^{-1}p_2 q_2}$. Under the null hypothesis that the proportions are the same, the overall proportion responding would be represented by the weighted average of the two proportions, $\bar{p} = (p_1 + r \cdot p_2) / (1 + r)$, with the corresponding contribution of a single observation in group 1 to the variance of an estimate of the effect, $\sigma_0 = \sqrt{pq}[1 + r^{-1}]$. Substituting into equation 11.4 yields

$$n = \frac{[z_{\alpha/2}\sqrt{1 + r^{-1})\,\overline{pq}} + z_\beta\sqrt{p_1 q_1 + r^{-1}\,p_2 q_2}]}{[p_1 - p_2]^2}$$

for the number in group 1, with the corresponding number in group 2 given by rn.

Example 11–3 (continued)   In this example, we reconsider the design for the study from the previous section in which the relative risk of interest is 2.0 and the proportion diseased among the unexposed is expected to be 0.1. Hence, our alternative hypothesis is that $p_1 = 0.1$ and $p_2 = 0.2$, and we still plan to use half as many subjects in group 2, or, $r = 0.5$. To test this hypothesis, we plan to use a two-tailed test with a significance level $\alpha = .05$, which has the corresponding standard normal deviate, $z_{\alpha/2} = 1.96$. In addition, we wish to have 80% power or a Type II error rate of $\beta = 0.20$, with normal deviate, $z_\beta = 0.84$. Hence, the required sample size for group 1 is

$$n_1 =$$

$$\frac{[(1.96)\sqrt{(1 + (0.5)^{-1})(0.133)(0.867)} + (0.84)\sqrt{(0.1)(0.9) + (0.5)^{-1}(0.2)(0.8)}]^2}{[0.2 - 0.1]^2}$$

$$= 286.2$$

which rounds up to 287, and $n_2 = 143.1$, which rounds up to 144. Notice that the number of observations required to just reject the null hypothesis is considerably less than the number required to achieve the fairly accurate estimate of risk that was stipulated in the earlier calculation. In fact, we are often limited by ethical considerations in human studies to simply demonstrating that risk is increased in a particular group. To improve an estimate beyond what is required to achieve statistical significance necessitates still more data collection, thus exposing more subjects to what has become a known etiologic agent. In these situations we must clearly limit our knowledge to the point of knowing that an agent causes harm.

Rate comparisons

To set up a study designed to compare two rates, one can either set up the null hypothesis as a test of the log rate ratio being zero or the difference in the two rates being zero. In the first instance, we have $H_0: \log(\psi) = \log(\lambda_2/\lambda_1) = \log(\lambda_2) - \log(\lambda_1) = 0$, compared to the alternative, $H_a:$

$\log(\psi) \neq 0$. Let $r = n_2/n_1$ be the number of observations in group 2 for each observation in group 1. The variance of the log rate ratio is given by

$$
\text{Var}(\log \psi) = \frac{1}{m_1} + \frac{1}{m_2} = \frac{1}{n_1 \varphi(\lambda_1)} + \frac{1}{n_2 \varphi(\lambda_2)}
$$

$$
= \frac{\varphi^{-1}(\lambda_1) + r^{-1}\varphi^{-1}(\lambda_2)}{n_1}
$$

where m_i is the expected number of failures, and $\varphi(\lambda_i)$ is the probability that subjects in the study are observed to failure; that is, the observations are complete. Hence, the contribution to the variance of a single observation in group 1 is $\varphi^{-1}(\lambda_1) + r^{-1}\varphi^{-1}(\lambda_2)$. Using this information in our sample size formula (2, 3) given in equation 11.4, we obtain

$$
n = \frac{(z_{\alpha/2} + z_\beta)^2 [\varphi^{-1}(\lambda_1) + r^{-1}\varphi^{-1}(\lambda_2)]}{[\log(\psi)]^2} \tag{11.6}
$$

Example 11–4 (continued)   In this example we reconsider the comparison of rates in two populations in which the values considered under the alternative hypothesis are $\lambda_1 = 0.3$ and $\lambda_2 = 0.2$, with the ratio of the number of observations in group 2 to each one in group 1, $r = 1.5$. As before, we assume a uniform recruitment of patients for 2 years, with a study end at 4 years. As we saw earlier, this gives rise to the contribution of a single observation in group 1 to the variance of 3.1924. We intend to employ a two-tailed test using a 5% significance level ($z_{\alpha/2} = 1.96$), and we seek 80% power ($z_\beta = 0.84$). From equation 11.6 we obtain the required sample size in group 1,

$$
n = \frac{(1.96 + 0.84)^2 [3.1924]}{[\log(0.3/0.2)]^2} = 152.2
$$

or 153. Correspondingly, we would recruit 229 subjects for group 2, for a total of 382 subjects in the study.

Another way of expressing, the null and alternative hypotheses for the two groups is in terms of the difference in the untransformed rates, $\lambda_1 - \lambda_2$, in which the contribution to the variance of each observation in group 1 under the alternative hypothesis is $\sigma_a^2 = [\lambda_1^2/\varphi(\lambda_1)] + [\lambda_2^2/r\,\varphi(\lambda_2)]$. If we assume that the corresponding variance under the null hypothesis is approximately the same, the sample size expression (2, 3) becomes

$$
n = \frac{(z_{\alpha/2} + z_\beta)^2 \{[\lambda_1^2/\varphi(\lambda_1)] + [\lambda_2^2/\varphi(\lambda_2)]\}}{(\lambda_1 - \lambda_2)^2} \tag{11.7}
$$

Survival curves

As we learned in Chapter 5, the log-rank test offers a nonparametric approach to the comparison of two survival curves, thus avoiding the strong assumption of a hazard independent of time that was required to justify the failure rate. We also noted that a rationale for this method was that of a score test of the parameter that related the hazards in two groups, the rate ratio $\psi = \lambda_2(t)/\lambda_1(t)$, or H_0: $\psi = 1$. A feature of the log-rank test is the fact that complete observations drive the power, and Schoenfeld (4) has derived an asymptotic formula for the required total number of failures needed, based on the log-rank statistic,

$$m_+ = \frac{(z_{\alpha/2} + z_\beta)^2[1 + r]^2}{[\log \psi]^2 \, r} \tag{11.8}$$

where m_+ is the total number of failures and r is the ratio of the number of observations in group 2 for each one in group 1. If φ represents the proportion of the total number of observations that fail, then the total sample size will be $n_+ = m_+/\varphi$ and, hence, $n_1 = n_+/(1 + r)$ and $n_2 = r \, n_+/(1 + r)$.

Freedman (5) provides an alternative expression for the total sample size based on the log-rank test,

$$m_+ = \frac{(z_{\alpha/2} + z_\beta)^2 \, [1 + \psi r]^2}{[1 - \psi]^2 \, r} \tag{11.9}$$

Hsieh (6) did a Monte Carlo simulation study of sample size formulae for the log-rank test, including the two given above. These results seem to suggest that equation 11.8 is best for predicting the power of a study when there are equal numbers in the two groups, but equation 11.9 performs better in other situations.

Example 11–5 A study has been proposed to determine the efficacy of a new treatment. The funding mechanism for the study allows for 2 years of recruitment, with 2 additional years of follow-up before the end of data collection. Hence, the range of follow-up is from 2 to 4 years. Patients receiving the best current therapy experience 20% mortality in the first 2 years and 25% mortality after 4 years. Therefore, if the rate of recruitment is uniform, we can expect about 22.5% mortality overall, the average of the experience at 2 and 4 years. We wish to design a study that will reduce the mortality rate by 50% ($\psi = 0.5$), using a two-tailed test with 5% significance ($z_{\alpha/2} = 1.96$) and 80% power ($z_\beta = 0.84$). If we assume that the proportional hazards model applies to the data to be collected in this study, then the patients receiving the new treatment would be expected to have $1 - (1 - $

$0.20)^{0.5} = 0.1056$ mortality at 2 years and $1 - (1 - 0.25)^{0.5} = 0.1340$ at 4 years, or an average of 0.1198.

Let us first consider a design in which each group is the same size, $r = 1$. We would then expect that the overall mortality experience for the study to be the average of what would occur in each group, $\phi = 0.1724$. Because of the equal sample size in each group, we can use equation 11.8 to determine the overall number of deaths required

$$m_+ = \frac{(1.96 + 0.84)^2 [1 + 1]^2}{[\log(0.5)]^2 (1)} = 65.27$$

which necessitate the recruitment of $n_+ = 65.27/0.1724 = 378.6$ subjects. Therefore, we would enroll at least 190 patients in each treatment group.

Suppose that instead of recruiting an equal number of subjects for each group, we plan to recruit twice as many in the group receiving the new treatment, $r = 2$. We can use equation 11.9 to obtain the total number of deaths that need to be observed:

$$m_+ = \frac{(1.96 + 0.84)^2 [1 + (0.5)(2.0)]^2}{[1 - 0.5]^2 (2.0)} = 62.72$$

Because we are now taking more subjects into the second group, the overall mortality experience would be the weighted average of the anticipated experience in each group,

$$[1(0.2250) + 2(0.1198)]/[1 + 2] = 0.1549$$

Hence, the total number of subjects required is $n_+ = 62.72/0.1549 = 405.04$, thus providing a goal of at least 136 subjects for the current treatment group and 271 for the new treatment.

Matched pairs

For the analysis of matched pairs, the unit of observation was, in effect, the pair, and the tabular summary of the results of such a study are usually laid out in the form shown in Table 10–2. Recall that conditional inference was an effective strategy for incorporating the design into the analysis, giving rise to McNemar's test when the response of interest was binary. To include the formulation of the sample size and power formulae in the framework used thus far in this chapter, we employ the square root of the usual representation of the test statistic,

$$Z = \frac{n_{12} - n_{21}}{\sqrt{n_{12} + n_{21}}}$$

which has a standard normal distribution under the null hypothesis of no effect. We have already noted the peculiar feature of the conditional analysis that results in only the discordant pairs entering into the calculation. Hence, the sample size problem will be to design the study in such a way as to end up with a sufficient number of discordant pairs.

If the null hypothesis is true, the probability that a pair will be tabulated in the cell above the diagonal is $\frac{1}{2}$, and the contribution of each pair to the standard deviation of the difference in the off-diagonal cell frequencies, the numerator of the test statistic, is $\sigma_0 = 1$. Likewise, under the alternative hypothesis we have $\sigma_a = 2\sqrt{\pi_{12}\pi_{21}}/(\pi_{12} + \pi_{21})$. Hence, an expression for the required number of discordant pairs, m, needed if we are to use an α significance level for a study with power $(1 - \beta)$ is

$$
m = \left\{ \frac{z_{\alpha/2} \cdot 1 + z_{\beta} \cdot 2 \cdot \sqrt{\pi_{12}\pi_{21}}/(\pi_{12} + \pi_{21})}{(\pi_{12} - \pi_{21})/(\pi_{12} + \pi_{21})} \right\}^2
$$

$$
= \left\{ \frac{z_{\alpha/2} \cdot (\pi_{12} + \pi_{21}) + z_{\beta} \cdot 2 \cdot \sqrt{\pi_{12}\pi_{21}}}{(\pi_{12} - \pi_{21})} \right\}^2 \tag{11.10}
$$

By dividing the numerator and denominator by π_{21}, we have an alternative representation in terms of the rate ratio, $\Omega = \pi_{12}/\pi_{21}$,

$$
m = \left(\frac{z_{\alpha/2} \cdot (\Omega + 1) + z_{\beta} \cdot 2 \cdot \sqrt{\Omega}}{\Omega - 1} \right)^2 \tag{11.11}
$$

Because only the proportion $\pi_d = \pi_{12} + \pi_{21}$ of the pairs enrolled in a study will be discordant, we will need to actually enroll m/π_d to arrive at the appropriate number on average (7).

A practical issue that we have ignored thus far is in finding a sensible realization for the proportions in the cells of Table 10–2, which, in turn, will yield the necessary proportion of discordant pairs. One idea is to propose values for the proportion of cases and controls who have been exposed, π_{+2} and π_{2+}, respectively, and derive the proportions for the interior cells by assuming that the probability that a case is exposed is independent of the probability that the corresponding control is exposed. This gives rise to $\pi_d = \pi_{1+}\pi_{+2} + \pi_{2+}\pi_{+1}$ (8). Unfortunately, if we really believe that exposure in the case and control members of a pair are independent, then this calls into question our whole rationale for matching in the first place. In general, we would choose as matching variables those that are related to both the disease and the exposure of interest; hence, if we have chosen these variables wisely, we would expect to see a dependence among the cells of Table 10–2.

A method that allows for a dependence between exposure among case and control members of the match pairs (7, 9, 10) can be derived from the proportion exposed among the controls, π_{2+}, the rate ratio of particular interest in the study, $\Omega = \pi_{12}/\pi_{21}$, and the case-control exposure odds ratio, $\psi = \pi_{11}\pi_{22}/\pi_{12}\pi_{21}$. It is sufficient to initially find π_{12}, which can be obtained by the solution to a quadratic equation in which $a = (\psi - 1)/\Omega$, $b = \pi_{2+} + (1 - \pi_{2+})/\Omega$, and $c = -\pi_{2+}(1 - \pi_{2+})$, thus

$$\pi_{12} = \frac{\sqrt{b^2 - 4ac} - b}{2a} \qquad (11.12)$$

The remaining cells can readily be filled in by using differences from the column totals and the rate ratio.

There is still another weakness in our design strategy, however. If we recruit the number of subjects that will give us the required number of discordant pairs on average, the actual number of discordant pairs obtained each time we conduct a study, m, is itself a random variable. Hence, the power we wish to achieve will not be realized because in practice we will often obtain fewer than the expected number of discordant pairs. Our first proposal for n is actually a first-order approximation, which can be improved by adopting Miettinen's second-order approach for determining the contribution to the variance under the alternative hypothesis (7, 11)

$$\sigma_a^2 = \frac{(\pi_{21} + \pi_{12})^2 - (\pi_{21} - \pi_{12})^2 (3 + \pi_{21} + \pi_{12})/4}{\pi_{21} + \pi_{12}} \qquad (11.13)$$

giving the corresponding second-order estimator of sample size,

$$n = \left[\frac{z_{\alpha/2} \sqrt{\pi_{21} + \pi_{12}} + z_\beta \sigma_a}{\pi_{12} - \pi_{21}} \right]^2 \qquad (11.14)$$

Example 11–6 We wish to design a matched case-control study that will detect a rate ratio of 2, using a significance level of 5% and power of 90%. In the general population, 20% are exposed to the factor of interest, so this is the proportion of controls we expect to see exposed. The variables used for matching are believed to be strongly effective, so that the cross product ratio for exposure in cases and controls is 3. Therefore, the conditions we have set are $\Omega = 2$, $\psi = 3$, and $\pi_{2+} = 0.2$. In addition, we have $z_{\alpha/2} = 1.96$ and $z_\beta = 1.28$, so that equation 11.11 yields the required number of discordant pairs,

$$m = \left(\frac{(1.96)(2 + 1) + 1.28 \cdot 2 \cdot \sqrt{2}}{2 - 1} \right)^2 = 90.26$$

To find the proportion of discordant pairs, we note that $a = (3 - 1)/2 = 1$, $b = 0.2 + (1 - 0.2)/2 = 0.6$, and $c = -0.2(1 - 0.2) = -0.16$, which gives

$$\pi_{12} = \frac{\sqrt{(0.6)^2 - 4 \cdot 1 \cdot (-0.16)} - (0.6)}{2 \cdot 1} = 0.2$$

The fact that $\pi_{11} + \pi_{12} = 0.8$ implies that $\pi_{11} = 0.6$. Because $\Omega = \pi_{12}/\pi_{21} = 2$, yields $\pi_{21} = 0.1$. Finally, we have $\pi_{22} = 1 - 0.2 - 0.6 - 0.1 = 0.1$, thus completing the table. Our first-order estimator of the odds ratio makes use of the fact that $\pi_d = \pi_{12} + \pi_{21} = 0.3$, so that the required number of pairs to be recruited is $n = m/\pi_d = 90.26/0.3 = 301$ pairs.

If we choose instead to use the second-order estimate of sample size, we use as the alternative variance the value obtained from using equation 11.13:

$$\sigma_a = \frac{(0.1 + 0.2)^2 - (0.1 - 0.2)^2 \, (3 + 0.1 + 0.2)/4}{0.1 + 0.2} = 0.2725$$

providing the second-order sample size estimate

$$n = \left[\frac{(1.96) \sqrt{0.2 + 0.1} + (1.28) \sqrt{0.2725}}{0.2 - 0.1} \right]^2 = 303.4$$

suggesting that 304 pairs should be recruited for study.

Extensions of these methods for estimating sample size in matched designs employing multiple controls per case are provided by Miettinen (11). Walter (12) further considers matched studies in which there is a variable number of controls selected for each case. The methods we have been considering here are based on large-sample approximations, so if they yield relatively small estimates of the required sample, they can be misleading. Royston (13) suggests that the normal approximation methodology not be used unless the number of discordant pairs is greater than 35 when the significance level is .05 and greater than 100 when the significance level is .01.

General Hypothesis Tests

To extend the idea of making sample size calculations to situations involving more complex phenomenon (like trends, adjustment for covariates, and interactions), it is convenient to work with the chi-square statistic generated by either the likelihood ratio, the Wald test, or the score statistics. The test only requires that we specify the distribution that arises under the null hypothesis, and the resulting chi-square distribution depends on the degrees of freedom, or the number of unique parameters being tested. In its more general formulation, the chi-square distribution depends not only on the degrees of freedom but also on a second variable called the non-centrality parameter, ν. Under the null hypothesis, $\nu = 0$, and this is by far the most familiar form for the chi-square distribution. However, under the alternative hypothesis the test statistic has a distribution in which the non-centrality parameter is greater than zero; thus, the calculation of power and sample size requires that we make use of the central chi-square to determine the rejection region for our hypothesis test, and then determine the probability that the test statistic does not fall in the rejection region using the noncentral chi-square distribution that arises under the alternative hypothesis.

Before specifying the calculation of the noncentrality parameter, let us consider in more detail a study that requires a significance test of four unique parameters using a likelihood ratio test. Under the null hypothesis, we would use a central chi-square distribution, $v = 0$, with 4 df, as shown in Figure 11–2. The critical value for the test at a significance level of .05 is 9.4877, and the values to the right represent the rejection region for the test. Notice that as the noncentrality parameter increases, the distribution shifts to the right, changing shape in part due to the boundary condition that does not allow the statistic to take negative values. The area under the noncentral chi-square distribution that lies to the left of the critical value represents the Type II error rate. When the noncentrality parameter is 11.9353, the area to the left of the critical value of 9.4877 is 0.20, the value required if we wish to design a study with 80% power. Therefore, we will seek the sample size required to provide a noncentrality parameter of 11.9353. Table 11–2 gives the necessary critical values for df = 1, 2, ... , 20, a variety of significance levels, and powers of 80% and 90%.

It turns out that the noncentrality parameter is proportional to sample size, $v = n\xi$, where ξ represents the contribution of a single observation to

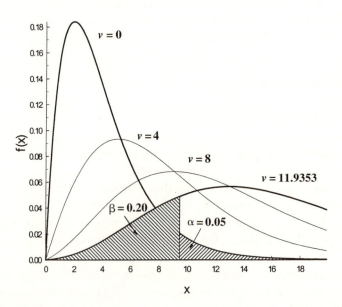

Figure 11–2 Chi-square distributions for df = 4 for various noncentrality parameters, including the central chi-square under H_0 ($v = 0$), and for the distribution that yields Type II error rate of 0.20, $v = 11.9353$.

Table 11-2. Critical noncentrality parameters by degrees of freedom, significance level for a two-tailed test (α), and power

			Significance level			
df	.100	.050	.020	.010	.002	.001
POWER = 0.8						
1	6.1822	7.8489	10.0360	11.6790	15.4595	17.0746
2	7.7105	9.6347	12.0808	13.8807	17.9471	19.6624
3	8.7977	10.9026	13.5385	15.4577	19.7488	21.5450
4	9.6827	11.9353	14.7294	16.7493	21.2334	23.1002
5	10.4469	12.8276	15.7604	17.8693	22.5258	24.4560
6	11.1287	13.6243	16.6821	18.8719	23.6856	25.6741
7	11.7500	14.3505	17.5231	19.7874	24.7470	26.7896
8	12.3244	15.0221	18.3015	20.6353	25.7313	27.8249
9	12.8610	15.6498	19.0294	21.4286	26.6533	28.7951
10	13.3665	16.2411	19.7154	22.1766	27.5236	29.7112
11	13.8456	16.8017	20.3661	22.8862	28.3500	30.5814
12	14.3021	17.3359	20.9864	23.5629	29.1384	31.4120
13	14.7390	17.8472	21.5801	24.2108	29.8938	32.2079
14	15.1584	18.3382	22.1505	24.8333	30.6200	32.9731
15	15.5624	18.8111	22.7000	25.4332	31.3200	33.7110
16	15.9526	19.2678	23.2307	26.0127	31.9966	34.4243
17	16.3302	19.7100	23.7446	26.5739	32.6520	35.1152
18	16.6965	20.1388	24.2431	27.1183	33.2879	35.7859
19	17.0523	20.5554	24.7274	27.6473	33.9061	36.4379
20	17.3985	20.9608	25.1988	28.1622	34.5080	37.0727
POWER = 0.9						
2	10.4579	12.6539	15.4138	17.4267	21.9314	23.8173
3	11.7964	14.1715	17.1181	19.2474	23.9706	25.9348
4	12.8827	15.4051	18.5083	20.7370	25.6495	27.6827
5	13.8190	16.4695	19.7106	22.0275	27.1102	29.2058
6	14.6534	17.4188	20.7846	23.1818	28.4203	30.5735
7	15.4129	18.2836	21.7640	24.2354	29.6186	31.8255
8	16.1145	19.0827	22.6699	25.2107	30.7296	32.9870
9	16.7695	19.8291	23.5166	26.1227	31.7699	34.0752
10	17.3861	20.5320	24.3144	26.9823	32.7515	35.1024
11	17.9703	21.1980	25.0707	27.7977	33.6832	36.0779
12	18.5267	21.8325	25.7914	28.5749	34.5721	37.0087
13	19.0588	22.4395	26.4811	29.3188	35.4234	37.9004
14	19.5697	23.0222	27.1435	30.0334	36.2416	38.7577
15	20.0615	23.5834	27.7815	30.7219	37.0303	39.5841
16	20.5364	24.1252	28.3976	31.3868	37.7924	40.3828
17	20.9959	24.6495	28.9939	32.0305	38.5303	41.1564
18	21.4414	25.1579	29.5723	32.6549	39.2464	41.9072
19	21.8741	25.6518	30.1341	33.2616	39.9424	42.6369
20	22.2951	26.1323	30.6809	33.8520	40.6199	43.3474

the test statistic. To find the contribution of a single observation, we can fit a generalized linear model in which (1) the response is generated by the conditions set out under the alternative hypothesis and (2) each observation is weighted by the relative frequency with which that combination of covariates occurs in the population being studied. The resulting test statistic is the contribution of a single observation, ξ. If we have n individuals in our study, then the noncentrality parameter is $v = n\xi$, and we would find the area to the left of the critical value for the test to determine the Type II error rate. Alternatively, if we wish to know the sample size necessary for a specified power, we would look up the necessary noncentrality parameter in Table 11–2, v_0, enabling us to find the necessary sample size, $n = v_0/\xi$ (14, 15).

Steps for calculating the noncentrality parameter

Determining power and sample size in the more complex situations that we are considering in this section requires that we specify much more detail about what we expect to find in the population to be studied. In particular, we will need to specify the distribution of risk groups that will be expected, along with the distribution of diseased subjects that would be implied by the model. These details can then be used to calculate the noncentrality parameter, if we are calculating power for an already identified study population, or the contribution of a single observation to the noncentrality parameter, if we wish to determine the sample size need to achieve a particular level of power. This can appear to be a fairly complex process, but it can be broken down into the following steps:

1. Specify the distribution of risk groups in the control population.
2. Find the distribution in the case population that would result from the model that has been proposed for describing the effect of exposure on disease, using the parameters specified by the alternative hypothesis.
3. Determine weights for each risk group by taking the sum of the proportion of cases and controls expected.
4. Fit the null and alternative models to these data, taking the difference in the likelihood ratio statistics, which yields the estimated contribution to the noncentrality parameter.
5. Calculate either the sample size or the power using the appropriate central and noncentral chi-square distributions.

We now use this approach to make sample size calculations in a number of specific situations.

Testing for trend

As we have seen from earlier examples, the effect of exposure to a risk factor can affect the response in a variety of ways. However, the framework of the generalized linear model provides a useful way of formulating scientifically meaningful questions. We now explore the ideas that were sketched in the preceding section and show how they can be used to determine the sample size or power. Broadly speaking, a dose–response relationship between exposure and disease can mean anything from a very specific linear form for the relationship to an ordinal pattern in which individuals with the highest levels of exposure have the highest risk. In the following example, we use the ways in which we framed these questions in earlier chapters and employ the generalized linear model to make the necessary intermediate calculations for determining either sample size or power.

Example 11–7 Suppose that we are planning a case-control study of non-Hodgkin's lymphoma (NHL), and the exposure of interest is exposure to a pesticide, as determined by a biomarker, serum levels of DDE. Our approach to the analysis will involve categorizing the continuous exposure measure into quintiles based on the distribution among the controls, thus estimating the quintiles of exposure in the general population. The use of quintiles means that 20% of controls will be in each exposure level. To determine the proportion of the overall study population in each exposure level for the controls, we need to specify the control to case ratio, r. If $r = 1$, then 10% of the overall study population will be in each control category, thus completing step 1.

For step 2, we shall assume that a log-linear model describes the relationship between quintile of exposure and the odds ratio. Hence, if the quintiles are represented by the regressor variable $X = -2, -1, 0, 1, 2$, the proportion of cases observed for a given exposure quintile can be described in terms of a linear logistic model

$$P(X) = \frac{\exp\{\alpha + X\beta\}}{1 + \exp\{\alpha + X\beta\}}$$

The magnitude of β, the parameter of interest, will be specified by our choice of an alternative hypothesis, or the value of interest. Suppose that the alternative hypothesis of interest results in an odds ratio for the comparison of the highest with the lowest quintiles of 2, or $\beta = \log 2/[2 - (-2)] = 0.1733$. What remains for step 2 is finding the value of α, which is implied by these assumptions. Given the log-linear odds and the proportion of controls, the proportion of the study population which are cases in the ith group are

$$\Pr(\text{Case and } i) = \frac{1}{5} \cdot \frac{r}{1 + r} \cdot \exp\{\alpha + X_i\beta\}$$

Solving for α yields $\alpha = \log[5/r \cdot \sum \exp\{X_i\beta\}] = -0.02984$.

For step 3, we sum the proportion of the hypothetical population that are controls and cases for each risk group, $w_i = r \cdot [1 + \exp\{\alpha + X_i\beta\}]/5$. Table 11–3 summarizes the resulting distribution, odds and weights implied by the conditions of our test.

Table 11.3. Population distribution, odds, and weights implied by conditions in Example 11.7

Quintile	X	Odds	Proportion controls	Proportion cases	w_i
1	−2	0.7071	0.2000	0.1373	0.3373
2	−1	0.8408	0.2000	0.1632	0.3632
3	0	1.0000	0.2000	0.1941	0.3941
4	1	1.1892	0.2000	0.2309	0.4308
5	2	1.4142	0.2000	0.2745	0.4745
Total		5.1514	1.0000	1.0000	2.0000

To accomplish step 4, we use the SAS program shown in Figure 11–3. Notice that the program itself has been designed to directly calculate the information in Table 11–3. Also, notice that we had to specify the link, the inverse link, and the deviance because the response was not an integer, as would be expected for a binomial distribution.

We now need to specify the particular hypothesis test that we wish to carry out. Unlike the simplicity of the two-group comparisons considered thus far, there are actually several alternatives that we might consider, including (a) the global test that the odds for disease among all five quintiles are identical (df = 4), (b) the test for linear trend among quintiles (df = 1), and (c) a comparison of the highest and the lowest quintiles (df = 1). Each of these can be tested using a likelihood ratio test, as we have seen earlier, and these are shown in the output results for the Type 3 tests in Figure 11–4.

Finally, the contribution of a single case to the noncentrality parameter for the test for linear trend is 0.0295, and we see from Table 11–2 that the noncentrality parameter required to achieve 80% power for a 5% significance level is 7.8489. Hence, the sample size required is $n_1 = 7.8789/0.0295 = 268$ cases, and an equal number of controls for a total study size of 536. Still, we may not wish to limit ourselves to a test for linear trend because it may not hold for these data. It turns out that the contribution of a single case to the likelihood ratio statistic (not shown) is also 0.0295 for the overall test of equality for the five quintiles. However, this is now a test with 4 df, so the corresponding noncentrality parameter for a test using the 5% significance criterion and 80% power is 11.9353, yielding a sample size for the cases of $n = 11.9353/0.0295 = 405$ and an identical number for the controls. Lastly, we might wish to consider just a comparison of the highest and lowest quintiles of exposure, a comparison represented by the coefficient for the regressor variable "X4." This is once again a test with 1 df, but the contribution of a single case is now 0.0233, as shown in Figure 11–4. Hence, the required sample size for cases and for controls is $n = 7.8489/0.0233 = 337$. Clearly, we have greatest efficiency for testing linear trend, because not only is this a focused hypothesis (df = 1), but also it uses all the data in that the comparison between high and low essentially ignores quintiles 2, 3, and 4. We now have a mechanism for considering alternative approaches to setting up the comparisons to be made, and we could consider still other alternative hypotheses.

As we have already noted, sample size and power are addressing closely related issues in study design. If there are essentially no limits to the size

```
%let r = 1.0;                *Ratio of controls to cases;
%let b = log(2)/4;           *Effect size;

data study;
sum = 0;                     *Intermediate calculation for alpha;
do x=-2 to 2;
sum = sum + exp(x*&b);
end;

alpha = log(5/(&r*sum));     *Estimate of alpha;

do x=-2 to 2;                *Create variable for analysis;
eta1 = alpha + x*&b;         *Linear predictor;
pr = exp(eta1)/(1+exp(eta1));  *Probability of case;
wt = .2*&r*(1 + exp(eta1));   *Weight;
x1=(x=-1);                   *Dummy variables for quintiles;
x2=(x= 0);
x3=(x= 1);
x4=(x= 2);
output;
end;

proc genmod data=study;      *Model for linear trend;
p = _mean_;  y = _resp_;
fwdlink link = log(p/(1-p));
invlink ilink = exp(_xbeta_)/(1+exp(_xbeta_));
variance var = p*(1-p);
deviance dev = 2*(y*log(y/p) + (1-y)*log((1-y)/(1-p)));
scwgt wt;
model pr = x / type3;
run;

proc genmod data=study;      *Model for categorical indicators;
p = _mean_;  y = _resp_;
fwdlink link = log(p/(1-p));
invlink ilink = exp(_xbeta_)/(1+exp(_xbeta_));
variance var = p*(1-p);
deviance dev = 2*(y*log(y/p) + (1-y)*log((1-y)/(1-p)));
scwgt wt;
model pr = x1 x2 x3 x4 / type3;
run;
```

Figure 11–3 SAS procedure for calculating contribution to the noncentrality parameter for a single case-control study in Example 11–7.

of the population that might be recruited, we generally seek the sample size necessary to achieve a specified level of power. Alternatively, once the sample size is fixed, the question is whether there is adequate power to address a particular research question. The following example considers such a comparison.

Example 11–7 (continued)   In our previous calculations related to NHL we considered as cases, everyone with disease at this site. In many ways, however, NHL is a mixture of different diseases, and tumor histology represents one approach to

```
                        The GENMOD Procedure

                  Criteria For Assessing Goodness Of Fit
               Criterion            DF        Value      Value/DF
               Scaled Deviance       3       0.0000       0.0000
               Pearson Chi-Square    3       0.0000       0.0000

                     Analysis Of Parameter Estimates
            Parameter    DF    Estimate    Std Err   ChiSquare  Pr>Chi
            INTERCEPT     1     -0.0298     1.4357      0.0004   0.9834
            X             1      0.1733     1.0151      0.0291   0.8645
            SCALE         0      1.0000     0.0000        .        .
NOTE:  The scale parameter was held fixed.

                      LR Statistics For Type 3 Analysis
                  Source       DF    ChiSquare  Pr>Chi
                  X             1      0.0295    0.8636


                        The GENMOD Procedure

                  Criteria For Assessing Goodness Of Fit
               Criterion            DF        Value      Value/DF
               Scaled Deviance       0       0.0000         .
               Pearson Chi-Square    0       0.0000         .

                     Analysis Of Parameter Estimates
            Parameter    DF    Estimate    Std Err   ChiSquare  Pr>Chi
            INTERCEPT     1  .  -0.3764     3.5050      0.0115   0.9145
            X1            1      0.1733     4.8385      0.0013   0.9714
            X2            1      0.3466     4.7367      0.0054   0.9417
            X3            1      0.5199     4.6494      0.0125   0.9110
            X4            1      0.6931     4.5747      0.0230   0.8796
            SCALE         0      1.0000     0.0000        .        .
NOTE:  The scale parameter was held fixed.

                      LR Statistics For Type 3 Analysis
                  Source       DF    ChiSquare  Pr>Chi
                  X1            1      0.0013    0.9714
                  X2            1      0.0054    0.9415
                  X3            1      0.0126    0.9105
                  X4            1      0.0233    0.8786
```

Figure 11–4 Output from the SAS procedure shown in Figure 11–3.

further classifying this disease. Of course, if the etiology varies by tumor histology, then an analysis that focuses on a particular histologic type would be more powerful, because the effect of exposure would not be diluted by mixing these cases with individuals with differing histologies. By considering subgroups, however, we are dealing with a smaller number of cases, and the question arises as to whether we have adequate power to meaningfully conduct an analysis of a subset of cases.

Suppose that we have decided on an overall design strategy that calls for 405 NHL cases and an identical number of controls, the number required for the global test. However, we are also interested in subjects with the follicular cell histology, which generally comprises about 20% of the cases. The analysis will involve a comparison of this subgroup of cases with the controls, so now the ratio of controls to

```
options nocenter;

%let r = 5.0;                   *Ratio of controls to cases;
%let b = log(2)/4;              *Effect size;
%let n = 81;                    *Sample size;

data study;

sum = 0;                        *Intermediate calculation for alpha;
do x=-2 to 2;
sum = sum + exp(x*&b);
end;

alpha = log(5/(&r*sum));        *Estimate of alpha;

do x=-2 to 2;                   *Create variable for analysis;
eta1 = alpha + x*&b;            *Linear predictor;
pr = exp(eta1)/(1+exp(eta1));   *Probability of case;
wt = .2*&r*(1 + exp(eta1));     *Weight;
output;
end;

proc genmod data=study;         *Model for linear trend;
p = _mean_;  y = _resp_;
fwdlink link = log(p/(1-p));
invlink ilink = exp(_xbeta_)/(1+exp(_xbeta_));
variance var = p*(1-p);
deviance dev = 2*(y*log(y/p) + (1-y)*log((1-y)/(1-p)));
scwgt wt;
model pr = x / type3;
make 'Type3LR' out=tests;
run;

data ss;  set tests;
test = cinv(0.95,DF);
power = 1-probchi(test,DF,&n*CHISQ);

proc print;  run;
```

Figure 11–5 SAS procedure for finding the power for the case-control study in Example 11–7 (continued).

cases will be 5. Clearly, we will not have adequate power for the global test with 4 df, but what is the power if we look at the much more focused test for linear trend?

Figure 11–5 shows a revision of the SAS program in Figure 11–3 and is designed to address the question of power for linear trend. We have, of course, added a macro for specifying the sample size, but, more important, we made use of the "MAKE" statement in PROC GENMOD to create a SAS file that adds the contribution of a single observation to the noncentrality parameter, which may be computed using the function for finding probabilities for the noncentral chi-square distribution. In the subsequent "DATA STEP" toward the end of the program, we use the noncentrality parameter to find the power, that is, the probability that the test statistic lies in the rejection region, given the alternative hypothesis. We compute the power by using the SAS function for finding probabilities for the non-

```
                          The GENMOD Procedure

                  Criteria For Assessing Goodness Of Fit

              Criterion            DF        Value      Value/DF
              Scaled Deviance       3       0.0000       0.0000
              Scaled Pearson X2     3       0.0000       0.0000
              Log Likelihood        .       0.0000          .

                     Analysis Of Parameter Estimates

         Parameter    DF    Estimate    Std Err   ChiSquare  Pr>Chi
         INTERCEPT     1     -1.6393     1.1229      2.1311   0.1443
         X             1      0.1733     0.7895      0.0482   0.8263
         SCALE         0      1.0000     0.0000         .        .
NOTE:  The scale parameter was held fixed.

                     LR Statistics For Type 3 Analysis

              Source        DF    ChiSquare  Pr>Chi
              X              1      0.0491    0.8247


OBS    SOURCE    DF      CHISQ     PVALC      TEST      POWER

 1       X        1     0.0491    0.8247    3.84146   0.51356
```

Figure 11–6 Output from the SAS procedure shown in Figure 11–5.

central chi-square distribution. The resulting output for this program in Figure 11–6 shows that the noncentrality parameter is $\nu = (81)(0.0491) = 3.98$, which yields a power of 51%. Clearly, we do not have adequate power to detect linear trend if the effect of exposure is such that the odds ratio comparing lowest to highest quintiles is 2.0. Further calculation suggests that if that odds ratio were 2.5 we would have 74% power, and 3.0 would have 88% power, somewhat higher effects than what we originally considered to be of interest. Hence, we must thoughtfully reconsider our overall design strategy, either by justifying consideration of the larger effect size or by increasing the number of cases and perhaps reducing the number of controls to save some of the costs of data collection. We should always be careful to be honest when introducing larger effects after an unfavorable power assessment. If smaller effects are indeed of great importance, then the unfavorable power result is really just preventing us from wasting our efforts on a study that is not likely to find an important result even if it were true.

As we well know at this stage, the generalized linear model framework does not limit us to the consideration of linear logistic models, but we can also consider alternative models for risk. In addition, we are not limited to the consideration of just a few categories when exposure is measured as a continuous variable, but, instead, we can include the actual level of the exposure variable. A continuous exposure requires that we specify the distribution of the measure in the population to be studied. To be completely rigorous in formulating our estimates of the noncentrality parameter would require an analytical approach, which is mathematically more difficult. However, we can obtain an excellent approximate result by taking a very fine categorization of that distribution, and then use results from fitting this model to make the sample size calculations.

Covariate adjustment

Because the methods employed in this section involve model fitting, they are extremely flexible in that they allow one to investigate the sample size or power for virtually any question that can be framed in the context of the generalized linear models we have discussed. Stratified analyses and covariate adjustment are among the most relevant questions that might be raised at the design phase of a study, and the effects that they can have on power can be explored using the methods described here. The most awkward part of making the sample size calculation is in specifying the distribution of the covariates or strata, and in identifying their effect on the response. If we are launching a new study on a population that has been studied before, we can use information on the distribution from the earlier study.

Suppose that we are planning to conduct a case-control study, and we know the distribution of covariate categories in the population at large. In the previous section, the categories were quintiles, or equal proportions in each group for the controls. However, in general, the proportion can vary, and we let w_i^*, $\sum_i w_i^* = 1$, represent the proportion of the general population that falls into the covariate and exposure category i, which we would expect to also reflect the distribution among the controls in our study. The ratio of controls to cases is r; therefore, the proportion of controls expected in the overall study population would be $r \cdot w_i^*/(1 + r)$. The overall proportion of cases in the study would be $1/(1 + r)$, but the proportion in the ith category would be governed by the model that defines the effect of the covariates on disease. If we have a log-linear odds model, then the ratio of cases to controls would be given by $\exp\{\alpha + \beta_i\}$. The β's would be determined by the effect of the covariates on disease, but the intercept, α, depends on the overall proportion of cases that we are trying to achieve. This can be found by solving

$$\sum_i \frac{r w_i^*}{1+r} \cdot \exp\{\alpha + \beta_i\} = \frac{r \exp\{\alpha\}}{1+r} \sum_i w_i^* \exp\{\beta_i\} = \frac{1}{1+r}$$

for α, yielding

$$\exp\{\alpha\} = (r \cdot \sum_i w_i^* \exp\{\beta_i\})^{-1}$$

The resulting proportion of cases in each category is

$$\Pr\{\text{Case} \mid i\} = \frac{\exp\{\alpha + \beta_i\}}{1 + \exp\{\alpha + \beta_i\}}$$

Finally, we also need to find overall weights for each stratum in the study population, which will reflect the proportion in each category that we expect to occur in our study,

$$w_i = w_i^* \cdot \frac{r\,(1 + \exp\{\alpha + \beta_i\})}{1 + r}$$

Example 11–8   Suppose that we are planning a case-control study in which we will need to control for age, because we know that age is associated with both the exposure of interest and disease. We are planning to employ five 10-year age categories, beginning with 20–29, coded by $X_a = -2, -1, 0, 1, 2$. The age distribution in the population is known to be 0.250, 0.225, 0.200, 0.175, and, 0.150. Exposure is coded as -0.5 and 0.5 for unexposed and exposed, respectively. The odds ratio for the association between age and exposure is given by $\gamma_{ae} * (\Delta e) * (\Delta a)$, where Δe and Δa represent the change in the dummy variable for exposure and decade of age, respectively. Therefore, the proportion exposed in each age group is given by

$$\Pr(X_e, X_a) = (\text{Proportion in age group}) \cdot \frac{\exp\{X_e X_a \gamma_{ae}\}}{1 + \exp\{X_e X_a \gamma_{ae}\}}$$

Figure 11–7 gives a SAS program for calculating the contribution of a single observation to the noncentrality parameter. The macros at the beginning define the association parameters that identify the effects of interest in the alternative hypothesis, along with those that determine the distribution of age and exposure. First, the program reads in the age distribution, calculating the initial weights, w_i^*, that would identify the distribution of exposure and age in the population at large, as well as the odds or case to control ratio. Next, we find the weighted sum of the odds using PROC MEANS, an intermediate calculation for determining the intercept term, α. This enables us to calculate the proportion of cases in each category, which is the response for the linear logistic model under H_a. The revised weights, w_i, reflect the distribution of the study population in each category. We double check the program by calculating the weighted mean of the proportion of cases using the new weight, which should give rise to the proportion sought in our design; thus, if $r = 2$, a third of the population should be cases. Finally, we use PROC GENMOD to fit the model, using the likelihood ratio statistic to determine the contribution of an observation to the likelihood ratio statistic.

Results from running the program in Figure 11–7 are shown in Figure 11–8. The PROC MEANS output are not shown to save space, but they revealed that we have indeed succeeded in achieving the desired ratio of controls to cases. Notice that in Example 11.7, we set up the weights so that they sum to 1 for cases, but

```
%let c_e_age = log(1.5);        *Association between exposure and age;
%let b_age = log(1.5);          *Association between age and disease;
%let b_e = log(2);              *Association between exposure and disease;
%let r = 2;                     *Ratio of controls to cases;
*                                                                      ;
*Enter age distribution and create population age/exposure distribution;
data one;  input age wt &&;
dummy=1;                        *Dummy variable used in merge
*                     ;
*Calculate odds and weight;
do e = -0.5 to 0.5 by 1;
        odds = exp(age*&b_age + e*&b_e);
        w_star = wt/(1+exp(-e*age*&c_e_age)); output;  end;
cards;
-2 0.250   -1 0.225    0 0.200    1 0.175    2 0.150
*                     ;
*Intermediate calculation for intercept;
proc means noprint;  var odds;  weight w_star;
output out=intercpt sum=wodds_t; run;
data intercpt(keep=dummy wodds_t);  set intercpt;
dummy=1;
*                     ;
*Calculate proportion cases and weights;
data two;
merge intercpt one; by dummy;
data two;  set two;
e_alpha = 1/(&r*wodds_t);            *Exponential of intercept;
pr = (e_alpha*odds)/(1+e_alpha*odds);  *Proportion cases;
w = w_star*&r*(1+e_alpha*odds)/(1+&r);  *Revised weight;
proc print;  run;                    *Display hypothetical population;
*                     ;
*Fit model to find contribution to noncentrality parameter;
proc genmod;
p = _mean_;  y = _resp_;
fwdlink link = log(p/(1-p));
invlink ilink = exp(_xbeta_)/(1+exp(_xbeta_));
variance var = p*(1-p);
deviance dev = 2*(y*log(y/p) + (1-y)*log((1-y)/(1-p)));
scwgt w;
model pr = age e / type3;
make 'Type3LR' out=tests noprint;
run;
proc print;  attrib chisq format=12.6;  run;
```

Figure 11–7 SAS procedure for finding the noncentrality parameter contribution for a case-control study with log-linear odds model with covariate in Example 11–8.

in this example the sum of all weights is 1. There is no practical difference in these two approaches, only that the former calculated the contribution of a case to the noncentrality parameter, while we are now considering a study subject. Hence, the contribution of a single observation to the noncentrality parameter is 0.022833 for the effect of exposure. If we are going to use a 5% level of significance, and wish to achieve 80% power, then from Table 11–2 we see that the overall noncentrality parameter required is 7.8489. Therefore, the total sample size needed is 7.8489/0.022833 = 343.8, or about 344. Hence, we need to recruit 115 cases and 230 controls.

OBS	WODDS_T	DUMMY	AGE	WT	E	ODDS	W_STAR	E_ALPHA	PR	W
1	1.14550	1	-2	0.250	-0.5	0.31427	0.15000	0.43649	0.12063	0.11372
2	1.14550	1	-2	0.250	0.5	0.62854	0.10000	0.43649	0.21529	0.08496
3	1.14550	1	-1	0.225	-0.5	0.47140	0.12386	0.43649	0.17065	0.09957
4	1.14550	1	-1	0.225	0.5	0.94281	0.10114	0.43649	0.29155	0.09517
5	1.14550	1	0	0.200	-0.5	0.70711	0.10000	0.43649	0.23585	0.08724
6	1.14550	1	0	0.200	0.5	1.41421	0.10000	0.43649	0.38168	0.10782
7	1.14550	1	1	0.175	-0.5	1.06066	0.07866	0.43649	0.31646	0.07672
8	1.14550	1	1	0.175	0.5	2.12132	0.09634	0.43649	0.48077	0.12370
9	1.14550	1	2	0.150	-0.5	1.59099	0.06000	0.43649	0.40984	0.06778
10	1.14550	1	2	0.150	0.5	3.18198	0.09000	0.43649	0.58140	0.14333

The GENMOD Procedure

Criteria For Assessing Goodness Of Fit

Criterion	DF	Value	Value/DF
Scaled Deviance	7	0.0000	0.0000
Scaled Pearson X2	7	0.0000	0.0000
Log Likelihood	.	-0.0000	.

Analysis Of Parameter Estimates

Parameter	DF	Estimate	Std Err	ChiSquare	Pr>Chi
INTERCEPT	1	-0.8290	2.3566	0.1237	0.7250
AGE	1	0.4055	1.6473	0.0606	0.8056
E	1	0.6931	4.6410	0.0223	0.8813
SCALE	0	1.0000	0.0000	.	.

NOTE: The scale parameter was held fixed.

OBS	SOURCE	DF	CHISQ	PVALC
1	AGE	1	0.064883	0.7989
2	E	1	0.022833	0.8799

Figure 11–8 Output from the SAS procedure shown in Figure 11–7.

Interactions

The variation of the effect of a factor over the levels of one or more co-variates can be described by the inclusion of interaction (or product) terms as the regressor variables in a model. This regression framework also enables us to make sample size and power calculations for interactions, as we can see in the following example.

Example 11–7 (continued)   Let us return to the previous example that considered exposure and the effect of age. Suppose that we are interested in whether the effect of exposure on disease risk varies with age. One way of addressing that question is to pose a situation in which the effect of exposure on the log odds for disease varies linearly with age, a hypothesis that can be tested by adding the product of exposure and age and making an inference on its corresponding parameter, β_{ae}. Using the same coding scheme as before, the difference between the odds for disease in the youngest age group and the oldest would be 4 β_{ae}. Suppose that the interaction effect is equal to the main effect for exposure, which was $\beta_e = \log(2)$ in the previous example. This would suggest a value for the interaction of $\log(2)/4$ under the alternative hypothesis. Modifying the SAS program shown in Figure 11–7 to include the interaction term (not shown) gives rise to the contribution of a single observation to the noncentrality parameter of 0.00254661, thus resulting in an overall sample size required to test this parameter using a two-tailed test with a 5% significance level and a power of 80% of $n = 7.8489/0.00254661 = 3,082.1$. This value is huge compared to the sample size we needed to look for the main effect of exposure. Of course, an interaction effect that is equal to a main effect of exposure is unusual, because it is often more likely that we will find interaction effects that are smaller than the main effects. Suppose that we are really interested in an interaction that is half as large as the main effect. Repeating the method just described indicates that we would need to recruit $n = 7.8489 / 0.00064727 = 12,126.2$ subjects.

As the previous example illustrates, the sample sizes required to investigate interactions are generally huge in comparison to what is needed for main effects. Even when the interaction effect is equal to the main effect, a much larger sample size is needed, so that the size of a study becomes gigantic when we propose an investigation of the much smaller effects that are often more realistic. It is usually beyond the resources of the typical epidemiologic study to set out to investigate the modification of a particular exposure by another factor, unless we are honestly looking for very large effects. Such an exception can arise in studies of gene–environment interactions, in which the regressor variables of interest are indicators of a particular gene polymorphism and exposure to some factor. In this situation, it is much more realistic to anticipate large interactions, which can often give rise to sample size estimates that are more in line with the resources that are typically available to a study.

Simulation

All of the techniques for estimating sample size that have been considered to this point involve the use of large-sample approximations, which may not work well, especially when the sample size is not large. Simulation offers a way of running literally thousands of studies using the conditions set out in a proposed study design, thus enabling one to see whether the approximations are sufficiently accurate. It also allows one to introduce new elements into the process that would be difficult to incorporate into the type of analytic approach that we have been using.

One of the most common questions we might wish to confirm is the power of the study. Recall that power is defined to be the probability that the null hypothesis is rejected if indeed the alternative hypothesis is true. We can directly estimate power in a simulation study by generating hypothetical data using the random mechanism that is appropriate, analyzing the results using the method established in the research protocol, and then determining the proportion of these studies that do in fact reject the null hypothesis.

Summary

In this chapter, we have considered the sample size and power aspects of study design. Before these calculations can be made, one must first consider other aspects of design, especially the study aims, which can help clarify whether it is sufficient to demonstrate an effect or whether one needs to estimate effect with some precision. Other fundamental design choices are whether a cohort study is needed, instead of the generally more efficient case-control approach, or whether matching would be appropriate. Once these have been decided, one can proceed with some of the details of sample size calculations.

We first considered sample size from the perspective of estimation, in which the confidence interval indicated the level of precision desired for the study. This required the introduction of an additional arbitrary element into the calculation, the confidence level. Values of 90% and 95% are commonly employed, but occasionally one might use 99% if it is critical to know a particular parameter with considerable precision. Hypothesis testing, by contrast, also requires that we specify the power or, equivalently, the Type II error rate, which is the complement of power. In these instances, values of 80% and 90% are most commonly employed, but one should not necessarily be held to these values if there is good reason to employ another value. One should avoid confusing a study's aims by pretending that estimation is the objective, when, in fact, hypothesis testing is more appropriate. This often amounts to setting $z_\beta = 0$ in the formulae given above, which corresponds to 50% power. An agency that is investing in an expensive epidemiologic study will generally not be favorably impressed if they understand that the odds for a successful outcome is similar to that of a coin toss.

The study designs for hypothesis testing that were considered here first involved two group comparisons. In the case of proportions, the sample size calculation required that we know what proportions to expect in the two groups, values that are clearly unknown before the study is carried out. Approximate values can sometimes be gleaned from published studies of similar populations or a small pilot study, but each would provide highly uncertain values for the population to be studied. Hence, one should repeat the calculation for a range of plausible values in order to determine the sensitivity of the estimate to a particular assumption. One should generally err on the side of planning a larger study, which would result in greater precision, than to be caught short at the end of a study with vague conclusions simply due to a lack of sufficient precision.

Sample size calculations involving rates, survival curves, and matching require more detailed assumptions about the level of censoring that will occur or the level of control that will be achieved by the matching. Once again, these are impossible to know with certainty in advance, but exploring a range of values can be very suggestive of the chances of success in a study, and they can point to potential weak links that can be monitored during the course of data collection. Sometimes, procedures can be modified to bring the reality in line with the assumptions that went into the design. For example, if censoring is excessive due to subjects dropping out of a study, one might explore incentives or improvements in follow-up procedures to reduce the number lost to follow-up.

The final approach to power and sample size calculation involved the use of the generalized linear models that we have seen to be extremely powerful methods of data analysis. This technique allows us to explore issues of power, not only for the comparison of more than two groups and trend, but we can also investigate the effect of covariate adjustment and interactions on the power and sample size needs of a study. On the practical side, this requires that we specify a great deal about what is likely to occur in the proposed study. In the case of covariates, not only do we need to give the strength of their association with the outcome, but also we need to specify how they are associated with each other. At some point, these calculations can become so speculative that they will be almost meaningless. Fortunately, covariate adjustment often has little effect on the overall results, so one can have a good estimate of the chance of success for a study by avoiding overly complex conjectures on the effect of many parameters.

Exercises

11.1. An accident has occurred at a chemical plant, and the local health department is planning a survey to estimate the extent of significant exposure to the pesticide that was produced. The level of exposure of interest has been identified, and it is thought that the proportion exposed might be as high as 30%. How many subjects should be sampled so that the width of the 90% confidence limit for the estimate is 5%?

11.2. The director of student health at a college wants to estimate the rate of occurrence for a particular infection among first-year students. Assume that the incidence rate is constant over the academic year, which is 9 months long. How many students should be recruited into the study if the rate is around 0.15 and the 95% confidence boundary is within 5% of the rate?

11.3. In an industrial plant with 1,500 employees, one in three are exposed to high levels of dust which are thought to be related to illness. A 1-year study is being considered to determine whether the incidence rate for a specified disease is the same for those exposed to the dust as those who are not. A 5% level of significance will be used for the test, and there is interest in detecting a rate ratio of 2 or more. How much power does this study have if the rate among the unexposed is 0.1?

11.4. A case-control study is being planned to study an unusual disease for which there are only 100 cases available for study. The strategy to be adopted calls for the use of three times as many controls as cases. The usual 5% significance level will be used to conduct a two-tailed test of the null hypothesis of no difference between the exposure in controls and cases.

   a. What power is available to detect an odds ratio of 2, if the proportion exposed to the factor of interest is 25%?
   b. Holding the exposure proportion fixed at 25%, prepare a graph showing the relationship between power and the odds ratio.
   c. Holding the odds ratio fixed at 2, prepare a graph showing the relationship between power and the exposure prevalence in controls.
   d. Holding the power fixed at 80%, find the minimal detectable odds ratio for an exposure prevalence of 5%, 10%, 15%, . . . , 70%. Draw a graph showing the relationship.

11.5. A matched case-control study is being planned to find a rate ratio of 1.5 for those exposed to those unexposed.

   a. How many discordant pairs will be needed if a significance level of 1% will be used for a two-tailed test with power of 90%?
   b. How many matched pairs will be needed to conduct this study if the prevalence of exposure in controls is 25% and the case-control exposure odds ratio is 4?
   c. Repeat (b) assuming that the case-control exposure odds ratio is 0.25.

11.6. To study the association between pesticide exposure and risk of lymphoma, a case-control study is being planned in which subjects will be divided into quartiles of exposure based on the distribution in controls. A two-tailed significance level of 5% will be used, and 80% is desired.

   a. How many subjects will be required to detect a linear trend with quartile of exposure if the odds ratio for lowest and highest levels of exposure is 1.8?

   b. Another major hypothesis of this study is that of a gene–exposure interaction. Suppose that there is no effect of exposure for those without polymorphism A which occurs in 67% of subjects, but there is a linear trend with quartile of exposure for those with A. How many subjects will be needed for a 5% two-tailed test with power of 80% if the odds ratio for highest versus lowest quartile is 2?

References

1. Fleiss JL. *Statistical Methods for Rates and Proportions.* New York: Wiley, 1981.
2. Friedman LM, Furberg CD, DeMets DL. *Fundamentals of Clinical Trials.* Littleton, MA: PSG Publishing, 1985.
3. Lachin JM. Introduction to sample size determination and power analysis for clinical trials. *Controlled Clinical Trials* 1981;2:93–113.
4. Schoenfeld D. The asymptotic properties of nonparametric tests for comparing survival distributions. *Biometrika* 1981;68:316–319.
5. Freedman LS. Tables of the number of patients required in clinical trials using the logrank test. *Statistics in Medicine* 1982;1:121–129.
6. Hsieh FY. Comparing sample size formulae for trials with unbalanced allocation using the logrank test. *Statistics in Medicine* 1992;11:1091–1098.
7. Lachin JM. Power and sample size evaluation for the McNemar test with application to matched case-control studies. *Statistics in Medicine* 1992;11:1239–1251.
8. Breslow NE, Day NE. *Statistical Methods in Cancer Research.* Lyon: International Agency for Research on Cancer, 1987.
9. Fleiss JL, Levin B. Sample size determination in studies with matched pairs. *Journal of Clinical Epidemiology* 1988;41:727–730.
10. Dupont WD. Power calculations for matched case-control studies. *Biometrics* 1988;44:1157–1168.
11. Miettinen OS. Individual matching with multiple controls in the case of all-or-none responses. *Biometrics* 1969;25:339–355.
12. Walter SD. Matched case-control studies with a variable number of controls per case. *Applied Statistics* 1980;29:172–179.
13. Royston P. Exact conditional and unconditional sample size for pair-matched studies with binary outcome: a practical guide. *Statistics in Medicine* 1993;12:699–712.
14. Agresti A. *Categorical Data Analysis.* New York: Wiley, 1990.
15. Lubin JH, Gail, MH. On power and sample size for studying features of the relative odds of disease. *American Journal of Epidemiology* 1990;131:552–566.

12

Extending Regression Models

Epidemiology continues to use rapidly developing new technologies, and creative approaches to data analysis offer just one aspect of the changes that continue to emerge. In this final chapter, we briefly consider some new directions that are emerging as important tools for the analysis of epidemiological data and which offer extensions to the approaches used in earlier chapters of this text. Some of these methods have been better developed than others, but they are active areas of research that should ultimately provide essential tools to the analytic epidemiologist. We have seen the progression from analytic strategies for comparing groups to the use of regression methods, and, in a real sense, the ideas presented here provide the next logical step in our thinking of approaches to looking at data. In particular, the new directions offer ways of exploring risk without making very restrictive parametric assumptions at the outset, and they provide more ways of accounting for the underlying structure in epidemiologic data by allowing for the imprecision in our estimates of exposure or by allowing for strong relationships among the exposures themselves.

In our discussion of approaches to the analysis of epidemiologic data, we began by considering the comparison of proportions, rates, and times to failure among various risk groups. This could be accomplished either by considering exposure by itself or by stratifying the data based on other known risk factors. We saw that all of these methods could be derived from the perspective of a specified mathematical form for the way in which these factors affect the fundamental quantities in the disease process. In each instance, the equations that specified the form for the relationship could be expressed as a generalized linear model, so the extension to considering analyses in the regression framework was a natural one.

The goal of all of the methods we have considered is to obtain summaries that accurately reflect the data obtained from a study. So it is critical that we get the equation right, or else we will be in danger of being misled by our calculations. In the regression framework, we suggested the strategy of tentatively entertaining a model and then evaluating its fit to the data. If the agreement is poor, we may need to modify the model by including another important covariate, by transforming either the response or a covariate, or by considering the possibility that the effect of one factor is modified by another. This process of trial and validation should proceed until the data analyst is satisfied with the quality of the data description.

An alternative strategy is to establish a flexible analytic framework that allows the form for the relationship between exposure and response to emerge from the data itself. This approach avoids the problem of forcing a specific parametric form for the relationship, thus providing very useful tools for understanding epidemiological data. We shall obtain the flavor of some of these approaches by considering classification trees and spline regression.

A fundamental axiom that underlies the classical approaches to regression analysis is the assumption that the covariates are known without error. However, in the case of exposure, it has now become a fact of life for an epidemiologist that exposure measurements are never fully accurate, even with the increasingly sophisticated measurements that are now feasible to conduct on a routine basis. Even the diagnoses used to classify the outcome for study subjects are prone to error. In addition, the measures themselves can be highly correlated, introducing collinearity among the possible effects, thus making the results difficult to interpret. We shall also discuss some of these issues that are now becoming much more widely addressed at the analysis phase of a study.

Some of the awkwardness of applying these methods arises from the lack of easy access to the techniques in currently available statistical software. Much of this will certainly be resolved in the near future, especially as a consensus begins to develop around the approaches and algorithms that are most promising.

Classification and Regression Trees (CART)

One important problem in epidemiology is the identification of groups who are at very high risk of disease. CART offers one such useful approach to the classification of subjects. The underlying strategy in analyzing data using classification and regression trees is to identify subgroups of the population that are at similar risk to the response of interest. These techniques are based on the work of Brieman et al. (1), who were primarily concerned with applications in which the response was continuous, as in the case of standard regression analysis. However, the essential idea can be directed toward the analysis of any type of outcome, so extensions now include the analysis of epidemiologic data. Hence, a familiar evolution has taken place, beginning with development of these ideas in the context of least squares that are optimal when the response has a normal distribution and are now being extended to other outcomes, including binary responses and censored survival data. A much more detailed discussion of current ideas on these methods of analyses is provided in the text by Zhang and Singer (2).

As we shall see, CART provides simple rules for identifying high- and low-risk groups, unlike a regression method that requires that we first calculate the parameters for a specified combination of regressor variables. This can provide a practical advantage if we are trying to develop a public health strategy that will focus on high-risk subgroups in a population. However, this can also be useful in the formation of strata of individuals with similar levels of risk. Once this has been accomplished, we can employ stratified data analyses, using such techniques as the Mantel–Haenszel statistic and the log-rank test.

Growing trees

The first step in CART is to divide the population into groups with very different levels of the outcome. To draw a diagram of the process, such as the one shown in Figure 12–1, we would start with the entire population, which is represented by the first node, and then draw lines or branches to two daughter nodes which then represent the first partition. We proceed to partition these daughter nodes, continuing this process for as long as we like or until we effectively run out of information so that we cannot partition the data further. The result of this process obviously resembles the formation of a family tree, except that in this formulation each node can only result in two daughters. We have already taken note of the fact that an effect can be missed if we do not control for an important confounder. In the context of forming trees, a similar phenomenon is manifested by the possibility of missing important nodes if we have not first identified nodes that partition the population by these important confounding variables. Hence, it is best to adopt a less rigid stopping rule when growing trees, which can give rise to an overgrown tree with far more nodes than are reasonable for a particular data set. Once such a tree has been grown to its fullest extent, we prune it back because in the process we hope to have stratified the data by all the important confounders that are available in the data set.

Recursive partitioning. Splitting a node results in two daughters, which we can arbitrarily refer to as the left and right daughters. We refer to the criterion for splitting the data into daughter nodes as the combined impurity

$$e_s(i) = p_{i_L}\, e(i_L) + p_{i_R}\, e(i_R) \qquad (12.1)$$

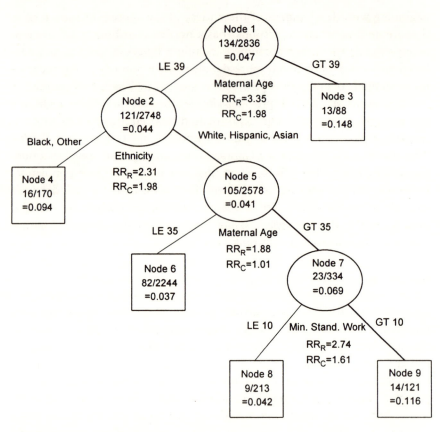

Figure 12–1 Classification tree for factors identifying differential risks of spontaneous abortion.

where p_{i_L} and p_{i_R} are the proportion of subjects in the left and right daughter nodes, respectively, and $e(\cdot)$ is an impurity function that seeks to refine
the daughter nodes by making them more nearly alike and thus more different from each other. In searching for optimal partitions of the data we
will be trying to minimize the combined impurity, e_s.

As an alternative approach to splitting the data based on an impurity
measure, we might think of using a test statistic such as one of those from
Chapter 3. However, the magnitude of a test statistic depends on both the
difference between groups and the sample size. In contrast, the impurity
index given in equation 12.1 only depends on the distribution of subjects
between the daughter nodes, not the actual numbers of subjects. One way
of obtaining a disparity index for the magnitude of difference between two
groups that is not dependent on sample size is to take a chi-square test of
significance and divide it by the number of observations in the parent node.
In this case, we would try to maximize the disparity index, which would

be equivalent to finding the split that maximized the chi-square statistic at a particular node. Often there is a close relationship between a disparity index and a particular impurity index, so that splitting the data to minimize combined impurity is equivalent to splitting to maximize disparity.

Possible subsets that are to be considered as optimal splits of a node may be identified from either ordinal or nominal factors. If the ith factor, x_i, is ordinal, then we must find the constant c, such that subsets, $x_i \leq c$ and $x_i > c$ minimize the combined impurity index, e_s. On the other hand, if x_i represents nominal categories, then we must search for the optimal two-group partition among all possible such subsets of these categories, giving rise to the two daughters, $x_i \in \beta$ and $x_i \notin \beta$. Depending on results of an exhaustive search that identifies the split that yields the most homogeneous two subgroups based on the impurity criterion, we would assign each observation to either the left or the right daughter nodes. It is important to emphasize the fact that a variable is not removed from the analysis once it is used to form a partition. After all, if it is a ordinal variable, there may still be subsets from among those with high or low levels of the factor that have different risks of disease. Likewise, there may still be subsets among the levels of nominal categories that provide additional partitions that are useful risk group classifications.

The process of partitioning the data can continue until (1) all nodes contain only one subject, (2) all subjects at a node exhibit the same response, or (3) all subjects have an identical level for all of the covariates under study. However, we may choose to stop the splitting process before we have reached that point, at which time it is no longer possible to further subdivide the population. For example, we might choose a critical value for the combined impurity score, and once the largest score from among all possible splits is smaller than this value, we would terminate the process. Anytime we stop the process, we must not forget the aforementioned danger of missing important factors that could have been identified when important confounding variables have been allowed to emerge. We have already seen in our discussion of stratified data in Chapter 3 that it is impossible to determine on the basis of a univariate analysis whether a factor may be either a confounding variable or an effect modifier. Hence, the very real possibility exists that we may miss a useful split that would have emerged had we allowed the tree to grow further. It is best to use a very weak stopping rule for tree growing, in an effort to provide every opportunity for important subgroups to emerge, remembering that superfluous branches can always be pruned at a later stage.

Pruning trees. Because of concern about the appropriateness of forward stopping rules that would be applied during the growing phase (1, 2), we choose instead to apply backward stopping rules to the task of pruning an overgrown tree. One suggested approach is to use a conventional significance test with an arbitrary significance level (3, 4). However, the fact that the branches of the tree are selected because they are, in a sense, extreme, we cannot interpret the separate nodes that remain as being statistically significant at the level α. The problem is related to the multiple comparisons problem, although it remains unclear as to what correction would be appropriate. In any case, the spirit of this technique falls into the realm of exploratory data analysis, and firm conclusions about the subsets would generally require the confirmation of further work.

Any automatic method for selecting important risk factors inherently suffers from the fact that the comparisons have not been specified a priori, and thus must be used with caution. Often, alternative splits that make more sense biologically have only slightly different values of the impurity index, a value that could easily be a result of random variation. Hence, we should thoughtfully consider the various splits and not be afraid to intervene by imposing an alternative split when appropriate. In addition, we need to recognize that sometimes additional data may be required before we can confidently conclude that a node has a different level of risk.

Uses of trees. One of the most straightforward uses of trees is in determining estimates of the response of interest in the terminal node. However, we must keep in mind that our final tree was grown by selecting branches that maximized differences between the daughter nodes, which is similar and sometimes identical to choosing daughters that minimize p values, depending on the splitting criterion. So in a sense, our raw results will provide relative risk estimates that are biased away from the null, and we need to consider introducing a necessary correction.

Another use of the terminal nodes is in identifying strata that have relatively homogeneous levels of risk. Once these groups have been identified, we can employ a stratified method of analysis to summarize the final results. In the case of a binary outcome, this might entail the use of Mantel–Haenszel methods, or for survival analysis we might make use of stratification extensions to the log-rank test.

Trees for binary responses

The first application we shall consider involves the use of data with a binary outcome, which is not unlike the situation considered in Chapters 3 and 7. If this outcome is an indicator of disease occurrence, then we need to assume that the time under observation is identical for all subjects.

Criteria for partitioning and pruning binary data. To split the observations at a given nodes, we need to first adopt an optimization criterion. As we already noted, CART was first developed in the standard regression framework (1), which led to the use of the error mean square as the measure of impurity within the daughter nodes. However, for a binary outcome we prefer to use a different measure of impurity. Two commonly used impurity measures for categorical responses are the entropy criterion and the Gini diversity index.

The entropy criterion at the ith node is $e(i) = -p_i \log(p_i) - (1 - p_i) \log(1 - p_i)$, where p_i is the proportion of failures at the ith node. If N_i is the number of observation at the ith node, then

$$N_i \, e(i) = \log[p_i^{N_i p_i} (1 - p_i)^{N_i (1 - p_i)}]$$

Because $N_i p_i$ is the expected number of failures, we can see a direct relationship between this measure of impurity and the log likelihood. In fact, we can readily show that the criterion of minimizing the total impurity at a given node is equivalent to maximizing the significance level based on a likelihood ratio test.

The Gini diversity index considers the sum of squared differences between the observed and expected proportions. For a binary outcome, the mean proportion for responders and non-responders is

$$\frac{p_i + (1 - p_i)}{2} = \frac{1}{2}$$

Hence, the total sum of squares becomes

$$(p_i - \tfrac{1}{2})^2 + (1 - p_i - \tfrac{1}{2})^2 = 2(p_i - \tfrac{1}{2})^2$$
$$= 2 \, p_i \, (1 - p_i) + \tfrac{1}{4}$$

The added constant will not influence the selection of subgroups, thus we can reduce this impurity criterion to $e^*(i) = 2 \, p_i \, (1 - p_i)$. The fact that we can motivate this criterion on the basis of the difference between the observed and expected proportions squared, points to the fact that the measure is related to the Pearson chi-square statistic.

Figure 12–2 plots both the entropy and the Gini diversity index as a function of p, and we can see that the shapes are very similar, with the entropy criterion being only slightly flatter. Hence, it should not be surprising that the results from growing trees based on either criterion are often consistent. In fact, the results from this method tend to be insensitive with respect to most reasonable choices of a convex function for the impurity index.

Trees are grown by using software specifically designed for the purpose. In the following example, a program described in detail by Zhang and Singer (2) was used for the growing a tree.

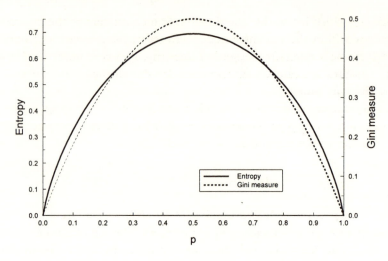

Figure 12–2 Plot of entropy and Gini measures of impurity.

Example 12–1 Bracken et al. (5, 6) conducted a cohort study of factors associated with increased risk of spontaneous abortion. In this analysis, 13 candidate factors were used to identify the risk groups: maternal age, alcohol consumption, used birth control, chronic health problems, used cocaine, coffee consumption, commuted to work, education, ethnicity, number of times reached over shoulder at job, smoked, minutes per day of standing at work, and weight at last menstrual period. After the tree is grown and then pruned, we have the result shown in Figure 12–1. Starting at node 1, which includes all subjects, the first split is based on maternal age, in that mothers who were older than 39 had 3.35 times the rate of spontaneous abortion when compared to younger women. The next split divided those 39 or younger on the basis of ethnicity, indicating that those who identified themselves as black or other had 2.31 times the risk of those who were white, Hispanic, or Asian. Node 5 is once again split on the basis of maternal age, only this time the cut point is at age 35, thus illustrating the way in which continuous variables can enter into the classification procedure more than once, which is the way in which more than one level of risk can be identified for a single factor.

Notice that in this approach, the terminal nodes that identify different risk groups are reached by traversing a decision tree based on the factors of interest. In the context of a regression model, we would have had to identify these groups using not only main effects, but higher order interactions. For example, nodes 8 and 9 are reached through a set of conditions that depend on a combination of maternal age, ethnicity, and the length of time spent standing at work.

Estimating effects for categories. We have already noted the problem with using a significance tests when comparing the risk between two daughter nodes due to the fact that the comparison was not specified a priori, but arose instead from the impurity criterion. Similarly, a bias will be present in an estimate of relative risk between two daughter nodes. This arises because in trying to minimize the impurity index we tend to select splits that have odds ratios different from the null value, 1. Suppose that we represent the observed results of a split as here:

Node	Healthy	Diseased
Left	a	b
Right	c	d

in which the crude odds ratio given by

$$OR = \frac{a\,d}{c\,d} \tag{12.2}$$

Without loss of generality, we shall assume that OR is greater than 1. Let the true frequencies be represented by a^*, b^*, c^*, and d^*, respectively. Because of the criterion for selecting the splits, the tendency is for $E[a] > a^*$, $E[b] < b^*$, $E[c] < c^*$, and $E[d] > d^*$. Hence, the crude odds ratio will tend to be biased, or larger than the true odds ratio.

Cross-validation offers one approach for correcting the bias that arises from the process of growing a tree (4). The population is divided at random into I subpopulations, with $I = 5$ being a typical number. Let P_i ($i = 1,2, \ldots, I$) denote each of these subpopulations and $P_{[-i]}$ its corresponding complement. We can use $P_{[-i]}$ as a training sample to select the split based on a selected covariate. The resulting frequencies are $a_{[-i]}$, $b_{[-i]}$, $c_{[-i]}$, and $d_{[-i]}$. We then apply the split obtained from the training sample to the ith sample, resulting in the tabulated frequencies a_i, b_i, c_i, and d_i. This process is repeated for all subsamples, and we estimate the bias in a by finding

$$\text{Max}\left\{ \frac{1}{4} \sum_{i=1}^{I} a_{[-i]} - \sum_{i=1}^{I} a_i, a - \frac{1}{2} \right\}$$

The bias for c is the negative of the bias estimate for a, and a similar technique is used to estimate the biases for b and d. The observed frequencies are corrected accordingly, followed by a recalculation of the odds ratio using these adjusted estimates of the cell frequencies used in equation 12.2.

Example 12–1 (continued) We continue to consider the study investigating the groups with excess risk of spontaneous abortion. The crude relative risk for each for each node, RR_R, is calculated in the usual way by taking the observed tabulated values formed by the split. Along with the estimate RR_R, Figure 12–1 shows the five-fold cross-validation estimate, RR_C, which corrects for the bias that results from using the tree-growing algorithm. Notice that in each case the cross-validation estimator has been attenuated; that is, it is nearer to the null value of 1.

Forming strata with homogeneous risks. CART offers a powerful technique for forming strata that have similar levels of disease risk. In Chapter 3 we discussed methods for analyzing stratified data, thus combining these techniques with a tree-based method for forming strata offers an alternative to the regression approach for obtaining adjusted estimates of risk (6). In this approach to data analysis, we first form strata with similar levels or disease risk, by forming a tree based on the set of potential confounding variables, using disease status as the response.

As before, we first grow an extended tree and then prune the branches that did not offer subgroups that were truly different. The terminal nodes from this tree will provide us with strata with similar levels of risk for developing disease based on the set of potential confounding variables. We now introduce the J-level factor of interest, and obtain a $2 \times J$ table that can be analyzed using a stratified method of analysis. From this point, the analysis follows the ideas we developed in Chapter 3, in that we can employ Mantel–Haenszel techniques for estimating and testing overall adjusted estimates of the odds ratio. As before, we also need to consider whether the odds ratio is homogeneous over the strata by evaluating the odds ratios within each strata, and perhaps conducting a significance test for homogeneity.

The formation of strata with similar levels of disease risk is reminiscent of Miettinen's method of multivariate confounder scores (7). In this approach, linear discriminant analysis was used to obtain a score, which was then categorized to form subgroups with similar estimates of the probability of developing disease. A major difference with the use of CART is that linear discriminant analysis relies on a highly parametric model that is closely related to logistic regression, while CART does not.

One of CART's strengths arises because there is no need for a priori specification of a formal model for the association between the factors of interest and the response. If we were to try to describe the types of exposure–response relationships allowed by this approach using a regression model, we would need to not only include a nonparametric form for the effect of each factor but would need to allow for high-level interactions. Yet with the efficient software that has been developed for ever more powerful computers, we are able to handle large numbers of factors in the analysis. Hence, this method appears to be especially useful for exploratory analyses, in that it is a good way to identify subsets of the data with exceptionally high or low risk of disease.

There remain certain aspects of commonly used statistical ideas that do not currently transfer easily into tree-based methods. In a well-designed study, we specify the primary hypotheses about the exposure–response association before we have begun to collect data, and the data analysis is directed toward answering that question. If we were to just include this factor along with many others in CART, we might never see an estimate of the association of primary interest, and we would thus be derelict in our mission to address a primary study aim. In addition, part of this aim may require a formal significance test to determine whether the evidence for an association had achieved a specified standard. The primary value of CART lies in its ability to offer a potentially useful way of forming strata in order to adjust for potential confounding variables, and in secondary analyses of data that can be important for generating hypotheses that merit further study in the search for the etiology of a disease.

The investigation of whether the odds ratios are in fact homogeneous among strata identified by terminal nodes may suggest that the association is different between low- and high-risk subgroups. This is related to the idea of looking at interactions between exposure and the covariates, although it is conceptually quite different. In forming the interactions, we must specify in our model that the modification of effect is identified with one or more factors, rather than the level of risk. For example, suppose that we are evaluating a particular treatment, and we are adjusting for several factors associated with disease risk. If the treatment had greater efficacy among high-risk patients, then we might need to include many interaction terms in a regression model in order to adequately describe that phenomenon. A tree-based method, however, would produce subsets with a range of risks, and we might expect the pattern to emerge quite readily. Nevertheless, if the underlying pharmacology for the treatment was modified by just one of the potential confounding variables, then a regression model would be a more direct method for investigating the modified effect.

CART for survival data

In our discussion of the analysis of failure-time data, we noticed that several of the methods of analysis bore a strong resemblance to methodology used in the analysis of contingency tables. Hence, it should not surprise us that we can extend some of the basic approaches we have just discussed to the analysis of survival data. The basic concepts for growing and pruning trees remain unchanged, but the choice of the splitting criterion must be modified to incorporate the censored failure-time data. The application of tree methods for survival data are described by a number of authors (3, 8–11), including the text by Zhang and Singer (2).

Splines

We have seen that regression models offer a great deal of flexibility in formulating and testing a hypothesis, as discussed in Chapter 7. They can even be used to represent polynomial effects for continuous measures of exposure, thus avoiding the restriction to effects that are straight lines. While it is true that any set of responses associated with a set of exposures can be exactly fitted with a polynomial curve, we also saw an example in which a high-degree polynomial was required to fit the observed data, and the resulting fitted curve could be very unstable and unrealistic, especially at the ends. Splines offer an alternative representation for the effect of a continuous exposure that is both more flexible and more stable than high-degree polynomials, and as such they can provide a useful way for providing a visual display of the relationship between dose and response.

Linear splines

The most basic spline representation of the effect of a continuous variable is a broken line or linear spline. Fitting such a model is a bit like trying to make a plastic straw conform to a complicated curve. The straw essentially remains straight but will crimp at some point when it is forced to bend, thus forming an angle at various points along the straw with straight sections in between, rather than forming a smooth curve. A similar exercise with a dry stick might result in line segments that were discontinuous, but the plastic straw does not physically disconnect between straight line segments, providing instead a continuous line from beginning to end.

To represent a linear spline, we must first specify the points along the x axis at which the bends occur, called *knots*, which can be represented by $\xi_1, \xi_2, \ldots \xi_I$. The spline function is given by

$$\zeta(z) = \beta_0 + z\beta_1 + \sum_{i=1}^{I} (z - \xi_i)_+ \gamma_i \qquad (12.1)$$

where z is the continuous regressor variable of interest, and $(z - \xi_i)_+$ is a special function that takes the value $(z - \xi_i)$ when the difference is positive and is 0 otherwise. For values of z to the left of the first knot ($z < \xi_1$), the function is described by the straight line, $\zeta(z) = \beta_0 + z\beta_1$. Also, at the knot itself there is no discontinuity, but instead the change in slope becomes $\beta_1 + \gamma_1$; thus, the interpretation of the first parameter in the summation is the change in slope at the knot. Similar phenomena occur at the subsequent knots, so that the continuity is maintained and the slope changes by an amount indicated by the introduction of the next parameter, γ_i.

The adoption of linear splines clearly offers a flexible framework for describing a relationship between dose and response. In addition, once the knots have been identified, the process reduces to one in which the researcher creates a set of variables that enter the regression model as additive terms associated with a parameter that is to be estimated. Hence, the framework of generalized linear models is easily adapted to the problem of fitting models of this kind.

Polynomial splines

An obvious disadvantage to linear splines is that nature usually does not behave in a way that results in sudden changes in slope. Instead, we are more likely to encounter a relationship that is represented by smooth curves instead of series of sharp angles. To begin the process of describing a more complex curve, one can extend the linear spline to the case of a second-order polynomial. In this case, we wish to have the second-order polynomial be continuous at the knot, but we do not wish to see a sharp angle at that point. The angle is produced by a sudden change in the slope, which can be represented quantitatively by specifying that a graph of the slope itself be continuous. (In the terminology of calculus, this is referred to as a condition of continuous first derivatives.) A second-order or quadratic spline may be expressed as

$$\zeta(z) = \beta_0 + z\beta_1 + z^2\beta_2 + \sum_{i=1}^{I} (z - \xi_i)^2_+ \, \gamma_i \tag{12.2}$$

Similarly, one can continue the process of constructing higher-order splines, although in general, cubic splines have been found to work very well in practice:

$$\zeta(z) = \beta_0 + z\beta_1 + z^2\,\beta_2 + z^3\,\beta_3 + \sum_{i=1}^{I} (z - \xi_i)^3_+ \, \gamma_i \tag{12.3}$$

This curve can be fitted using the standard regression model software we have been using throughout this text by introducing the regressor variables:

$$X_1 = z$$
$$X_2 = z^2$$
$$X_3 = z^3$$
$$X_4 = (z - \xi_1)_+{}^3$$
$$\dots X_{I+3} = (z - \xi_I)_+{}^3$$

In general, one does not attempt to interpret the individual regression co-efficients from this model, but to draw a graph of the curve as a way of offering a description of the dose–response relationship.

The parts of the spline curve that remain somewhat unstable for cubic splines are the ends, which have a tendency to bend either up or down to a greater extent than would be expected. A further restriction that has been found to be helpful in alleviating this problem, forces the beginning and end of the curve to be a straight line, as suggested by Durrleman and Simon (12).

In principle, one can construct a hypothesis test in the usual way by adding or dropping the spline regressor variables from the model, but care must be exercised when interpreting these results because a potentially large number of parameters may not offer a sufficiently focused hypothesis to provide reasonable power, and there may be issues of multiple comparisons if multiple sets of spline parameters were considered in the fitting process. An exception to this rule arises in linear splines, in which the parameters are much more readily interpreted. For example, in examining the effect of age on disease risk in women, an a priori point to place a knot is around 50, when menopause often occurs. The spline parameter in this case could suggest that a change in trend might be related to the hormonal changes associated with menopause. Zhou and Shen (13) provide an algorithm for selecting the location of knots.

One practical difficulty in the use of the polynomial splines we have considered arises when we have a large number of knots. This results in covariates that are highly correlated, which can result in numerical instability for the estimates. B splines offer an alternative way of specifying the covariates to be used in the regression and will alleviate the numerical difficulties (14). The fact that the regression parameters associated with each of these regressor variables are difficult to compute does not matter, in a way, because we will actually be basing our conclusions on the curve that estimates the effect of the factor and not on individual parameters that identify the curve.

Example 12–1 Hairston (15) provides data on the age-specific prevalence of *Schistosoma haematobium* in subjects participating in the Egypt-49 project, and the results are displayed in Figure 12–3. A cubic spline was used to describe this curve, placing knots at years 10 and 20, and the fitted curve is also presented in the graph. Overall, the goodness of fit is excellent ($\Delta G^2 = 11.14$, df $= 19$, $p = .919$), and the largest standardized residual was -1.51, indicating that in no particular age group was there evidence of a lack of fit. Hence, by using splines, we were able to obtain a good description of the relationship between age and disease prevalence in this population, even though the curve itself is fairly complex.

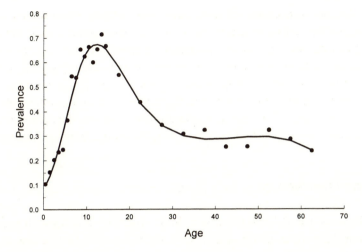

Figure 12-3 Observed and fitted prevalence of *Schistosoma haematobium* by age.

GAMS and MARS

In the previous sections, we have seen that the advantage of adopting a nonparametric approach to data analysis lies in the fact that a strong assumption has not been used in formulating the method. This is especially useful in exploratory approaches to data analysis in which the form for the dose–response relationship emerges from the data, instead of an explicit mathematical form that has been specified a priori. One such set of methods is known as *generalized additive models* (GAMS), in which the form for the effect of regressor variables on the response is given by

$$E[y] = \beta_0 + \zeta_1(X_1) + \zeta_2(X_2) + \cdots + \zeta_I(X_I) \tag{12.4}$$

where $\zeta_i(\cdot)$ is a function to be estimated. Splines offer one possibility, but other options are also available. Hastie and Tibshirani (16, 17) provide a much more complete discussion of this approach to the analysis of multiple covariates.

While GAMS allow complete flexibility for the effect of covariates, it is important to note that the effects are still additive, which implicitly introduces the assumption that the effect of one factor is not modified by another. For two factors, in which one modifies the effect of another, we can represent the result by a surface in a three-dimensional graph. As the number of factors increases, it becomes impossible to represent the joint effects on the response visually, because it becomes a dose–response surface in hyperspace. One approach to fitting such surfaces is to consider covariates that take the form described in the previous section, along with products (or interaction terms) between the regressor variables for two or more factors. This method of analysis is referred to as *multivariate adaptive regression splines* (MARS). Obviously the number of possible regression variables grows enormously in this approach, so considerable care is required in selecting the optimal set of covariates. Recursive partitioning offers one such approach to fitting these models, and a more complete discussion of these methods are described by Freedman (18, 19) and Zhang and Singer (2).

Missing Observations

In Chapters 4 and 5 we discussed the problem of dealing with censored or incomplete data that resulted from individuals being withdrawn from observation prior to the occurrence of the event of interest, or being lost to follow-up. Potentially even more serious to the validity of a study is the situation in which data are missing altogether, so that one cannot even identify a range in which observations might occur. Such instances are not uncommon in epidemiologic studies because they rely very heavily on the cooperation of subjects. Hence, an investigator may find that data are missing due to non-response to part of a questionnaire, or to inability on the part of a lab to obtain a valid measurement. This can occur either for the response, or for the regressor variables.

At first, it might seem that dealing with missing data would pose an impossible problem for the analyst, because any approach would appear to be creating data out of thin air. It is clearly best to minimize the amount of incomplete data, but if one has some understanding of the mechanism that gave rise to the missing observations, then one can sometimes glean some useful information that is relevant to the population as a whole. This depends on an accurate understanding of the conduct of the study, otherwise the assumptions involved in applying these methods could invalidate the results. The nomenclature used to characterize the most common mechanisms that are thought to give rise to missing data is described in the texts by Little and Rubin (20) and Schafer (21).

Data that are *missing completely at random (MCAR)* occur when the reason that an observation is missing is independent of both the response and the regressor variables. For example, suppose that a particular variable of interest depends on the analysis of a blood sample determined by a lab, but somehow the test tubes containing the blood were broken in shipment. It is hard to see that the breaking of the tube was the result of anything but an accident, and thus independent of all variables recorded in the study. Hence, the missing lab values would be regarded as MCAR. The most common way for statistical software to deal with missing data is to drop the observation from the analysis, which provides a valid analysis when the MCAR condition holds.

A less restrictive mechanism for the missing data process is referred to as *missing at random (MAR)*, in which the probability that an observation is missing is conditionally independent of the unobserved data given the observed data. Of course, it could still be dependent on either the response or other observed covariates, and the next step in the process would involve the search for a way of characterizing that association among the complete observations. The resulting model would provide a way for imputing a value for each of the missing observations. In this way we can glean additional information on the associations of interest, and thus improve our estimates of association reducing bias and the standard error of the estimator. The advantage we would have in this instance over the case in which the reason for missing data depended on unobserved data is that we can actually use the observed data to formulate some information about the missing observations.

One practical way of dealing with missing data is through multiple imputation (22, 23). The scenario envisioned by this approach arises from a conceptually complete set of data, in which we have only observed a subset of the observations, $\mathbf{Y} = (\mathbf{Y}_{obs}, \mathbf{Y}_{mis})$. By using the observed data, we develop a prediction model that enables us to impute a value for each of the missing observations, $\mathbf{Y}^{(k)} = (\mathbf{Y}_{obs}, \mathbf{Y}_{mis}^{(k)})$, where k(= 1, . . . m) refers to one realization of the imputation process. If this prediction is based on a regression model, the imputed values are not just fitted values, but they would also include an added random error which has mean 0 and standard deviation equal to the root mean square error. Because of this random component in the imputation process, we would obviously obtain a different set of imputed variables each time it was repeated. For each simulated set of complete data obtained by this imputation process, one would carry out the analysis as if the data were complete, thus giving rise to a different set of parameter estimates for each imputation, $b_j^{(k)}$ in the case of the kth estimate of the jth model parameter. Let m represent the number of times this process is carried out. The final estimate would be the average of these estimates, $\bar{b}$. Of course, our estimate of the variance of this quantity would have to reflect the fact that we had simulated the "complete" data, thus giving rise to the standard error

$$\text{se}(\bar{b}_j) = \sqrt{(1 + m^{-1})\, B + \overline{W}_j}$$

where $\overline{W}_j$ is the mean of the within sample variances obtained for each imputed sample, and B is the between sample variance, $B = (m - 1)^{-1} \sum_k (b_j^{(k)} - \bar{b}_j)$. In general, the method works well when m is between 5 and 10.

Other alternatives for dealing with this important problem include the use of maximum likelihood estimation through the use of the EM algorithm (24). One approach for implementing this algorithm is the method of weights, described by Horton and Laird (25). In this approach, the combinations of possible realizations of the missing observations are added to form an augmented data set, and each of these is given a weight that corresponds to the probability that it occurs. These weights depend on parameters that are estimated at each cycle of the iterative process, which is repeated until the estimates converge. Still another alternative involves the use of Bayesian methods, and can be implemented using Markov chain Monte Carlo (MCMC) techniques (26). For many years Bayesian approaches to inference were avoided because of the difficulty in obtaining computationally effective ways of conducting the analysis. The rapid increase of computing power along with the development of effective simulation algorithms have made these techniques much more accessible to the data analyst, thus providing effective ways of handling many problems that arise in epidemiology, including missing data.

The final group of missing data approaches arises when we have neither MCAR nor MAR, that is they are said to be missing not at random (MNAR). These are the most difficult situations to deal with analytically because they depend on strong assumptions, that may be impossible to verify due to the fact that the reason the observation is missing may depend on information that is itself missing. These issues can be especially critical when repeated observations are taken longitudinally on each subject in a study. A review of some models for dealing with incomplete data in these situations are discussed in the text by Diggle, Liang and Zeger (27) and by Kenward and Molenberghs (28).

Variance Components

The simpler statistical models used in data analysis involve just a single component of random variation which is characterized by its variance. For example, if blood pressure is to be compared among two or more groups then one might take one measurement for each individual, and compare the means among the populations. If we were to modify this hypothetical experiment by taking more than one blood pressure measurement for each subject, we would see that the variability in each group actually has more than one component, that is variation from individual-to-individuals and variation among the repeated observations taken on each individual. The former is summarized by between subjects variance, and the latter by within subjects variance. In the early statistics literature, this was referred to as a variance components problem, but in the current literature on statistical methods in epidemiology is may be called hierarchical or multi-level modeling.

To see more clearly how this hierarchy of variation can be important to the understanding of the development of disease, consider attempts to model the effect of CD4 lymphocyte counts on risk of developing AIDS. At one level, one would need to develop a model that described the CD4 trends within each individual along with their underlying variability, and then we would need to use this information to estimate the association between these model parameters and risk of developing AIDS, which would in itself include a random component. Reviews of some of the approaches that have been used in dealing with these complex statistical models are provided by Boscardin, Taylor and Law (29) and Hogan and Laird (30).

The need to deal with these different levels of variation can arise whenever we combine data in which each observation is itself determined with a level of precision that can be estimated. Meta-analysis offers a useful way of summarizing various clinical trials that have been conducted to address a particular clinical question. Each trial estimates the effect of treatment with a reported precision, but the effect in each trial may also have its own component of random variation about a hypothetical super population of all possible clinical trials that could be modeled with a hierarchical model (31, 32). Similarly, disease mapping can give rise to models with multiple levels of random error that would include not only to the error associated with estimates of rates for each defined geographic region, but a component due to a spatially related component. In this case, the random spatial components may not be independent, complicating the model still further. For example, if exposure to a causal agent varied among regions, it may be plausible that disease rates for regions that are close together are more highly correlated than are regions that are far apart. Methods for dealing with these types of data are described by (33–37). In addition, a review of the various methods that can be used for this class of models is provided by Breslow, Leroux and Platt (38).

Errors in Variables

The assessment of exposure has become increasingly sophisticated, enabling epidemiologists to more closely determine the basic chemicals or agents that may cause disease. However, in many instances, this added detail has brought home the fact that inherent difficulties remain, which can cause considerable instability in the estimates of risk associated with those exposures. One source of instability arises from inaccuracies of measurement, or measurement error. In the simplest case in which the error is random and unbiased, this often will attenuate the estimates of risk—introduce a bias in the estimate that tends toward the null value. On the one hand, this could be viewed as providing a conservative estimate of risk, so that if an association is found it will tend to be real, and thus increase confidence in the result. But on the other hand, there is a real possibility that an association will be missed, leaving us unaware of factors that really do affect disease risk.

In more complex situations in which exposure to multiple factors are under consideration in the same study, it is not necessarily true that the estimator will always be attenuated, even when the measurement is random. There are now a variety of methods available for correcting estimates of association for measurement error, and these are described in the text by Carroll, Rupert, and Stephanski (39). Some of these methods introduce correction factors for the estimated regression parameters, and others require simulation methods that are incorporated into the regression procedures. What is essential in each approach is knowledge about the structure of the measurement error. Obtaining information about the behavior of error in measurements of exposure usually requires careful and imaginative planning. Often, it can be incorporated into the overall study design in which the study is conducted in what amount to two stages, one of which will result in the necessary information related to measurement error.

One approach that can sometimes be applied calls for repeated measurement of an exposure, the variability or variance providing an estimate of precision, assuming that there is no bias in the estimates. For example, if the average blood pressure during the course of a day is a putative risk factor of interest, then using just one measurement in our analysis would suffer from the fact that it could be at a low or high point in the data for the individual. Presumably, we could improve our estimate by taking additional measurements at random times during the day, thus obtaining not only an improved estimate of the mean for that individual but also an estimate of the variability. While it may not be cost effective to obtain multiple measures on each individual, one could conduct this precision study on just a subset of individuals and then incorporate the information in the final results.

Sometimes, measurement error arises from the need to reduce cost in a study due to the expense of laboratory procedures for the best estimates of exposure. In these instances, one can obtain information from either an independent study or a study of a subset of the population on both the relatively inexpensive estimate and the best estimate of exposure. The objective would be to try to predict the best estimate by developing an appropriate regression model. Of course, it would also be possible to include other covariate information, along with the inexpensive estimator in the model. The result would provide not only an expression for predicting the best estimate of exposure for each individual but also the precision or standard deviation of that estimator. Hence, we would once again have an exposure estimate that was determined with error, and it would be essential to take that into account in the analysis by not simply treating the predicted value as the true exposure. Such an approach is called regression calibration, and Carroll et al. (39) described an approach for conducting the appropriate analysis.

Collinearity

Variables that are strongly related to each other can cause difficulties of interpretation for regression methods, including those that we have discussed; such variables cause a type of confounding that is difficult to resolve. The problem is broadly referred to as *collinearity*, and a trivial example of this would be the case in which we have two measures of the same quantity using different units of measure. Weight in pounds and in kilograms would be one such example, and it would obviously be silly to try to extract more information from a regression analysis when one was already in the model. However, in other situations, very similar phenomena can occur, especially when several variables are involved in some form of mutual dependence.

One example involves the analysis of disease trends as a function of age at diagnosis (A), year of diagnosis which is called period (P), and year of birth or cohort (C). If we know a subject's age at a particular point in time, then their year of birth is a simple calculation, $C = P - A$. Therefore, analyses that attempt to consider all three factors simultaneously are bound to cause difficulty in interpreting the results because in one very real sense there are but two variables that completely describe the temporal space. For a further discussion of the analysis of age, period, and cohort effects, see Holford (40–43).

In the two examples we just considered, a perfect algebraic relationship exists among the variables, but it is also not uncommon to come across situations in which relationships are not perfect, yet there is a high degree of interrelationships, giving rise to high levels of correlation among two or more variables or some combination thereof. When computers were first being used routinely in data analysis, collinearity caused some algorithms to produce numerically spurious results. Currently available software is much less likely to produce numerically inaccurate results, but the results can be difficult to interpret.

One reason that collinearity is likely to remain an important issue in the analysis of epidemiologic data is in part due to the large number of agents of interest and the way in which exposures occur. For example, one group of chemicals that have been thought to be related to cancer risk are PCBs, which for many years were marketed by the proportion of chlorine by weight. However, there are 209 different congeners for this group of chemicals, some of which have very different hormonal effects on an individual, so it would ultimately be of interest to evaluate the congeners separately. The way these chemicals were manufactured and ultimately made their way into the environment resulted in exposures to a mixture of different congeners, so that exposure to one is likely to be highly correlated with exposure to others that happened to be in the same product. The resulting high correlation among the exposure levels for individual congeners can result in the type of collinearity that is of concern. For example, if the exposure to an estrogenic congener was highly correlated with an anti-estrogenic congener and we are studying risk for breast cancer, then the effect of either one might not be apparent because when one was high, the other would also be high and their combined effect could tend to cancel each other out. In this hypothetical case, a better analysis might be to evaluate the effect of the difference in exposure levels for these two congeners.

Two common ways of dealing with large numbers of variables that are highly correlated are the following:

> *Variable reduction*, in which one drops redundant variables from the regression model using a variable selection algorithm; this approach is predicated on the idea that only a subset of variables are needed to describe disease risk. If we have two chemicals that have highly correlated exposure levels, and they both affect the risk of disease, it may not be possible to accurately determine their separate effects. Dropping one of the chemicals from a model may not change the accuracy of the prediction, but it forces that regression coefficient to be zero, thus providing a biased estimate of effect for both chemicals.

> *Principal components* offer an alternative to dropping variables from the analysis by considering linear combinations of the variables that will hopefully make scientific sense. One of the simplest and most commonly used summaries in the analysis of PCBs is to analyze the effect of their total. Principal components analysis offers another approach for identifying different combination of the exposures that are identified in terms of their components of variation in the environment. However, this is often predicated on the idea that there are common unmeasured factors giving rise to an observed joint distribution of exposures, and not their biochemical action within the individual. Hence, this does not necessarily address the scientific question of interest.

The following example illustrates the use of ridge regression, which is one alternative way of dealing with the problem of collinearity. However, it is not meant as necessarily being the ideal approach, as it clearly involves a certain amount of art in its application.

Example 12–3   Zhang et al. (44, 45) conducted a case-control study of the effect of a variety of organochlorine compounds, including PCB exposure, on breast cancer risk. In this analysis we consider the joint effect of nine PCB congeners measured in breast adipose tissue. The exposure levels for individual congeners were highly correlated, as seen in Table 12–1. Hence, collinearity could have a profound effect on the estimated associations. Of primary interest in this analysis were the joint effects of individual PCB congeners on risk of breast cancer and whether the effect of each congener was the same. Table 12–2 shows some summary results from fitting a linear logistic model to these data. The results of an analysis of total PCB exposure suggested a neutral effect, $OR = 0.97$ (95% CI = 0.90–1.05) for a 100-ppb change in exposure that did not achieve nominal statistical significance ($p = .498$), and this implicitly assumed that the contribution of PBCs to the overall model is $X_+\beta = X_1\beta + X_2\beta + \cdots + X_9\beta$; that is, the effect of each congener is the same. Table 12–2 presents estimates of the relative risk for breast cancer associated with a 10-ppb change in exposure to individual congeners, obtained by fitting a linear logistic model to the data. Notice that some congeners are positively associated with breast cancer risk while others are negative, and the global test of all congeners entered simultaneously was nominally significant ($p = .034$). Comparing the fit of this model to the one in which separate regressor variables are included for each congener provides a test of equality among the effects, $\Delta G^2 = 17.63$, df = 8 ($p = 0.024$), which provides fairly strong evidence for different effects among the congeners.

Ridge regression offers one approach for dealing with instability of parameter estimates in the presence of collinearity (46). Extensions of this idea to binary outcomes and/or the generalized linear model are provided by Schaefer (47, 48) and Segerstedt (49). To employ this method, we first normalized the exposure measures for each congener by subtracting the mean for the study population and dividing the result by the standard deviation for the congener. Maximum likelihood esti-

Table 12–1. Summary statistics and correlation coefficients for PCB congeners

Congener	74	118	138	153	156	170	180	183	187
118	0.68								
138	0.67	0.82							
153	0.58	0.66	0.86						
156	0.40	0.52	0.58	0.54					
170	0.52	0.59	0.80	0.78	0.71				
180	0.45	0.43	0.67	0.87	0.47	0.79			
183	0.46	0.53	0.70	0.77	0.65	0.77	0.69		
187	0.53	0.50	0.68	0.84	0.47	0.74	0.83	0.75	
Mean	36.16	52.39	95.04	143.29	24.80	37.73	110.32	14.52	34.58
SD	30.11	52.28	64.61	76.50	16.15	22.24	58.09	8.98	22.21

Table 12-2. Estimates of the relative risk for breast cancer associated with a 10-ppb change in exposure to individual congeners by type of model; numbers in parentheses are 95% CIs

Congener	Standardized coefficient[1]	All congeners[*]	Ridge[†] (age only)
74	−0.21	0.93(0.84–1.04)	0.98(0.92–1.04)
118	0.19	1.04(0.96–1.12)	0.99(0.96–1.03)
138	0.28	1.04(0.94–1.16)	1.00(0.97–1.03)
153	−1.04	0.87(0.78–0.98)	0.98(0.96–1.00)
156	−0.37	0.79(0.64–0.99)	0.87(0.77–0.98)
170	−0.36	0.85(0.65–1.11)	1.00(0.91–1.09)
180	0.74	1.14(1.00–1.29)	1.04(1.01–1.07)
183	0.54	1.82(1.12–2.98)	1.22(0.98–1.54)
187	0.24	1.11(0.90–1.37)	1.04(0.95–1.14)
LR χ^2	18.09 (df = 9)		

[*] Adjusted for age and months of lactation, body mass index, fat consumption, age at menarche, number of live births (none, <3, and ≥3), age at first full pregnancy (<25 and ≥25), income (<$8,750, 8,750–14,284, 14,396–24,999, ≥25,000, and unknown), fat levels of DDE (<435.2, 435.2–784.3, 784.4–1437.3, ≥1437.4).

[†] Ridge regression estimate of OR for a 10-ppb change in exposure for $k = 20$.

mates of the logistic regression parameters for each congener were obtained using PROC GENMOD in SAS, first adjusting for age alone, and then the remaining covariates. These results were then used to obtain ridge regression estimators for a particular ridge coefficient, $k (\geq 0)$, by implementing the formulae described in Appendix of Holford et al (46).

A fundamental issue in ridge regression is the selection of the ridge coefficient, k. When $k = 0$, the result is the usual maximum likelihood estimator, and as k becomes large the ridge estimators eventually go to 0, although before reaching the limit they can change sign. Parameter estimates that are heavily influenced by collinearity tend to change rapidly for small values of k and become more stable as k increases. This phenomenon can be observed by creating a ridge trace, which plots the ridge estimators against k. The reported ridge estimator of a regression parameter uses a small value of k in the range in which the ridge trace has been stabilized. While the resulting estimator is no longer a maximum likelihood estimate, and is thus biased, it will generally have reduced variance. Our objective is to find estimates that have a reduced mean squared error, which is the sum of the variance and the square of the bias. The results from this approach are not unique, in the sense that a certain amount of judgment is necessary when interpreting the ridge trace, but the fact that the choice of k is in the range where the trace is stable means that some variation in this coefficient will not substantially change an estimate's effect.

The ridge trace for an analysis based on all congeners and adjusting for age only is shown in Figure 12-4. The logistic regression coefficients shown in the graph reflect the contribution of normalized exposures; that is, they represent the effect of 1 SD change in exposure. While some coefficients do change sign, most tend to

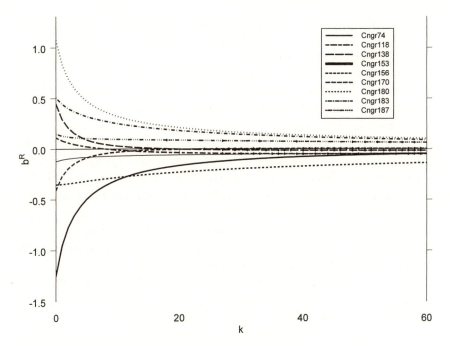

Figure 12–4 Ridge trace for individual congeners adjusted for age only.

be near the null value of zero. While 153 shows the largest protective effect, this effect largely disappears when the trace stabilizes as k nears 20, at which point 156 has a stronger protective effect. Congeners 180 and 183 have the largest adverse effect on breast cancer risk. Table 12–2 presents the ridge estimate ($k = 20$) for each congener, adjusted for age only. The ridge trace was also completed for an analysis that adjusted for the other covariates, and the results were very similar. Covariate adjusted ridge estimates for the congener effects are shown in Table 12–2.

Summary

In this text we have explored some of the fundamental ways in which epidemiologic data have been analyzed, and we have seen ways in which regression models have extended those ideas. All of these techniques require the careful specification of a set of assumptions that need to accurately reflect the conditions set out in the study design and the data. One of the themes seen in the tools that are currently being developed is the movement to avoid overly restrictive assumptions, thus providing every opportunity for the data to reveal the form for the relationships. These might include the formation of risk groups such as the approach we saw in CART, as well as the estimation of a dose–response relationship by using methods that are developed in the spirit of spline functions.

Other major areas of methodology that we have not discussed in detail, but which continue to undergo active development, are approaches for dealing with problems like measurement error in the exposure, errors of classification of disease, collinearity, and missing data. Many of the techniques that are being developed to deal with these issues make use of simulation methods that can broadly be referred to as Markov Chain Monte Carlo (MCMC) methods (50). These techniques enable one to develop methods under a more realistic set of assumptions than was previously possible. The rapid growth of computational power has now made these techniques feasible, where they were not really possible before. Currently, many of these ideas have not found their way into some of the standard software packages that are in common use, but that will certainly be resolved as a consensus develops as to the better approaches to these problems.

The statistical aspects of study design and analysis are usually just a tiny fraction of the cost of conducting epidemiologic research, but in the end, this part of the work can yield an enormous return.

References

1. Breiman L, Friedman JH, Olshen RA, Stone CJ. *Classification and Regression Trees*. California: Wadsworth, 1984.
2. Zhang H, Singer B. *Recursive Partitioning in the Health Sciences*. New York: Springer-Verlag, 1999.
3. Segal MR, Block DA. A comparison of estimated proportional hazards models and regression trees. *Statistics in Medicine* 1989;8:539–550.
4. Zhang H, Holford TR, Bracken MB. A tree-based method of analysis for prospective studies. *Statistics in Medicine* 1996;15:37–49.
5. Bracken MB, Belanger K, Hellenbrand K, Dlugosz L, Holford TR, McSharry JE, Addesso K, Leaderer B. Exposure to electromagnetic fields during pregnancy with emphasis on electrically heated beds: association with birth weight and intrauterine growth retardation. *Epidemiology* 1995;6:263–270.
6. Zhang H, Bracken MB. Tree-based, two-stage risk factor analysis for spontaneous abortion. *American Journal of Epidemiology* 1996;144:989–996.
7. Miettinen OS. Stratification by a multivariate confounder score. *American Journal of Epidemiology* 1976;104:609–620.
8. Davis RB, Anderson JR. Exponential survival trees. *Statistics in Medicine* 1989; 8:947–961.
9. LeBlanc M, Crowley J. Survival trees by goodness of split. *Journal of the American Statistical Association* 1993;88:457–467.
10. Segal MR. Regression trees for censored data. *Biometrics* 1988;44:35–47.
11. Kooperberg C, Stone CJ, Truong YK. Hazard regression. *Journal of the American Statistical Association* 1995;90:78–94.

12. Durrleman S, Simon R. Flexible regression models with cubic splines. *Statistics in Medicine* 1989;8:551–561.
13. Zhou S, Shen X. Spatially adaptive regression splines and accurate knot selection schemes. *Journal of the American Statistical Association* 2001;96:247–259.
14. de Boor C. *A Practical Guide to Splines.* New York: Springer-Verlag, 1978.
15. Hairston NG. An analysis of age-prevalence data by catalytic models. *Bulletin of the World Health Organization* 1965;33:163–175.
16. Hastie T, Tibshirani R. Generalized additive models. *Statistical Science* 1986; 1:297–318.
17. Hastie R, Tibshirani R. Generalized additive models for medical research. *Statistical Methods in Medical Research* 1995;4:187–196.
18. Friedman JH. Multivariate adaptive regression splines. *Annals of Statistics* 1991; 19:1–141.
19. Friedman JH, Roosen CB. An introduction to multivariate adaptive regression splines. *Statistical Methods in Medical Research* 1995;4:197–217.
20. Little LJA, Rubin DB. *Statistical Analysis with Missing Data.* New York: John Wiley & Sons, 1987.
21. Schafer JL. *Analysis of Incomplete Multivariate Data.* London: Chapman & Hall, 1997.
22. Rubin DB. *Multiple Imputation for Nonresponse in Surveys.* New York: John Wiley & Sons, 1987.
23. Schafer JL. Multiple imputatioin: a primer. *Statistical Methods in Medical Research* 1999;8:3–15.
24. Dempster AP, Laird NM, Rubin DB. Maximum likelihood from incomplete data via the EM Algorithm. *Journal of the Royal Statistic Society,* Series B 1977;69:1–38.
25. Horton NJ, Laird NM. Maximum likelihood analysis of generalized linear models with missing covariates. *Statistical Methods in Medical Research* 1999;8:37–50.
26. Gilks WR, Richardson S, Spiegelhalter DJ. *Markov Chain Monte Carlo in Practice.* London: Chapman and Hall, 1996.
27. Diggle PJ, Liang K-Y, Zeger SL. *Analysis of Longitudinal Data.* Oxford: Clarendon Press, 1994.
28. Kenward MG, Molenberghs G. Parametric models for incomplete continuous and categorical longitudinal data. *Statistical Methods in Medical Research* 1999; 8:51–83.
29. Boscardin WJ, Taylor JMG, Law N. Longitudinal models for AIDS marker data. *Statistical Methods in Medical Research* 1998;7:13–27.
30. Hogan JW, Laird NM. Increasing efficiency from censored survival data by using random effects to model longitudinal covariates. *Statistical Methods in Medical Research* 1998;7:28–48.
31. Dersimonian R, Laird NM. Meta-analysis in clinical trials. *Controlled Clinical Trials* 1986;7:177–188.
32. Berkey CS, Hoaglin DC, Mosteller F, G.A. C. A random-effects regression model for meta-analysis. *Statistics in Medicine* 1995;14:395–411.
33. Clayton D, Kaldor J. Empirical Bayes estimates of age-standardised relative risks for use in disease mapping. *Biometrics* 1987;43:671–681.
34. Bernardinelli L, Montomoli C. Empirical Bayes versus fully Bayesian analysis of geographical variation in disease risk. *Statistics in Medicine* 1992;11:983–1007.

35. Clayton DG, Bernardinelli L, Montomoli C. Spatial correlation in ecological analysis. *International Journal of Epidemiology* 1993;22:1193–1202.
36. Bernardinelli L, Clayton D, Pascutto C, Montomoli C, Ghislandi M. Bayesian analysis of space-time variation in disease risk. *Statistics in Medicine* 1995;14: 2433–2443.
37. Mollié A. Bayesian mapping of disease. In: Gilks WR, Richardson S, Spiegelhalter DJ, eds. *Markov Chain Monte Carlo in Practice*. London: Chapman & Hall, 1996:359–379.
38. Breslow NE, Leroux B, Platt R. Approximate hierarchical modelling of discrete data in epidemiology. *Statistical Methods in Medical Research* 1998;7: 49–62.
39. Carroll RJ, Ruppert D, Stefanski LA. *Measurement Error in Nonlinear Models*. London: Chapman and Hall, 1995.
40. Holford TR. The estimation of age, period and cohort effects for vital rates. *Biometrics* 1983;39:311–324.
41. Holford TR. Understanding the effects of age, period and cohort on incidence and mortality rates. *Annual Reviews of Public Health* 1991;12:425–457.
42. Holford TR. Analyzing the temporal effects of age, period and cohort. *Statistical Methods in Medical Research* 1992;1:317–337.
43. Holford TR. Age-period-cohort analysis. In: P Armitage and T. Colton (eds.) *Encyclopedia of Biostatistics*, 1998:82–99.
44. Zheng T, Holford TR, Mayne ST, Ward B, Carter D, Owens PH, Dubrow R, Zahm S, Boyle P, Archibeque S, Tessari. DDE and DDT in breast adipose tissue and risk of female breast cancer. *American Journal of Epidemiology* 1999; 150:453–458.
45. Zheng T, Holford TR, Mayne ST, Tessari J, Ward B, Owens PH, Boyle P, Dubrow R, Archibeque-Engle S, Dawood O, Zahm SH. Risk of female breast cancer associated with serum polychlorinated biphenyls and 1,1-dichloro-2,2'-bis(*p*-chlorophenyl)ethylene. *Cancer Epidemiology, Biomarkers and Prevention* 2000;9:167–174.
46. Holford TR, Zheng T, Mayne ST, Zahm SH, Tessari JD, Boyle P. Joint effects of nine polychlorinated biphenyl (PCB) congeners on breast cancer risk. *International Journal of Epidemiology* 2000;29:975–982.
47. Schaefer RL, Roi LD, Wolfe RA. A ridge logistic estimator. *Communications in Statistics—Theory and Methods* 1984;13:99–113.
48. Schaefer RL. Alternative estimators in logistic regression when the data are collinear. *Journal of Statistical Computation and Simulation* 1986;25:75–91.
49. Segerstedt B. On ordinary ridge regression in generalized linear models. *Communications in Statistics—Theory and Methods* 1992;21:2227–2246.
50. Gilks WR, Richardson S, Spiegelhalter DS. *Markov Chain Monte Carlo in Practice*. London: Chapman and Hall, 1996.

Appendix 1

Theory on Models for Disease

A more precise definition of the hazard function is given in terms of the probability of the occurrence of an event during a relatively short period of time $(t, t + \Delta t)$. The probability that a person who is healthy at t will become diseased by $(t + \Delta t)$ is $\lambda(t)\Delta t + o(\Delta t)$, where $o(\Delta t)$ represents terms such that $o(\Delta t)/\Delta t \to 0$ as $\Delta t \to 0$; that is, the instantaneous transition probability is essentially proportional to the interval width and the hazard function.

The definition of the survival function, $\mathcal{F}(t)$, refers to the overall outcome probability rather than the instantaneous conditional probabilities given by the hazard function, but they are directly related (1). We can see this by noting that

$$\mathcal{F}(t + \Delta t) = \Pr\{\text{Healthy at } (t)\} \cdot [1 - \Pr\{\text{Diseased at } (t + \Delta t) \mid \text{Healthy at } t\}]$$

$$= \mathcal{F}(t) \left[1 - \lambda(T) \cdot \Delta t + o(\Delta t)\right]$$

which can be rearranged to yield

$$\frac{\mathcal{F}(t + \Delta t) - \mathcal{F}(t)}{\Delta t} = -\lambda(t)\,\mathcal{F}(t) + \frac{o(\Delta t)}{\Delta t}$$

Taking the limit as $\Delta t \to 0$ results in the differential equation,

$$\frac{d\mathcal{F}(t)}{dt} = -\lambda(t)\,\mathcal{F}(t)$$

The particular solution to this differential equation, subject to the initial condition that one begins life healthy, $\mathcal{F}(0) = 1$, is

$$\mathcal{F}(t) = \exp\left\{-\int_0^t \lambda(\tau)d\tau\right\} \tag{A1.1}$$

Conversely, one can derive the hazard function from the survival function from the expression,

$$\lambda(t) = \frac{d\{-\log \mathcal{F}(t)\}}{dt} \tag{A1.2}$$

so that to know one expression is to know the other.

The probability density function of time to death or disease is represented by $f(t)$. From the properties of probability density functions, we know that its relationship to the distribution function is given by

$$f(t) = \frac{dF(t)}{dt}$$

Because the distribution function is in turn related to the survival function by $F(t) = 1 - \mathcal{F}(t)$, we have

$$f(t) = -\frac{d\{\mathcal{F}(t)\}}{dt}$$

$$= \lambda(t) \cdot \exp\left\{-\int_0^t \lambda(\tau) \, d\tau\right\}$$

which depends on either the survival or the hazard functions. Likewise, we can express the survival function by

$$\mathcal{F}(t) = \int_t^\infty f(\tau) \, d\tau$$

and the hazard by

$$\lambda(t) = \frac{f(t)}{\displaystyle\int_t^\infty f(\tau) \, d\tau}$$

It is clear that if any one of these three fundamental quantities is known, then the other two can be derived by a specified mathematical maneuver, so that these are essentially different summaries of the same underlying phenomenon. This is important to realize because the models considered in this book deal with different fundamental quantities; because they are mathematically related, however, we can understand the effect of a risk factor by formulating a result based on any one of them.

Constant Rates in Time

The simplest form for a disease model is to assume that the hazard rate is constant over time, $\lambda(t) = \lambda$. Under this model the survival function is represented by $\mathcal{F}(t) = \exp\{-\lambda t\}$, which implies that the logarithm is linear in t, with a slope of $-\lambda$. The disease density function has an exponential distribution (2): $f(t) = \lambda \exp\{-\lambda t\}$. These functions are plotted in Figure A1–1, and one sees that the survival function steadily decreases to 0 over time, t. The shape of the disease density function is the same as the survival function, only it is λ at its highest point when $t = 0$ instead of 1.

For some applications, the constant hazard assumption may be realistic. For example, survival after a diagnosis of lung cancer is one such case; because the prognosis is very poor for these patients, there is little time for a change in factors that might affect the mortality rate. In many applications it is not reasonable to assume a constant hazard over the entire range of follow-up, however. For instance, the hazard rate for most cancers increases with age, so that an assumption of constant hazard over the entire lifetime would be quite unrealistic. In the absence of more precise knowledge, we might limit our observations to only a short time interval, during which the constant hazard model may give a satisfactory approximation. In general, however, we need an approach that gives greater flexibility.

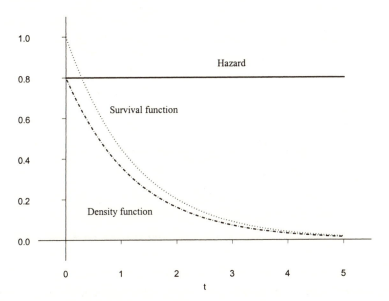

Figure A1–1 Plot of the hazard, the survival, and the density function for the constant hazards model.

Idealized Model for Rates Changing over Time

While the assumption of constant hazards is likely to be unrealistic in describing real data, we might approach the problem by defining a model that specifies a particular way in which the hazard varies with time. The Weibull model is one attempt to introduce flexibility in the hazard function. This model gives the hazard rate as $\lambda(t) = \lambda \gamma t^{\gamma-1}$, where $\lambda, \gamma > 0$ (2). The possible shapes for the hazard are shown in Figure A1–2, and these include the constant hazard as a special case, $\gamma = 1$. For other values of γ, the hazard may be either strictly increasing ($\gamma > 1$) or strictly decreasing ($\tau < 1$), as seen in Figure A1–2.

In some cases, we might consider a particular form for the hazard because of theoretical considerations that allow us a way of incorporating knowledge about the underlying biology of a disease. Armitage and Doll (3) propose a multistage model for carcinogenesis in which ($\gamma - 1$) changes are required to transform a normal cell to one that is malignant. It turns out that this results in a cancer incidence rate that has the Weibull form where t represents age. However, a different set of assumptions about the underlying biology of disease can give rise to a very different form for the

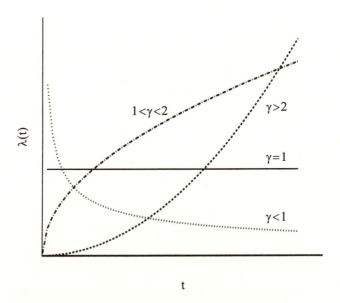

Figure A1–2 Plot of the Weibull hazard for alternative values of the shape parameter, γ.

model. For example, Moolgavkar and Venson (4) consider a two-stage model that gives rise to an age-dependant hazard that is very different from that described by the Weibull function.

While the flexibility of the Weibull function increases its applicability, by no means does this function fit every situation. For example, it cannot change from a decreasing to an increasing function of time. Hence, we would not expect it to accurately describe the effect that surgery might have in some instances, because initially there is often a high hazard because of risks associated with surgery itself. After a decline, the hazard might once again rise, from either a wearing off of the beneficial effect of surgery or the aging process itself. The following section demonstrates that, in reality, the shape of a hazard curve can be fairly complex.

The survival function for the Weibull hazard can be directly determined from the hazard itself: $\mathcal{F}(t) = \exp\{-\lambda t^{\gamma}\}$, in which $\log[-\log \mathcal{F}(t)] = \log \lambda + \gamma \cdot \log t$. Hence, $\log[-\log \mathcal{F}(t)]$ is linear in $\log t$, which provides a way of checking the assumption, as we shall see in a later chapter. The density function for the Weibull hazard is $f(t) = \lambda \gamma t^{\gamma-1} \exp\{-\lambda t^{\gamma}\}$.

Observed Effects of Age on Rates

The hazard rate for human mortality, which we usually call the age-specific mortality rate, decreases initially as an infant progresses beyond the neonatal period but increases again with the onset of old age. A typical curve is shown in Figure A1–3; this figure presents lifetable age-specific mortality rates, an estimate of the hazard function for all causes of death, for U.S. males and females in 1990 (5). This particular shape is very difficult to represent by a simple equation, and one usually would not try to do so. In specific studies it may not be possible or interesting to estimate the function, even though one suspects that the shape is not well defined by a simple model, such as the constant or Weibull hazard. It is for just these instances that nonparametric methods of analysis have been developed in which we do not employ a model that results in an explicit expression for the hazard.

Relationship between Models for Rates and Proportions

To derive a relationship between a model for rates and one for risk, let τ be the length of follow-up for a particular individual. The log-linear hazard model implies that

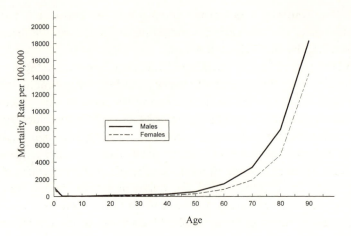

Figure A1–3 Mortality rate per 100,000 among U.S. whites in 1990.

$$\Pr(\mathbf{X}) = 1 - \mathscr{F}(\tau)$$

$$= 1 - \exp\left\{-\exp[\mathbf{X}\boldsymbol{\beta}]\int_0^\tau \lambda_0(u)\,du\right\} \qquad \text{(A1.3)}$$

$$= 1 - \exp\{-\exp[\alpha(\tau) + \mathbf{X}\boldsymbol{\beta}]\}$$

where

$$\alpha(\tau) = \log\int_0^\tau \lambda_0(u)\,du$$

The similarity of the linear logistic and the log-linear hazard models, when the probability of disease is small, can be shown analytically. To distinguish the two sets of parameters, let an asterisk be used for the linear logistic parameters. By considering the exponential series expansion for the log-linear hazards model in equation A1.3, we have

$$\Pr(\mathbf{X}) = 1 - [1 - \exp\{\alpha + \mathbf{X}\beta\} + \exp\{\alpha + \mathbf{X}\beta\}^2/2 - \cdots]$$

$$= \exp\{\alpha + \mathbf{X}\beta\} + o[\exp\{\alpha + \mathbf{X}\beta\}]$$

Similarly, by expanding the division in equation 2.1, we obtain a series for the linear logistic model:

$$\Pr(X) = \exp\{\alpha^* + \mathbf{X}\beta^*\} - \exp\{\alpha^* + \mathbf{X}\beta^*\}^2 + \cdots$$

$$= \exp\{\alpha^* + \mathbf{X}\beta^*\} + o[\exp\{\alpha^* + \mathbf{X}\beta^*\}]$$

Table A1–1. Percentage difference in odds ratio and hazard ratio by probability of disease in unexposed subjects and the relative risk

Probability of disease in unexposed subjects	*Hazard ratio* (R)				
	1.5	2.0	3.0	4.0	5.0
.005	0.1	0.3	0.5	0.8	1.0
.010	0.3	0.5	1.0	1.5	2.0
.050	1.3	2.6	5.4	8.2	11.1
.100	2.7	5.6	11.5	17.9	24.8
.150	4.3	8.8	18.7	29.7	42.1

Clearly, when $\Pr(\mathbf{X})$ is small, $\exp\{\alpha + \mathbf{X}\boldsymbol{\beta}\} \approx \exp\{\alpha^* + \mathbf{X}\boldsymbol{\beta}^*\}$, indicating that the models are nearly equal to the first order—that is, when $\exp\{\cdot\}$ is small.

One implication of this discussion is that the hazard ratio and the odds ratio will be in good agreement when the probability of disease in a fixed period is small. For positive risks, the odds ratio is generally larger than the hazard ratio. However, as one can see from Table A1–1, the percentage of difference is quite small unless the probability of disease for the unexposed or the hazard ratio becomes fairly large.

References

1. Gross AJ, Clark VA. *Survival Distributions: Reliability Applicatioins in the Biomedical Sciences.* New York: Wiley, 1975.
2. Johnson NL, Kotz S. *Continuous Univariate Distributions-1.* Boston: Houghton Mifflin, 1970.
3. Armitage P, Doll R. The age distribution of cancer and a multi-stage theory of carcinogenesis. *British Journal of Cancer* 1954;8:1–12.
4. Moolgavkar SH, Venson DJ. A stochastic two-stage model for cancer risk assessment: I. The hazard function and the probability of tumor. *Mathematical Biosciences* 1979;47:55–77.
5. National Center for Health Statistics. *Vital Statistics of the United States, 1990.* Washington, DC: Public Health Service, 1994.

Appendix 2

Theory on Analysis of Proportions

This appendix discusses some of the statistical theory behind the tests that were described in Chapter 3. We will focus on statistical inference for the regression parameter, β, in the linear logistic model, and the emphasis will be on methods that lend themselves to hand calculation. All of the methods described in Chapter 3 deal with the general problem of a trend that is logit linear in X, considering significance testing for a single $I \times 2$ table, as well as the special case of a binary exposure, $I = 2$. For this derivation the general $I \times 2$ table is considered, along with the particular case where $I = 2$. Finally, these tests are extended to the situation where the information is being combined over K such tables.

Likelihood for the Linear Logistic Model

The linear logistic model for trend in a single $I \times 2$ table may be written as

$$\pi_{j|i} = P\{Y|X_i\} = \frac{\exp\{Y(\alpha + X_i\beta)\}}{1 + \exp\{\alpha + X_i\beta\}} \tag{A2.1}$$

where the two possible observed responses are $Y = 0$ or 1 ($j = 1$ or 2, respectively), which represents a well or diseased outcome in the ith row of a table. These outcomes occur with observed frequencies, n_{i1} and n_{i2}, as shown in Table 3–9, and X_i is the ith exposure dose level. Each row of an $I \times 2$ table has an independent binomial distribution, $\text{Bin}(\pi_{j|i}, n_{i+})$, and the likelihood function is the probability of observing the particular outcome, which depends on the linear logistic model parameters, α and β:

$$\ell(\alpha,\beta) \propto \prod_i \pi_{1|i}^{n_{i1}} \cdot \pi_{2|i}^{n_{i2}}$$

$$= \prod_i \left[\frac{1}{1 + e^{\alpha + X_i\beta}} \right]^{n_{i1}} \cdot \left[\frac{e^{\alpha + \beta X_i}}{1 + e^{\alpha + X_i\beta}} \right]^{n_{i2}} \tag{A2.2}$$

$$= \frac{\exp\{n_{+2}\alpha + \beta \sum_i X_i n_{i2}\}}{\prod_i [1 + \exp\{\alpha + X_i\beta\}]^{n_{i+}}}$$

It is generally more convenient to work with the log likelihood:

$$L(\alpha,\beta) = \sum_i \left[n_{i1} \cdot \log \pi_{1|i} + n_{i2} \cdot \log \pi_{2|i} \right]$$

$$= n_{+2}\,\alpha + \beta \sum_i X_i\, n_{i2} - \sum_i n_{i+} \log(1 + e^{\alpha + X_i\beta}) \tag{A2.3}$$

because of its relative simplicity, and well known asymptotic properties (1). In addition to the log likelihood itself, it is necessary to also determine derivatives in order to derive various formulae for likelihood-based statistical inference. The vector of first derivatives for the log likelihood, $L(\cdot)$, is represented by $\mathbf{U}(\alpha,\beta)$ (2):

$$\mathbf{U}(\alpha,\beta) = \begin{bmatrix} \dfrac{\partial L}{\partial \alpha} \\[2mm] \dfrac{\partial L}{\partial \beta} \end{bmatrix}$$

$$= \begin{bmatrix} n_{+2} - \sum_i n_{i+}\left(\dfrac{\exp\{\alpha + X_i\beta\}}{1 + \exp\{\alpha + X_i\beta\}} \right) \\[4mm] \sum_i X_i\left(n_{i2} - \dfrac{n_{i+} \cdot \exp\{\alpha + X_i\beta\}}{1 + \exp\{\alpha + X_i\beta\}} \right) \end{bmatrix} \tag{A2.4}$$

To find the maximum likelihood estimators for α and β, $\mathbf{U}(\cdot)$ is set to $\mathbf{0}$ and solved for α and β. In general, a closed form solution is not available for the resulting $\hat{\alpha}$ and $\hat{\beta}$, but there is in the particular case where there are just two exposure categories, represented by $X = 0$ or 1:

$$\begin{bmatrix} \hat{\alpha} \\ \hat{\beta} \end{bmatrix} = \begin{bmatrix} \log(n_{12}/n_{11}) \\ \log(n_{11} \cdot n_{22}/n_{12} \cdot n_{21}) \end{bmatrix} \tag{A2.5}$$

Variance estimates can be obtained from the matrix found by evaluating the negative of the expectation for the matrix of second derivatives of the log likelihood at the maximum likelihood estimates (2):

$$\mathbf{I}(\hat{\alpha},\hat{\beta}) = -E \begin{bmatrix} \dfrac{\partial^2 L}{\partial \alpha^2} & \dfrac{\partial^2 L}{\partial \alpha \partial \beta} \\[2ex] \dfrac{\partial^2 L}{\partial \beta \partial \alpha} & \dfrac{\partial^2 L}{\partial \beta^2} \end{bmatrix}_{\alpha=\hat{\alpha},\beta=\hat{\beta}}$$

$$= \begin{bmatrix} \displaystyle\sum_i n_{i+}\,\pi_{1|i}\,\pi_{2|i} & \displaystyle\sum_i n_{i+}\,X_i\,\pi_{1|i}\,\pi_{2|i} \\[2ex] \displaystyle\sum_i n_{i+}\,X_i\,\pi_{2|i}\,\pi_{1|i} & \displaystyle\sum_i n_{i+}\,X_i^2\,\pi_{1|i}\,\pi_{2|i} \end{bmatrix}$$

(A2.6)

This matrix is known as the Fisher information matrix, and its inverse gives an estimate of the covariance matrix of the parameter estimates:

$$\mathbf{I}(\hat{\alpha},\hat{\beta})^{-1} = \begin{bmatrix} \mathrm{Var}(\hat{\alpha}) & \mathrm{Cov}(\hat{\alpha},\hat{\beta}) \\ \mathrm{Cov}(\hat{\alpha},\hat{\beta}) & \mathrm{Var}(\hat{\beta}) \end{bmatrix} = \mathbf{Var}(\hat{\alpha},\hat{\beta}) \qquad (A2.7)$$

In the particular case where the regressor variable is binary, $X = 0$ or 1, the variance of $\hat{\beta}$ reduces to

$$\mathrm{Var}(\hat{\beta}) = n_{11}^{-1} + n_{12}^{-1} + n_{21}^{-1} + n_{22}^{-1} \qquad (A2.8)$$

Wald Statistic for a 2 × 2 Table

In general, the Wald test for a subset of the full vector of regression parameters, β_1 where $\beta' = (\beta_1' \mid \beta_2')$, depends on the covariance matrix of the estimated parameters, $\mathrm{Var}(\beta_1)$. To test the null hypothesis, H_0: $\beta_1 = {}_0\beta_1$, one can use the quadratic form:

$$W^2 = (\beta_1 - {}_0\beta_1)' \cdot \mathrm{Var}(\beta_1)^{-1} \cdot (\beta_1 - {}_0\beta_1) \qquad (A2.9)$$

which is compared to a chi-square distribution with degrees of freedom equal to the dimension of β_1. In the particular situation where there is just one parameter of interest, this test becomes the square of the familiar z test:

$$W^2 = \frac{(\hat{\beta}_1 - {}_0\hat{\beta}_1)^2}{\mathrm{Var}(\hat{\beta}_1)}$$

Advantages of the Wald statistic include its ease of computation once the estimate and its variance have been obtained, allowing one to look not only at the significance test itself but also at the magnitude of the estimate and its precision. However, the computational effort involved in obtaining maximum likelihood estimates can be considerable if one is doing hand calculation, and it also requires the inversion of a matrix for hypotheses that involve more than one parameter. Hence, it is not uncommon to also see other, more convenient to implement, tests used in practice.

Likelihood Ratio Statistic for a 2 × 2 Table

The likelihood ratio statistic to test H_0: $\beta = 0$, for the simple two-parameter model shown in equation A2.1 compares the likelihood when both parameters, α and β, are estimated to the likelihood when β is restricted to its null value, 0. One can represent this as twice the difference between the two log likelihoods,

$$G^2 = 2\,[L(\hat{\alpha},\hat{\beta}) - L(\tilde{\alpha},0)] \tag{A2.10}$$

where $\hat{\alpha}$ and $\hat{\beta}$ are given in equation A2.5, and under H_0, $\tilde{\alpha} = \log(n_{+2}/n_{+1})$. In the first instance, $\hat{\alpha}$ and $\hat{\beta}$ may be substituted into equation A2.1 to obtain a fitted probability of disease, $\hat{\pi}_{j|i} = n_{ij}/n_{i+}$, and the maximum log likelihood may be expressed as

$$L(\hat{\alpha},\hat{\beta}) = \sum_{ij} n_{ij} \cdot \log(n_{ij}/n_{i+})$$

Similarly, the estimate $\tilde{\alpha}$ when $\beta = 0$ gives $\tilde{\pi}_2 = n_{+2}/n_{++}$, and the maximum log likelihood becomes

$$L(\tilde{\alpha},0) = \sum_{ij} n_{ij} \cdot \log(n_{+2}/n_{++})$$

By substituting these expressions into equation A2.10, one obtains the likelihood ratio statistic:

$$G^2 = 2 \cdot [L(\hat{\alpha},\hat{\beta}) - L(\tilde{\alpha},0)]$$

$$= 2 \cdot \sum_{ij} n_{ij} \cdot \log\left(\frac{n_{ij}}{n_{i+} \cdot n_{+j}/n_{++}}\right) \tag{A2.11}$$

$$= 2 \cdot \sum_{ij} n_{ij} \cdot \log\left(\frac{n_{ij}}{\tilde{m}_{ij}}\right)$$

which is the expression given in equation 3.14 (3).

Score Statistics for an $I \times 2$ Table

The score statistic is an efficient test described by Rao (4) that does not require maximum likelihood estimates for the full set of regression parameters. In fact, it is only necessary to obtain the estimates under the null hypothesis, H_0, which in some interesting special cases can be done using a closed-form solution. To obtain the score test of the general null hypothesis, $H_0: \beta_2 = {}_0\beta_2$, it is necessary to make use of the maximum likelihood estimates for β_1 assuming that H_0 is true, $\tilde{\beta}_1$. If

$$\mathbf{U}(\tilde{\beta}_1, {}_0\beta_2) = \begin{bmatrix} 0 \\ \mathbf{U}_1(\tilde{\beta}_1, {}_0\beta_2) \end{bmatrix}$$

is the vector of first partials evaluated under the condition of the null hypothesis and $I(\tilde{\beta}_1, {}_0\beta_2)$ is the corresponding information matrix, the score statistic is

$$S^2 = \mathbf{U}_1(\tilde{\beta}_1, {}_0\beta_2)' \cdot \mathbf{I}(\tilde{\beta}_1, {}_0\beta_2)^{-1} \cdot \mathbf{U}(\tilde{\beta}_1, {}_0\beta_2) \qquad (A2.12)$$

which has a chi-square distribution with degrees of freedom equal to the dimension of β_2. Two particular cases for the score test are especially noteworthy because they involve tests that are very common in practice. The test for linear trend considered in this subsection will be followed by the corresponding stratified analysis in the following subsection.

The test for linear trend in the linear logistic model involves the test of the single regression parameter, $H_0: \beta = 0$. As seen in the previous section, this yields $\tilde{\alpha} = \log(n_{+2}/n_{+1})$, with a vector of first partials:

$$\mathbf{U}(\tilde{\alpha}, 0) = \begin{bmatrix} 0 \\ \sum_i X_i \left(n_{i2} - \dfrac{n_{i+}n_{+2}}{n_{++}} \right) \end{bmatrix} \qquad (A2.13)$$

The corresponding information matrix becomes

$$\mathbf{I}(\tilde{\alpha}, 0) = \left(\frac{n_{+1}\, n_{+2}}{n_{++}^2} \right) \begin{bmatrix} n_{++} & \sum_i n_{i+}\, X_i \\ \sum_i n_{i+} X_i & \sum_i n_{i+}\, X_i^2 \end{bmatrix} \qquad (A2.14)$$

Because the first row of $\mathbf{U}(\tilde{\alpha}, 0)$ is 0, it is only necessary to determine the lower right element of $I(\tilde{\alpha}, 0)^{-1}$, giving

$$S^2 = \frac{n_{++}^3 \left[\sum_i X_i \, (n_{i2} - \tilde{m}_{i2}) \right]^2}{n_{+1}n_{+2} \left[n_{++}\sum_i X_i^2\, n_{i+} - (\sum_i X_i\, n_{i+})^2 \right]} \qquad (A2.15)$$

which is the test for linear trend described by Armitage (5). In the special case where there are just two categories described by the binary regressor variable $X = 0,1$, equation A2.15 simplifies to give

$$S^2 = \frac{n_{++}^2 [n_{11} \, n_{22} - n_{12} \, n_{21}]^2}{n_{1+} \, n_{2+} \, n_{+1} \, n_{+2}} \tag{A2.16}$$

which is the familiar Pearson chi-square test for 2×2 tables.

The parameter α is not of particular interest for the inference described here, but it is clearly necessary for the model in order for the probabilities of disease to take on the complete range of possible values. In the development just described, this "nuisance parameter" was estimated by using a maximum likelihood estimate under the restrictions of the null hypothesis. An alternative to finding an estimate for α is to use conditional inference as described by Cox (2). Notice that in the numerator for the likelihood, shown in equation A2.2, the contribution of α only depends on n_{+2}. In fact, n_{+2} is a minimal sufficient statistic for the parameter α (1). To perform conditional inference, it is necessary to find the probability of the observed combination of diseased and well individuals, conditional on the total number observed to be diseased, n_{+2}. This leads to a likelihood that depends only on the parameter of interest, β:

$$\ell_c(\beta) = \frac{\prod_i \binom{n_{i+}}{n_{i2}} \exp\{n_{i2} \, X_i \, \beta\}}{\sum_{\{u : u_+ = n_{+2}\}} \prod_i \binom{n_{i+}}{u_i} \exp\{u_i X_i \beta\}} \tag{A2.17}$$

where the sum in the denominator is taken over all possible combinations of $\mathbf{u}$ such that their total is n_{+2}. The log of the conditional likelihood is

$$L_c(\beta) = C + \sum_i n_{i2} \, X_i \, \beta - \log\left[\sum_{\mathbf{u}} \prod_i \binom{n_{i+}}{u_i} \exp\{u_i \, X_i \beta\} \right] \tag{A2.18}$$

giving a first derivative or score function of

$$U_c(\beta) = \sum_i n_{i2} \, X_i - \frac{\sum_{\mathbf{u}} \prod_i \binom{n_{i+}}{u} u_i \, X_i \, \exp\{u_i \, X_i \, \beta\}}{\sum_{\mathbf{u}} \prod_i \binom{n_{i+}}{u} \exp\{u_i \, X_i \, \beta\}} \tag{A2.19}$$

The negative of the second derivative of the conditional likelihood is

$$
-I_c(\beta) = \frac{\sum_{\mathbf{u}} \binom{n_{i+}}{u} \prod_i (u_i \, X_i)^2 \, \exp\{u_i \, X_i \, \beta\}}{\sum_{\mathbf{u}} \binom{n_{i+}}{u} \prod_i u_i \, \exp\{u_i \, X_i \, \beta\}}
$$

$$
- \frac{\left\{ \sum_{\mathbf{u}} \binom{n_{i+}}{u} \prod_i u_i \, X_i \, \exp\{u_i \, X_i \, \beta\} \right\}^2}{\left\{ \sum_{\mathbf{u}} \binom{n_{i+}}{u} \prod_i u_i \, \exp\{u_i \, X_i \, \beta\} \right\}^2}
\tag{A2.20}
$$

Conditional inference on the parameter β can be conducted by directly using the conditional log likelihood along with its derivatives. For instance, one might construct a score statistic by setting $\beta = 0$ and substituting into equation A2.19, yielding

$$
U_c(0) = \sum_i X_i \left(n_{i2} - \left[\frac{n_{i+} \, n_{+2}}{n_{++}} \right] \right) = \sum_i X_i \cdot (n_{i,2} - \tilde{m}_{i,2})
$$

Similarly, equation A2.20 reduces to

$$
I_c(0) = \frac{n_{+1} \, n_{+2}}{n_{++}^2 \, (n_{++} - 1)} \left\{ n_{++} \sum_i X_i^2 \, n_{i+} - \left(\sum_i X_i \, n_{i+} \right)^2 \right\}
$$

and the conditional score statistic becomes

$$
S_c^2 = \frac{n_{++}^2 \, (n_{++} - 1) \, [\sum_i X_i \, (n_{i2} - \tilde{m}_{i2})]^2}{n_{+1} \, n_{+2} \, [n_{++} \sum_i X_i^2 \, n_{i+} - (\sum_i X_i \, n_{i+})^2]}
\tag{A2.21}
$$

Score Statistics for Combining $I \times 2$ Tables

In equation 3.25, the model for stratified analyses using the linear logistic model was

$$
\pi_{j|ik} = P\{Y \,|\, k, X_i\} = \frac{\exp\{Y(\alpha_k + X_i\beta)\}}{1 + \exp\{\alpha_k + X_i\beta\}}
\tag{A2.22}
$$

where α_k represents the intercept for the kth stratum ($k = 1, \ldots K$). Letting n_{ijk} represent the observed frequency for the ith row of the jth column in the kth table, the likelihood takes the form

$$\ell(\boldsymbol{\alpha},\beta) \propto \prod_k \frac{\exp\{n_{+2k}\alpha_k + \beta \sum_i X_i\, n_{i2k}\}}{\prod_i[1 + \exp\{\alpha_k + X_i\beta\}]^{n_{i+k}}}$$

where $\boldsymbol{\alpha} = (\alpha_1, \alpha_2, \ldots, \alpha_K)$.

To compute the score statistic, we obtain the first derivatives of the log likelihood, evaluated at the maximum likelihood estimates for $\boldsymbol{\alpha}$, under H_0: $\beta = 0$:

$$\mathbf{U}(\tilde{\boldsymbol{\alpha}},0) = \begin{bmatrix} 0 \\ 0 \\ \vdots \\ \sum_{ik} X_i(n_{i2k} - \tilde{m}_{i2k}) \end{bmatrix} \tag{A2.23}$$

where $\tilde{m}_{i2k} = n_{i+k}n_{+2k}/n_{++k}$ and the corresponding information matrix is

$$
\hat{\mathbf{I}}(\tilde{\boldsymbol{\alpha}},0) = \begin{bmatrix}
n_{++1}p_1q_1 & 0 & \cdots & (\sum_i X_i n_{i+1})p_1q_1 \\
0 & n_{++2}p_2q_2 & \cdots & (\sum_i X_i n_{i+2})p_2q_2 \\
\vdots & \vdots & \ddots & \vdots \\
(\sum_i X_i n_{i+1})p_1q_1 & (\sum_i X_i n_{i+2})p_2q_2 & \cdots & \sum_k(\sum_i X_i n_{i+k})p_kq_k
\end{bmatrix}
$$

$$= \begin{bmatrix} \mathbf{A} & \mathbf{B} \\ \mathbf{B'} & \mathbf{D} \end{bmatrix} \tag{A2.24}$$

where $p_k = n_{+2k}/n_{++k} = 1 - q_k$. Rao (4) shows that the inverse of such a partitioned covariance matrix is

$$\begin{bmatrix} \mathbf{A}^{-1} + \mathbf{F}\,\mathbf{E}^{-1}\,\mathbf{F'} & -\mathbf{F}\,\mathbf{E}^{-1} \\ -\mathbf{E}^{-1}\,\mathbf{F'} & \mathbf{E}^{-1} \end{bmatrix} \tag{A2.25}$$

where $\mathbf{E} = \mathbf{D} - \mathbf{B'}\mathbf{A}^{-1}\mathbf{B}$ and $\mathbf{F} = \mathbf{A}^{-1}\mathbf{B}$. Because all but the kth elements of $\mathbf{U}(\cdot)$ are 0, the score statistic only involves the term in the lower right-hand corner of the information matrix, and the test reduces to

$$S^2 = \mathbf{U}(\tilde{\boldsymbol{\alpha}},0)'\, I(\tilde{\boldsymbol{\alpha}},0)^{-1}\, \mathbf{U}(\tilde{\boldsymbol{\alpha}},0)$$

$$= \frac{[\sum_{ik} X_i\, (n_{i2k} - \tilde{m}_{i2k})]^2}{E} \tag{A2.26}$$

where

$$E = \sum_k \frac{n_{+1k}\, n_{+2k}}{n_{++k}^3}\left[n_{++k}\sum_i X_i^2 n_{i+k} - \left(\sum_i X_i\, n_{i+k}\right)^2\right]$$

In the cases where one is just combining K 2×2 tables—that is, $X = 0$ or 1—this is identical to Cochran's test (6):

$$S^2 = \frac{[\sum_{ik}(n_{i2k} - \tilde{m}_{i2k})]}{\displaystyle\sum_k \frac{n_{+1k}\, n_{+2k}\, n_{1+k}\, n_{2+k}}{n_{++k}^3}} \tag{A2.27}$$

In the test for trend in the $I \times 2$ table it was noted that an alternative for estimating the nuisance intercept parameter was to use conditional inference. This concept extends directly to the situation where one is combining information in K tables, by conditioning on this a minimal sufficient statistic for α_k, n_{+2k}. The argument results in a contribution to the overall likelihood by a single table taking the form shown in equation A2.17 so that the overall conditional likelihood is

$$\ell_c(\beta) = \prod_k \frac{\prod_i \binom{n_{i+k}}{n_{i2k}} \exp\{n_{i2k}\, X_i\, \beta\}}{\displaystyle\sum_{\{u_k:\, u_{+k}=n_{2+k}\}} \prod_i \binom{n_{i+k}}{u_{ik}} \exp\{u_{ik}\, X_i\, \beta\}} \tag{A2.28}$$

The resulting score is

$$U_c(0) = \sum_{ik} X_{ik}(n_{i2k} - \tilde{m}_{i2k}) \tag{A2.29}$$

which is identical to the kth element of equation A2.23. The second derivative of the log likelihood at H_0 is

$$\hat{I}_c(0) = \frac{n_{+1k}\, n_{+2k}}{n_{++k}^2\,(n_{++k}-1)}\left\{ n_{++k}\sum_i X_i^2 n_{i+k} - \left(\sum_i X_i\, n_{i+k}\right)^2\right\} \tag{A2.30}$$

and the resulting score statistic is found in this unusual way. When I = 2

$$S_C^2 = \frac{U_C(0,\beta)^2}{I_C(0,\beta)}$$

$$= \frac{[\sum_{ik}(n_{i2k} - \tilde{m}_{i2k})]^2}{\displaystyle\sum_k \frac{n_{+1k}\, n_{+2k}\, n_{1+k}\, n_{2+k}}{(n_{++k}^2 - 1)}} \tag{A2.31}$$

which is the test proposed by Mantel and Haenszel (7).

References

1. Cox DR, Hinkley DV. *Theoretical Statistics*. London: Chapman & Hall, 1974.
2. Cox DR. *Analysis of Binary Data*. London: Methuen, 1970.
3. Bishop YMM, Fienburg SE, Holland PW. *Discrete Multivariate Analysis: Theory and Practice*. Cambridge, MA: MIT Press, 1973.
4. Rao CR. *Linear Statistical Inference and Its Applications*. New York: Wiley, 1973.
5. Armitage P. Test for linear trend in proportions and frequencies. *Biometrics* 1955; 11:375–386.
6. Cochran WG. Some methods for strengthening the common χ^2 tests. *Biometrics* 1954;10:417–451.
7. Mantel N, Haenszel W. Statistical aspects of the analysis of data from retrospective studies of disease. *Journal of the National Cancer Institute*. 1959;22: 719–748.

Appendix 3

Theory on Analysis of Rates

Here we consider some of the underlying theoretical issues for the various methods we have described in Chapter 4. The types of epidemiological studies that give rise to rates are time to failure at the outcomes, standardized morbidity estimates, and vital statistics. Even though these appear on the surface to have very different foundations, they do have elements that are sufficiently similar to enable us to make use of the same formulae for our analysis.

Likelihood Formation

We first consider three ways in which the likelihood can be formulated for these methods, all of which result in equivalent kernel log likelihoods, which is the part of the likelihood that affects the statistical inference. These three foundational distribution assumptions can then flow into a common set of analytical formulae that can be used for statistical inference.

Time to failure models

First let us formulate the likelihood for inference in a constant hazards model, in which the observed data consist of information on the length of follow-up for each individual, t_i, and the status of that individual at the time of last follow-up is $\delta_i = 1$ if they failed and $\delta_i = 0$ if they were censored. If an individual fails, their contribution to the likelihood is the probability density function, $f(t) = \lambda \cdot \exp\{-\lambda t\}$, and if they are censored the contribution is the survival function, $\mathcal{F}(t) = \exp\{-\lambda t\}$. We can represent the overall likelihood by introducing the appropriate contribution for each individual:

$$\ell = \prod_i f(t_i)^{\delta_i} \cdot \mathcal{F}(t_i)^{1-\delta_i}$$

$$= \lambda^{\sum_i \delta_i} \cdot \exp\{-\sum_i t_i\} \tag{A3.1}$$

$$= \lambda^n \cdot \exp\{-\lambda D\}$$

where $n = \sum \delta_i$ is the number of failures and $D = \sum t_i$ is the total follow-up time. For grouped data, in which the hazard for the jth group is given by λ_j and the corresponding summary statistics for the group are n_j and D_j, respectively, we shall assume that each group's contribution is independent, and the likelihood becomes $\ell = \prod_j \lambda_j^{n_j} \cdot \exp\{-\lambda_j D_j\}$. The corresponding log-likelihood is

$$L = \sum_j [n_j \cdot \log \lambda_j - D_j \lambda_j] \tag{A3.2}$$

which is the kernel of the log-likelihood on which we will base our statistical inference.

Counts of failures

As we have already mentioned, under fairly general conditions (1), counts of the number of failures, including the number of deaths and cases of disease in defined populations, can be thought of as having a Poisson distribution with a mean that is proportional to the denominator for the rate. If we let n_j represent the observed number of failures in the jth population where D_j represents the appropriate mid-period population, then the probability of observing this outcome is given by

$$\Pr\{n_j\} = \frac{\lambda_j^{n_j}}{n_j!} \cdot \exp\{-\lambda_j D_j\}$$

If we assume that the counts in all populations act independently, then the likelihood can be represented by

$$\ell = \prod_j \frac{\lambda_j^{n_j}}{n_j!} \cdot \exp\{-\lambda_j D_j\}$$

$$\propto \prod_j \lambda_j^{n_j} \cdot \exp\{-\lambda_j D_j\}$$

and the kernel of the log-likelihood obviously reduces to the expression we saw in equation A3.2.

Comparisons to standard rates

Breslow (2) showed that the SMR could be derived by considering a model in which the hazard for a particular population was proportional to a known or standard hazard. Hence, if we let the standard hazard be represented by $\lambda^*(t)$, the hazard for the group under consideration becomes $\psi\lambda^*(t)$, where ψ is an unknown parameter or a specified function of unknown parameters. We can use an idea from Chapter 2 to look at the density function for the event times

$$f(t) = \psi\,\lambda^*(t)\,\exp\left\{-\psi\int_{t_0}^{t}\lambda^*(u)du\right\}$$

If we introduce a transformation of variables, where

$$t^* = h(t) = \int_{t_0}^{t}\lambda^*(u)du$$

then the distribution of the transformed time becomes

$$g(t^*) = f(t^*) \cdot \frac{dt^*}{} = \psi \cdot \exp\{-\psi t^*\}$$

Notice that the observed transformed variable for the ith individual becomes Λ_i, and we have just shown that its distribution is exponential with parameter ψ, thus reducing the problem to one that is essentially the same as the analysis of a constant hazard model.

Estimation

From the kernel of the log-likelihood, shown in equation A3.2, we can obtain

$$\frac{\partial L}{\partial \lambda_j} = \frac{n_j}{\lambda_j} - D_j \tag{A3.3}$$

and

$$\frac{\partial^2 L}{\partial \lambda_j^2} = -\frac{n_j}{\lambda_j^2} \tag{A3.4}$$

Setting equation A3.3 to zero and solving for λ_j yields the maximum likelihood estimate:

$$\hat{\lambda}_j = \frac{n_j}{D_j}$$

We can obtain a variance estimate of this statistic by substituting $\hat{\lambda}$ into equation A3.4, in order to obtain the negative information, giving

$$\text{Var}(\hat{\lambda}_j) = \left[-\frac{\partial^2 L}{\partial \lambda_j^2} \right]_{\lambda_j = \hat{\lambda}_j}^{-1} = \frac{\hat{\lambda}_j^2}{n_j}$$

from which we can readily use the delta method to obtain the expression for the variance of $\text{Var}(\log \hat{\lambda}_j)$ shown in equation 4.3.

Score Test for Nominal Categories

In the case of the SMR, the simplest hypothesis becomes relevant, H_0: $\lambda_j = 1$, and the score or the first derivative of the log-likelihood evaluated under this condition is $(n_j - D_j)$. The information is

$$-E \left[\frac{\partial^2 L}{\partial \lambda_j} \right] \Bigg|_{\lambda_j = 1} = D_j$$

which results in the statistics shown in equation 4.5.

To compare two or more groups, we can represent the problem by establishing a log-linear model for the rate

$$\lambda(\mathbf{X}) = \alpha + X_2 \cdot \beta_2 + \cdots + X_{\mathcal{J}} \cdot \beta_{\mathcal{J}} = \alpha + \mathbf{X}\boldsymbol{\beta}$$

in which $X_j = 0$ for the reference group $j = 1$, and $X_j = 1$ if the individual is in the jth exposure group, and $\mathbf{X} = (X_2, X_3, \ldots, X_{\mathcal{J}})$. The test of equality of the hazard for the groups is given by H_0: $\boldsymbol{\beta} = \mathbf{0}$, and we can set up the test by using the log-likelihood in equation A3.2, which becomes

$$L = \sum_j [n_j \cdot (\alpha + \beta_j) - D_j \cdot \exp\{\alpha + \beta_j\}]$$

where $\beta_1 = 0$. Under H_0, α is the overall log failure rate, which is estimated by $\hat{\alpha} = \log(n_+/D_+)$ and the expected number of failures in the jth group becomes $m_j = (D_j n_+)/D_+$. In contrast, the alternative hypothesis is saturated, so the expected number of failures is estimated by the observed number, n_j. We can set up a likelihood ratio test by

$$G^2 = 2 \cdot [L(\hat{\alpha}, \hat{\beta}) - L(\tilde{\alpha}, 0)]$$

$$= 2 \cdot \left\{ \sum_j [n_j \cdot \log n_j - D_j \cdot (n_j/D_j)] - \sum_j [n_j \cdot \log m_j - D_j \cdot (n_+/D_+)] \right\}$$

$$= 2 \cdot \left\{ \sum_j n_j \cdot \log(n_j/m_j) \right\}$$

which is the test given in equation 4.13.

For the score test, we need to specify the vector of first partial derivatives evaluated at the maximum likelihood estimates under the null hypothesis

$$U(\tilde{\alpha}, 0) = \begin{bmatrix} n_+ - \sum_j D_j \cdot \exp\{\alpha + \beta_j\} \\ n - D_2 \cdot \exp\{\alpha + \beta_2\} \\ \vdots \\ n_J - D_J \cdot \exp\{\alpha + \beta_J\} \end{bmatrix}_{\alpha = \tilde{\alpha}, \beta_2 = \cdots = \beta_J = 0} = \begin{bmatrix} 0 \\ n_2 - m_2 \\ \vdots \\ n_J - m_J \end{bmatrix}$$

(A3.5)

and the corresponding information matrix is

$$I(\tilde{\alpha}, 0) =$$

$$\begin{bmatrix} \sum_j D_j \cdot \exp\{\alpha + \beta_j\} & D_2 \cdot \exp\{\alpha + \beta_2\} & \cdots & D_J \cdot \exp\{\alpha + \beta_J\} \\ D_2 \cdot \exp\{\alpha + \beta_2\} & D_2 \cdot \exp\{\alpha + \beta_2\} & \cdots & 0 \\ \vdots & \vdots & \ddots & \vdots \\ D_J \cdot \exp\{\alpha + \beta_J\} & 0 & \cdots & D_J \cdot \exp\{\alpha + \beta_J\} \end{bmatrix}_{\alpha = \tilde{\alpha}, \beta_2 = \cdots = \beta_J = 0}$$

$$= \begin{bmatrix} m_+ & m_2 & \cdots & m_J \\ m_2 & m_2 & \cdots & 0 \\ \vdots & \vdots & \ddots & \vdots \\ m_J & 0 & \cdots & m_J \end{bmatrix}$$

(A3.6)

The score test only depends on the inverse of the matrix formed by deleting the first row and first column of equation A3.6, which is

$$I^{-1}(\tilde{\alpha}, 0) = \begin{bmatrix} m_2^{-1} & 0 & \cdots & 0 \\ 0 & m_3^{-1} & \cdots & 0 \\ \vdots & \vdots & \ddots & \vdots \\ 0 & 0 & \cdots & m_J^{-1} \end{bmatrix} + m_1^{-1} \cdot \mathbf{1}_{(J-1) \times (J-1)}$$

and the test statistic becomes

$$S^2 = \mathbf{U}'(\tilde{\alpha},0)\cdot\mathbf{I}^{-1}(\tilde{\alpha},0)\cdot\mathbf{U}(\tilde{\alpha},0) = \sum_j \frac{(n_j - m_j)^2}{m_j}$$

which has a chi-square distribution with (J-1) df under H_0, and it is identical to the Pearson chi-square presented in equation (4.14).

Score Test Controlling for Strata

To develop a score test for a stratified analysis comparing two groups, we assume a log-linear model for the hazard function for a table of rates with j rows and two columns:

$$\lambda_{ij} = \exp\{\alpha_j\} \qquad \text{for } i = 1$$
$$= \exp\{\alpha_j + \beta\} \qquad \text{for } i = 2$$

where α_j represents the log rate for the jth stratum for group 1, and β represents the log hazard ratio, which is clearly homogeneous across all the strata. We wish to test the null hypothesis, H_0: $\beta = 0$. The kernel of the log-likelihood can be expressed as

$$L = \sum_j [n_{+j}\alpha_j + n_{2j}\beta - \exp\{\alpha_j\}(D_{1j} + D_{2j}\exp\{\beta\})]$$

and the score is given by

$$\mathbf{U}(\tilde{\alpha},0) = \begin{bmatrix} \partial L/\partial\alpha_1 \\ \vdots \\ \partial L/\partial\alpha_J \\ \partial L/\partial\beta \end{bmatrix}_{\alpha=\tilde{\alpha},\beta=0} = \begin{bmatrix} n_{+1} - m_{+1} \\ \vdots \\ n_{+J} - m_{+J} \\ \sum_j(n_{2j} - m_{2j}) \end{bmatrix}$$

where $m_{ij} = n_{+j}D_{ij}/D_{+j} = n_{+j}P_{ij}$. We can obtain the information matrix from

$I(\tilde{\alpha},0) =$

$$\begin{bmatrix} e^{\alpha_1}\cdot(D_{11} + D_{21}e^{\beta}) & 0 & \cdots & 0 & D_{21}e^{\beta} \\ 0 & e^{\alpha_2}\cdot(D_{12} + D_{22}e^{\beta}) & \cdots & 0 & D_{22}e^{\beta} \\ \vdots & \vdots & \ddots & \vdots & \vdots \\ 0 & 0 & \cdots & e^{\alpha_J}\cdot(D_{1J} + D_{2J}e^{\beta}) & D_{2J}e^{\beta} \\ D_{21}e^{\beta} & D_{22}e^{\beta} & \cdots & D_{2J}e^{\beta} & \sum_j D_j\cdot e^{\alpha_j+\beta} \end{bmatrix}_{\alpha=\tilde{\alpha},\beta=0}$$

$$= \begin{bmatrix} n_{+1} & 0 & \cdots & m_{21} \\ 0 & n_{+2} & \cdots & m_{22} \\ \vdots & \vdots & \ddots & \vdots \\ 0 & 0 & \cdots & m_{2j} \\ m_{21} & m_{22} & \cdots & m_{2+} \end{bmatrix}$$

To construct the score test, we only require the lower right element of the inverse of the information matrix, which can be expressed as

$$V = \sum_j m_j - \sum_j (m_j^2/n_{+j})$$

$$= \sum_j n_{+j} \cdot \left(\frac{D_{2j}}{D_{+j}} \right) \cdot \left(1 - \frac{D_{2j}}{D_{+j}} \right)$$

$$= \sum_j n_{+j} \cdot P_{2j} \cdot (1 - P_{2j})$$

where $P_{2j} = (D_{2j}/D_{+j})$. It is interesting to note that the form for this variance is essentially the same as the expression given by Cochran's method for combining 2×2 tables, only here we introduce the proportion of follow-up time observed in group 2 for the jth stratum, rather than the proportion of subjects in group 2. Thus, the score test becomes

$$S^2 = \frac{(n_{2+} - m_{2+})^2}{\sum_j n_{+j} \cdot P_{2j} \cdot (1 - P_{2j})}$$

References

1. Brillinger DT. The natural variability of vital rates and associated statistics. *Biometrics* 1986;42:693–734.
2. Breslow N. Some statistical models useful in the study of occupational mortality. In: A Whittamore (ed.) *Environmental Health: Quantitative Methods.* Philadelphia: SIAM, 1977.

Appendix 4

Theory on Analysis of Time to Failure

In this appendix we consider some of the theoretical issues that underlie the methods for analyzing survival curves discussed in Chapter 5.

Actuarial Estimate

The first step in formulating an actuarial estimate is to divide the period of follow-up into intervals at cutpoints: $x_1, x_2, \ldots, x_I$. If we adopt the piece-wise exponential model, then the hazard is given by equation 5.1. The contribution to the likelihood for an individual who is observed until failure in the ith interval is

$$
\begin{aligned}
f(t) &= \lambda(t) \, \exp\left\{ -\int_0^t \lambda(u)\,du \right\} \\
&= \lambda_i \exp\left\{ -\sum_{\{j:x_i<t\}} \lambda_{j-1}(x_j - x_{j-1}) - \lambda_i(t - x_i) \right\} \\
&= \lambda_i \prod_{j=0}^{i} \exp\{-\lambda_j \, t_j\}
\end{aligned}
$$

where

$$
\begin{aligned}
t_j &= x_j - x_{j-1} & &\text{if } x_j < t \\
&= t - x_{j-1} & &\text{if } x_{j-1} < t < x_j \\
&= 0 & &t < x_{j-1}
\end{aligned}
$$

the corresponding quantity for a censored individual is

$$\mathcal{F}(t) = \exp\left\{-\int_0^t \lambda(u)du\right\}$$

$$= \prod_{j=0}^{i} \exp\{-\lambda_j\, t_j\}$$

If we let $\delta_j = 0$ for an observation that does not fail in the jth interval, and $\delta_j = 1$ if it does, then the overall likelihood can be expressed as

$$\ell = \prod_{n=1}^{N} \prod_{j=0}^{\mathcal{J}} \lambda_j^{\delta_{nj}} \exp\{-\lambda_j \cdot t_{nj}\}$$

and the log likelihood is

$$L = \sum_{n=1}^{N} \sum_{j=0}^{\mathcal{J}} [\delta_{nj} \log(\lambda_j) - t_{nj}\,\lambda_j]$$

$$= \sum_{j=0}^{\mathcal{J}} [d_j \log(\lambda_j) - T_j\,\lambda_j]$$

where $d_j = \sum_n \delta_{nj}$ is the total number of deaths, and $T_j = \sum_n t_{nj}$ is the total observed follow-up time during the jth interval of follow-up. To find the maximum likelihood estimate of the hazard for the jth interval, we set the partial derivative,

$$\frac{\partial L}{\partial \lambda_j} = \frac{d_j}{\lambda_j} - T_j$$

to zero and solve, yielding

$$\hat{\lambda}_j = \frac{d_j}{T_j}$$

The matrix of second partial derivatives of the log likelihood is a diagonal matrix, hence the variance for our estimator is

$$\mathrm{Var}(\hat{\lambda}_j) = \frac{\lambda_j^2}{d_j}$$

and all covariances are zero.

The conditional probability of surviving the jth interval, given a subject is alive at the beginning of the interval, can be expressed as

$$p_j = \exp\left\{ -\int_{x_j}^{x_{j+1}} \lambda(u)du \right\} = \exp\{-\lambda_j (x_{j+1} - x_j)\}$$

The invariance property of maximum likelihood estimators implies that we can obtain maximum likelihood estimators for the p_j's by substituting our estimates for the hazard. The probability of surviving until the ith cutpoint of the follow-up time, x_i, is found by multiplying over the conditional probabilities of surviving each of the previous intervals:

$$\hat{\mathcal{F}}_i = \prod_{j=0}^{i-1} \hat{p}_j \tag{A4.1}$$

One way of establishing the actuarial estimator is to consider the number of failures in an interval as arising from a multinomial distribution, which is directly applicable if no individuals are lost to follow-up. If l_i subjects are alive and under active follow-up at the beginning of the ith interval, then a failure during the interval represents a binary outcome. Thus, the number of failures during an interval would have a binomial distribution with parameters l_i and p_i, and the obvious estimator for the probability of surviving the interval is also the maximum likelihood estimator, $\hat{p}_i = 1 - d_i/l_i$, where d_i is the number of failures during the interval. Under this derivation, the variance for this estimator is $\text{Var}(\hat{p}_i) = p_i(1 - p_i)/l_i$. Suppose that we adopt a somewhat heuristic approach for the censored observation case, and we treat the number of failures as if they behaved like a binomial random variable drawn from a sample of size equal to the effective number at risk, $l'_i = l_i - \frac{1}{2} \cdot W_i$. Thus, we have the estimator for the conditional probability of surviving the interval, $\hat{p}_i = 1 - d_i/l'_i$. The variance for the estimate of p_i is $\text{Var}(\hat{p}_i) = p_i(1 - p_i)/l'_i$. The survival curve would once again be estimated using equation A4.1, which can be introduced into the Taylor series expansion formula for the variance yielding

$$\text{Var}(\hat{\mathcal{F}}_i) \simeq \hat{\mathcal{F}}_i^2 \sum_j \frac{\text{Var}(\hat{p}_j)}{\hat{p}_j^2} = \hat{\mathcal{F}}_i^2 \sum_j \frac{d_j}{l'_j \cdot (l'_j - d_j)}$$

which is Greenwood's formula (1).

Product Limit Estimate

To formulate the product limit estimator, we selected a large number of small intervals, and we adopted the convention that ties between failure and censoring times are broken so that the censored observations are moved to the next interval. Focusing on just the jth interval, the conditional distribution for d_j failures out of l_j entering the interval has a binomial distribution with parameters l_j and $(1 - p_j)$.

We can readily show that the maximum likelihood estimator is given by

$$\hat{p}_j = \frac{l_j - d_j}{l_j}$$

with variance

$$\mathrm{Var}(\hat{p}_j) = \frac{p_j (1 - p_j)}{l_j}$$

For two different intervals, j and $j^* > j$, the expectation of the product is

$$E[\hat{p}_j \cdot \hat{p}_{j^*}] = E[\hat{p}_j \cdot E[\hat{p}_{j^*}|l_{j^*}]] = E[\hat{p}_j \cdot p_{j^*}] = p_j \cdot p_{j^*}$$

which implies that $\mathrm{Cov}(\hat{p}_j, \hat{p}_{j^*}) = 0$. To estimate the survival function, we need to consider only the intervals in which deaths occur, because $\hat{p}_j = 1$ for the others, yielding the expression in equation 5.2. The variance can be directly obtained by applying the Taylor series expansion formula, yielding equation 5.3.

Two-Sample Score Test for Piecewise Constant Hazards

To construct a two-sample score test for a piecewise constant hazards models we will assume that the hazards are proportional; that is, the hazard for group 2 is related to group 1 by

$$\lambda_{2j} = \exp\{\beta\} \lambda_{1j}$$

The null hypothesis of interest is: H_0: $\beta = 0$. For this case, the log likelihood becomes

$$L = \sum_{k=1}^{2} \sum_{j=0}^{\mathcal{J}} [d_{jk} \log(\lambda_{jk}) - T_{jk} \lambda_{jk}]$$

$$= \sum_{j=0}^{\mathcal{J}} [d_{j+} \log(\lambda_{j1}) + d_{j2} \beta - T_{j1} \lambda_{j1} - T_{j2} \lambda_{j1} \exp\{\beta\}]$$

where d_{jk} and T_{jk} are the number of deaths and the total follow-up times for group k during interval j. The partial derivatives of the log likelihood are

$$\frac{\partial L}{\partial \lambda_{j1}} = \frac{d_{j+}}{\lambda_{j1}} - T_{j1} - T_{j2} \exp\{\beta\} \tag{A4.2}$$

for the interval parameters, and

$$\frac{\partial L}{\partial \beta} = \sum_{j=0}^{\mathcal{J}} d_{j2} - \sum_{j=0}^{\mathcal{J}} T_{2j} \lambda_{j1} \exp\{\beta\} \tag{A4.3}$$

for the log hazard ratio. We can find the maximum likelihood estimates of the interval parameters under H_0 by first letting $\beta = 0$, setting the resulting equation A4.2 to 0, and solving, giving

$$\tilde{\lambda}_{j1} = \frac{d_{j+}}{T_{j+}}$$

Substituting this value into equation A4.3 yields the score under the null hypothesis:

$$\frac{\partial L}{\partial \beta} = \sum_{j=0}^{\mathcal{J}} d_{j2} - \sum_{j=0}^{\mathcal{J}} \frac{T_{2j} d_{j+}}{T_{j+}} = \sum_{j=0}^{\mathcal{J}} [d_{j1} - d_{j+} P_{j2}]$$

where P_{j2} is the proportion of the total follow-up time during interval j that is observed in group 2, and $d_{j+}P_{j2}$ can be regarded as an "expected" number of failures. Thus, the score statistic reduces to considering the total difference between the observed number of deaths in group 2 and the expected number under the null hypothesis.

Second partial derivatives of the log likelihood are as follows:

$$\frac{\partial^2 L}{\partial \lambda_{j1} \partial \lambda_{j*1}} = \frac{-d_{j+}}{\lambda_{j1}^2} \qquad \text{for } j = j^*$$

$$= 0 \qquad \text{for } j \neq j^*$$

$$\frac{\partial^2 L}{\partial \lambda_{j1} \partial \beta} = -T_{j2} \exp\{\beta\}$$

and

$$\frac{\partial L^2}{\partial \beta^2} = \sum_{j=0}^{\mathcal{J}} T_{j2} \lambda_{j1} \exp\{\beta\}$$

Substituting the null value of $\beta = 0$ into the matrix of second partials yields the information matrix, and inverting this yields the variance for the score itself in the corner for the second partial derivative with respect to β:

$$V = \sum_{j=0}^{\mathcal{J}} d_{j+} P_{j2} (1 - P_{j2})$$

The resulting score test for H_0: $\beta = 0$ is

$$S^2 = \frac{\left[\sum_{j=0}^{\mathcal{J}} (d_{j1} - d_{j+} P_{j2}) \right]^2}{\sum_{j=0}^{\mathcal{J}} d_{j+} P_{j2} (1 - P_{j2})}$$

which is compared to a chi-square distribution with 1 df.

Log-Rank Test

As with the estimators for the survival curve, we can also develop our two-sample test for the case in which we take many small intervals, thus effectively relaxing the assumption of the piece-wise constant hazards model. As before, we move censored observations that are tied with a failure to the next interval. Likewise, for simplicity we shall assume that deaths are observed for the entire interval, thus the total follow-up time for the jth interval of width Δ is $l_j \Delta$. Hence, the expected number of failures for the jth interval is

$$E[d_{j2}] = d_{j+} P_{j2} = \frac{d_{j+} l_{j2} \Delta}{l_{j+} \Delta} = \frac{d_{j+} l_{j2}}{l_{j+}}$$

and the variance reduces to

$$\text{Var}(d_{j2}) = \sum_{\mathcal{J}=1}^{\mathcal{J}} \frac{d_{j+} l_{j1} l_{j2}}{l_{j+}^2} \tag{A4.4}$$

Notice that only in those intervals in which failures occur do we have a contribution to the expected and variance totals. Hence, we only need to consider the results at the times at which failures occur, $\tau_{[1]}, \tau_{[2]}, \ldots, \tau_{[\mathcal{I}]}$, and the test statistic becomes

$$S^2 = \frac{(\sum_j d_{j2} - \sum_j E[d_{j2}])^2}{\sum_j \mathrm{Var}(d_{j2})}$$

which is compared to a chi-square distribution with 1 df.

We can readily see the relationship between the log-rank test and the tests for combining information across a series of 2×2 tables, and indeed Mantel (2) proposed a version of this test, based on a rationale similar to what he had used in developing the Mantel–Haenszel test (3). Not surprisingly, alternative forms for the variance for this statistic have also been proposed (4), including the use of a marginal likelihood approach (5), that gives rise to the expression

$$\mathrm{Var}^*(d_{j2}) = \sum_{j=1}^{\mathcal{I}} \frac{d_{j+} \, l_{j1} \, l_{j2}}{l_{j+}^2} \cdot \frac{(l_{j+} - d_{j+})}{(l_{j+} - 1)} \tag{A4.5}$$

Notice that no difference between the variance formulae in equations A4.4 and A4.5 exists when there are no ties in the failure times, or when $d_{j+} = 1$ for all j. In addition, we would usually have few failure time ties relative to the number at risk of failing at most times, or when $d_{j+} \ll l_{j+}$, in which case any difference between these two formulae is small.

Because of the relationship between the hazard and the survival functions, we can also express the model on which this test is based as a test of $H_0: \theta = 1$, where the survival functions for the two groups are related by

$$\mathcal{F}_2(t) = \mathcal{F}_1^\theta(t)$$

Under the null hypothesis the survival functions are identical, and the relationship between the two is called the Lehman alternative. Savage (6) proposed a test that was optimal for testing such an alternative, and the log-rank test can be regarded as an extension of the Savage test to the case in which there are censored observations. Other tests have been derived that are optimal for different alternatives, for example the Wilcoxon rank sum test is optimal for an alternative, in which the survival functions for the two groups are related by

$$\mathcal{F}_2(t) = \mathcal{F}_1(t + \varphi)$$

A version of this test for censored data has been described by Gehan (7), and Peto and Peto (4) develop these ideas further, showing the relationship between these methods. Of course, these are just two of many different ways of expressing the alternative hypothesis, and Harrington and Fleming (8) consider such tests that can arise under a very general class of alternatives.

References

1. Greenwood M. A report on the natural duration of cancer. *Reports on Public Health and Medical Subjects* 1926;33:1–26.
2. Mantel N. Chi-square tests with one degree of freedom: Extensions of the Mantel–Haenszel procedure. *Journal of the American Statistical Association* 1963; 58:690–700.
3. Mantel N, Haenszel W. Statistical aspects of the analysis of data from retrospective studies of disease. *Journal of the National Cancer Institute* 1959;22: 719–748.
4. Peto R, Peto J. Asymptotically efficient rank invariant procedures (with discussion). *Journal of the Royal Statistical Society, Series A* 1972;135:185–206.
5. Kalbfleisch JD, Prentice RL. *The Statistical Analysis of Failure Time Data.* New York: Wiley, 1980.
6. Savage IR. Contributions to the theory of rank order statistics—the two sample case. *Annals of Mathematical Statistics* 1956;27:590–615.
7. Gehan EA. A generalized Wilcoxon test for comparing arbitrarily singly-censored samples. *Biometrika* 1965;52:203–223.
8. Harrington DP, Fleming TR. A class of rank test procedures for censored survival data. *Biometrika* 1982;69:553–566.

Appendix 5

Theory on Regression Models for Proportions

The approach for fitting generalized linear models is based on work by Nelder and Wedderburn (1) and McCullagh and Nelder (2), which provides a powerful synthesis of regression methodology, thus unifying various techniques that had previously been considered separately. The elements of a generalized linear model that need to be identified in order to obtain maximum likelihood estimates are the distribution of the response and the relationship between the mean, μ, and the linear predictor, η, which introduces the regressor variables into the analysis. These elements are then used to derive the necessary information for statistical inference on the model parameters.

Distribution for Binary Responses

As we saw in Chapter 3, the total number of responders in a group of n individuals with a common probability of the outcome has a binomial distribution in which

$$
\begin{aligned}
\Pr\{Y = y\} &= \binom{n}{y} \pi^y \, (1 - \pi)^{n-y} \\
&= \binom{n}{y} n^{-n} \, \mu^y \, (n - \mu)^{n-y}
\end{aligned}
\tag{A5.1}
$$

One of the required elements for fitting a generalized linear model is the variance of the response, expressed as a function of the mean, which in this case is given by

$$
\mathrm{Var}(Y) = n \, \pi(1 - \pi) = \frac{\mu \, (n - \mu)}{n}
$$

The likelihood, $\ell(\mu)$, is given by the probability of observing the response. If we have I independent samples, then

$$\ell \propto \prod_{i=1}^{I} \pi_i^{y_i} (1 - \pi_i)^{n_i - y_i}$$

and the log likelihood is

$$L = \sum_{i=1}^{I} [y_i \log \pi_i + (n_i - y_i) \log(1 - \pi_i)]$$

Maximum likelihood estimates can be found by solving the normal equations, which were formed by setting the partial derivatives of L with respect to the model parameters to zero. For models belonging to the exponential class, it is convenient to employ the chain rule (2):

$$\frac{\partial L}{\partial \beta_r} = \sum_{i=1}^{I} \frac{\partial L}{\partial \pi_i} \cdot \frac{\partial \pi_i}{\partial \beta_r} = \sum_{i=1}^{I} \left[\frac{y_i - n_i \pi_i}{\pi_i (1 - \pi_i)} \right] \cdot \frac{\partial \pi_i}{\partial \beta_r} \tag{A5.2}$$

If all of the parameters are the regression terms in the linear predictor, then we can conveniently carry the chain rule one step further, by noting that

$$\frac{\partial \pi_i}{\partial \beta_r} = \frac{\partial \pi_i}{\partial \eta_i} \cdot \frac{\partial \eta_i}{\partial \beta_r} = \frac{\partial \pi_i}{\partial \eta_i} \cdot x_{ir}$$

where x_{ir} is the rth regressor variable for the ith subject.

A final term that is often used when formulating likelihood-based inference for binary responses is the deviance, which is defined as twice the logarithm of the ratio of the likelihood evaluated at the observed response to that of the expected response. For the ith subject this becomes

$$\text{Dev}(y_i, \mu_i) = 2 \cdot \log \left(\frac{\ell(y_i)}{\ell(\mu_i)} \right)$$

$$= 2 \cdot \log \left(\frac{y_i^{y_i} (n_i - y_i)^{n_i - y_i}}{\mu_i^{y_i} (n_i - \mu_i)^{n_i - y_i}} \right)$$

$$= 2 \cdot \left[y_i \log \left(\frac{y_i}{\mu_i} \right) + (n_i - y_i) \log \left(\frac{n_i - y_i}{n_i - \mu_i} \right) \right]$$

and the overall deviance is found by summing over I. Maximizing the likelihood is equivalent to minimizing the deviance, but the deviance is especially useful in the present context because when n_i is large, it can be interpreted as an overall goodness of fit statistic, which can be compared to a chi-square distribution with $I - p$ df, where p is the number of parameters in our model.

Functions of the Linear Predictor

The relationship between the proportion responding and the linear predictor is defined by the link function, $\eta = g(\pi)$, which gives the transformation of the probability of the response that leads to the linear portion of the model. It is also necessary to be able to reverse the process by determining π as a function of the linear predictor, $\pi = g^{-1}(\eta)$, called the inverse link. Some software also requires that we specify the derivative of the linear predictor with respect to π,

$$\frac{d\eta}{d\pi} = \frac{dg(\pi)}{d\pi}$$

Table A5–1 gives some useful link functions along with their corresponding inverses and derivatives. Some of these are commonly included in software as built in options, including logit, complementary log-log, and probit.

Example A5–1. Suppose we are interested in fitting a model in which the odds for disease is a linear function of the regression parameters. Let π represent the

Table A5–1. Commonly used link functions, inverse links, and derivatives for binary response data

Model	Link function $g(\pi)$	Inverse link $g^{-1}(\eta)$	Derivative $\dfrac{dg(\pi)}{d\pi}$
Logit	$\log\left(\dfrac{\pi}{1-\pi}\right)$	$\dfrac{\exp\{\eta\}}{1+\exp\{\eta\}}$	$\dfrac{1}{\pi(1-\pi)}$
Complementary log-log	$\log[-\log(1-\pi)]$	$(1 - \exp[-\exp\{\eta\}])$	$\left[\dfrac{-1}{(1-\pi)\cdot\log(1-\pi)}\right]$
Probit	$\Phi^{-1}(\pi)$	$n \cdot \Phi(\eta)$	$\dfrac{d[\Phi^{-1}(\pi)]}{d\pi}$
Linear odds	$\dfrac{\pi}{1-\pi}$	$\left(\dfrac{\eta}{1+\eta}\right)$	$\dfrac{1}{(1-\pi)^2}$
Power odds $(\gamma \neq 0)$ $(\gamma = 0;$ see Logit$)$	$\left(\dfrac{\pi}{1-\pi}\right)^{\gamma}$	$\dfrac{\eta^{1/\gamma}}{1+\eta^{1/\gamma}}$	$\left(\dfrac{\gamma}{\pi^2}\right)\cdot\left(\dfrac{\pi}{1-\pi}\right)^{\gamma+1}$

probability that disease occurs, and let the response, Y, represent the number of cases that occur out of n observed in a particular risk group. Hence, the mean response is $\mu = n\pi$, and the link function is given by

$$\eta = \frac{\pi}{1 - \pi} = \frac{\mu}{n - \mu} = g(\mu)$$

This can be rearranged to give the inverse link

$$\pi = \frac{\eta}{1 + \eta} = g^{-1}(\eta)$$

and the derivative of the link function is given by

$$\frac{d\eta}{d\pi} = \frac{1}{(1 - \pi)^2}$$

Using Results to Conduct Inference

Typical output from statistical software includes computations involving the functions defined here, which are evaluated at various values of the underlying model parameters. Let us now consider how these elements are typically used in conducting statistical inference.

First, we are given the maximum likelihood estimates of the model parameters, β, along with the estimated covariance matrix, calculated from

$$\mathbf{Var}(\hat{\boldsymbol{\beta}}) = -E\left[\frac{\partial^2 L(\mu)}{\partial \boldsymbol{\beta}^2}\right]^{-1}_{\beta=\hat{\beta}}$$

and the square root of the diagonal elements yield the estimated standard errors of the model parameters, $\text{SE}(\hat{\beta}_r)$, for the rth parameter. If we apply the chain rule to equation A5.1, then the information matrix is

$$\begin{aligned}
\mathbf{I} &= -E\left[\frac{\partial^2 L}{\partial \beta_r \partial \beta_s}\right] \\
&= -\sum_{i=1}^{I} E\left[\frac{\partial^2 L}{\partial \pi_i^2} \cdot \frac{\partial \pi_i}{\partial \beta_r} \cdot \frac{\partial \pi_i}{\partial \beta_s} + \frac{\partial L}{\partial \pi_i} \cdot \frac{\partial \pi_i^2}{\partial \beta_r \partial \beta_s}\right]
\end{aligned}$$

(A5.3)

The partial derivative of L with respect to π_i has expectation zero, so we can drop the second term in brackets, and write the information matrix as

$$\mathbf{I} = \sum_{i=1}^{I}\left[\frac{n_i}{\pi_i(1 - \pi_i)} \cdot \frac{\partial \pi_i}{\partial \beta_r} \cdot \frac{\partial \pi_i}{\partial \beta_s}\right]$$

Perhaps the most familiar way in which the covariance matrix can be used is in constructing a Wald test

$$W = \frac{\hat{\beta}_p - \beta_{0p}}{\text{SE}(\beta_{\hat{p}})}$$

which is compared to a standard normal deviate, or its square, W^2, which is compared to a chi-square distribution with 1 df. A generalization of this test can also be constructed if we wish to consider a p^* vector of parameters containing a subset of all parameters in the model, $H_0\colon \boldsymbol{\beta}^* = \boldsymbol{\beta}_0^*$,

$$W^2 = (\hat{\boldsymbol{\beta}}^* - \boldsymbol{\beta}_0^*)'\, \text{Var}(\hat{\boldsymbol{\beta}}^*)^{-1}\, (\hat{\boldsymbol{\beta}}^* - \boldsymbol{\beta}_0^*)$$

which is compared to a chi-square distribution with p^* df.

An alternative approach for constructing a significance test is to use the log likelihood or the scaled deviance to construct a likelihood ratio test of whether a set of regression parameters has no effect, $H_0\colon \boldsymbol{\beta} = \mathbf{0}$, which yields the fitted mean, $\boldsymbol{\mu}_0^*$. Typically, we are given the log likelihood, so that the test is given by

$$G^2 = -2 \cdot \log\left(\frac{\ell(\hat{\boldsymbol{\mu}}_0)}{\ell(\hat{\boldsymbol{\mu}})}\right)$$

$$= 2 \cdot [L(\hat{\boldsymbol{\mu}}) - L(\hat{\boldsymbol{\mu}}_0)]$$

An equivalent test can be constructed using the scaled deviance, which is often given as an alternative to the log likelihood:

$$G^2 = -2 \cdot \log\left(\frac{\ell(\hat{\boldsymbol{\mu}}_0)/\ell(\boldsymbol{y})}{\ell(\hat{\boldsymbol{\mu}})/\ell(\boldsymbol{y})}\right)$$

$$= \text{Dev}(\hat{\boldsymbol{\mu}}_0) - \text{Dev}(\hat{\boldsymbol{\mu}})$$

Finally, we consider the construction of interval estimates of the model parameters. The simplest approach is to make use of the parameter estimates and their standard errors, so that the $100(1 - \alpha)\%$ confidence interval for the pth parameter is

$$\hat{\beta}_p \pm z_{\alpha/2} \cdot \text{SE}(\hat{\beta}_p)$$

which are by definition symmetric about the parameter estimates. This approach works well for large samples in which the distribution of the maximum likelihood estimates are well approximated by normal distributions. We can also see that this approach is similar in spirit to the Wald test, so we might also consider an analogous procedure that reminds us of the likelihood ratio statistic, by finding the value of the parameter that reduces the maximum of the log-likelihood by the half the corresponding critical value of the chi-square distribution, $\frac{1}{2} \cdot \chi_{1,\alpha}^2$. In order to construct such a confidence interval consider the *profile likelihood* in which we fix one or more parameters and maximize the likelihood for the remaining parameters. We can express the resulting linear predictor as

$$\eta^*(\beta_p) = x_p\beta_p + \hat{\beta}_0 + x_1\hat{\beta}_1 + \cdots + x_P\hat{\beta}_P$$
$$= x_p \cdot \beta_p + \hat{\eta}_{-p}$$

where the subscript $-p$ indicates that the pth regressor variable has been dropped from the linear predictors. Notice that the form for the linear predictor is the same, only now, $x_p \beta_p$ is a specified constant, or *offset*. The inverse link function yields the linear predictor, μ_{-p}, which, in turn, gives us the profile log likelihood, $L^*(\beta_p)$, and the confidence limits are found by solving

$$L^*(\beta_p) = L(\hat{\mu}) - \frac{1}{2} \cdot \chi_{1,\alpha}^2$$

for β_p, which typically has two solutions giving the lower and upper limits.

A model is always proposed as a possible candidate for describing a set of data, hence, it is important that we be sure that it provides an adequate description of the data. One way in which this can be accomplished is to conduct a goodness of fit test. When the number of subjects at each of the I independent samples is reasonably large, say about 10 or more, then we already noted that the deviance can be used for this purpose, comparing it to a chi-square distribution with $I - p$ df, where p is the number of parameters estimated. Alternatively, we can use the Pearson chi-square statistic:

$$X^2 = \sum_{i=1}^{n} (Y_i - \hat{\mu}_i)^2 \cdot \left[\frac{1}{\hat{\mu}_i} + \frac{1}{n_i - \hat{\mu}_i} \right]$$

Example A5–2.   One approach we might employ when trying to decide among alternative models for the odds for disease is to consider a general family of regression models that includes both the linear odds model and the linear logistic model as special cases. Such a family is one in which a power transformation of the odds for disease is a linear function of the regressor variables

$$
\begin{aligned}
\eta = g(\mu) &= \left(\frac{\mu}{n - \mu}\right)^{\gamma} = \left(\frac{\pi}{1 - \pi}\right)^{\gamma} && \text{if } \gamma \neq 0 \\
&= \log\!\left(\frac{\mu}{n - \mu}\right) = \log\!\left(\frac{\pi}{1 - \pi}\right) && \text{if } \gamma = 0
\end{aligned}
\tag{A5.4}
$$

Alternatively, we can express the probability of disease by

$$
\begin{aligned}
\pi &= \frac{\eta^{1/\gamma}}{1 + \eta^{1/\gamma}} && \gamma \neq 0 \\
&= \frac{\exp\{\eta\}}{1 + \exp\{\eta\}} && \gamma = 0
\end{aligned}
\tag{A5.5}
$$

If the parameter γ is known, then this reduces to a generalized linear model in which the only parameters to be estimated assess the association between the regressor variables and the outcome. However, we can also regard γ as another parameter to be estimated, so that the model is now a conditionally linear model in which the condition depends on this unknown parameter. We can find the maximum likelihood estimate of γ by fitting the model in equation A5.4 for specified values of γ and then searching for the one that maximizes the likelihood.

While this approach will indeed determine the maximum likelihood estimates of the parameters, the variance estimators provided by the software will not take into account the fact that γ was estimated from the data and is not a known constant. Hence, we will need to correct the covariance matrix for the parameters by considering the resulting information matrix, which can be partitioned as

$$
\begin{aligned}
\mathbf{I} &= \begin{bmatrix}
\left[\sum_i \dfrac{n_i}{\pi_i(1 - \pi_i)} \cdot \left(\dfrac{\partial \pi_i}{\partial \eta_i}\right)^2 \cdot x_{ir} \cdot x_{is}\right]_{p \times p} & \left[\sum_i \dfrac{n_i}{\pi_i(1 - \pi_i)} \cdot \left(\dfrac{\partial \pi_i}{\partial \eta_i}\right) \cdot x_{ir} \cdot \left(\dfrac{\partial \pi_i}{\partial \gamma}\right)\right]_{p \times 1} \\[3ex]
\left[\sum_i \dfrac{n_i}{\pi_i(1 - \pi_i)} \cdot \left(\dfrac{\partial \pi_i}{\partial \gamma}\right) \cdot \left(\dfrac{\partial \pi_i}{\partial \eta_i}\right) \cdot x_{ir}\right]_{1 \times p} & \left[\sum_i \dfrac{n_i}{\pi_i(1 - \pi_i)} \cdot \left(\dfrac{\partial \pi_i}{\partial \gamma}\right)^2\right]_{1 \times 1}
\end{bmatrix} \\[3ex]
&= \begin{bmatrix} \mathbf{A} & \mathbf{B} \\ \mathbf{B'} & \mathbf{D} \end{bmatrix}
\end{aligned}
$$

where

$$
\frac{\partial \pi_i}{\partial \eta_i} = \frac{\pi_i^2}{\gamma} \cdot \left(\frac{1 - \pi_i}{\pi_i}\right)^{\gamma + 1}
$$

and

$$
\frac{\partial \pi_i}{\partial \gamma} = \frac{\pi_i(1 - \pi_i)}{\gamma} \cdot \log\!\left(\frac{1 - \pi_i}{\pi_i}\right)
$$

The last row and column contain the covariance term involving γ, and $\mathbf{A}$ is the information matrix for the regression parameters that are part of the linear predictor. As the software is treating the maximum likelihood estimate of γ as fixed, it provides as an estimate of the covariance matrix, $\mathbf{A}^{-1}$. Using the form for the inverse of a partitioned symmetric matrix given by Rao (3), we can write the covariance of all estimated parameters as

$$\mathbf{I} = \begin{bmatrix} \mathbf{A}^{-1} + \mathbf{F} \cdot \mathbf{E}^{-1} \cdot \mathbf{F}' & -\mathbf{F} \cdot \mathbf{E}^{-1} \\ -\mathbf{E}^{-1} \cdot \mathbf{F}' & \mathbf{E}^{-1} \end{bmatrix}$$

where $\mathbf{E} = \mathbf{D} - \mathbf{B}' \cdot \mathbf{A}^{-1} \cdot \mathbf{B}$ and $\mathbf{F} = \mathbf{A}^{-1} \cdot \mathbf{B}$. Notice that we must add a correction, $\mathbf{F} \cdot \mathbf{E}^{-1} \cdot \mathbf{F}'$, to the covariance matrix generated by the software, and as the diagonal elements of this correction are positive, it is clear that if we ignore the fact that γ is estimated, then we will always underestimate the standard errors of our estimates of association with the response.

References

1. Nelder JA, Wedderburn RWM. Generalized linear models. *Journal of the Royal Statistical Society, Series A* 1972;135:370–384.
2. McCullagh P, Nelder JA. *Generalized Linear Models*. London: Chapman and Hall, 1989.
3. Rao CR. *Linear Statistical Inference and Its Applications*. New York: Wiley, 1973.

Appendix 6

Theory on Parametric Models for Hazard Functions

Here we consider some theoretical issues involved in conducting maximum likelihood inference on generalized linear models used in the analysis of rates. As we have already noted, the data that give rise to rates usually are comprised either of counts that have a Poisson distribution or of failure times that may include censoring. We begin by discussing log-linear models for a constant hazard which has a log-likelihood kernel that is identical to a Poisson distribution. We then move on to discuss the Weibull hazard, in which the covariates affect the hazard log-linearly. Finally, we consider a model in which some power of a rate is linearly related to the regressor variables. As we shall see, both of these latter two cases involve the estimation of a parameter that is not included with the linear predictor, which offers a useful extension to our class of linearizable models.

Poisson Regression

In Appendix 3, we saw that the likelihood for a rate could be derived from the standpoint of time to failure for a constant hazard model or Poisson distributed counts in which the mean was proportional to population size. In either case, the kernel of the log likelihood can be represented by

$$L = \sum_i [n_i \log \lambda(\mathbf{X_i}) - D_i \lambda(\mathbf{X_i})]$$

where n_i is the number of failures in group i and D_i is the corresponding total person-years of follow-up or rate denominator, which has the form for the log likelihood of a Poisson distribution with mean $D_i \cdot \lambda(\mathbf{X_i})$.

If we assume that a log-linear hazards model applies to a particular set of data, the likelihood becomes

$$L = \sum_i [n_i \, \mathbf{X_i}\boldsymbol{\beta} - \exp\{\mathbf{X_i}\boldsymbol{\beta} + \log D_i\}]$$

in which the mean of the Poisson for the ith observation can be expressed as $\mu_i = \exp\{\mathbf{X_i}\boldsymbol{\beta} + \log D_i\}$ and the linear predictor is obtained through the log link $\eta_i = \log \mu_i = \mathbf{X_i}\boldsymbol{\beta} + \log D_i$. We can see that in addition to the typical regression component of the linear predictor, we also have the known added constant, $\log D_i$, which is an offset term.

An alternative way of expressing the log likelihood is by factoring out the denominator, yielding

$$L = \sum_i D_i \left[\left(\frac{n_i}{D_i} \right) \cdot \log \lambda(\mathbf{X_i}) - \lambda(\mathbf{X_i}) \right]$$

In this formulation, we see the log likelihood expressed in terms of the observed rate, n_i/D_i, and once again it resembles one arising from a Poisson distribution. The difference in this case is that each contribution to the log likelihood is weighted by D_i, thus providing a rationale for our second approach to finding the maximum likelihood estimates (1, 2).

To find maximum likelihood estimates of the model parameters, we can apply the approaches used for fitting generalized linear models (2). The first partial derivative of the log likelihood with respect to the model parameters is

$$\frac{\partial L}{\partial \beta_r} = \sum_i \frac{\partial L}{\partial \lambda_i} \cdot \frac{\partial \lambda_i}{\partial \beta_r} = \sum_i \left[\frac{n_i}{\lambda_i} - D_i \right] \cdot \frac{\partial \lambda_i}{\partial \beta_r}$$

Parameter estimates can then found by setting this expression to zero and solving for the β's. The Hessian matrix has elements

$$\frac{\partial^2 L}{\partial \beta_r \partial \beta_s} = -\sum_i \frac{n_i}{\lambda_i^2} \cdot \frac{\partial \lambda_i}{\partial \beta_r} \cdot \frac{\partial \lambda_i}{\partial \beta_s} + \sum_i \left[\frac{n_i}{\lambda_i} - D_i \right] \cdot \frac{\partial^2 \lambda_i}{\partial \beta_r \partial \beta_s}$$

Because the expectation of the second term on the right is zero, the elements of the information matrix reduce to

$$E \left[-\frac{\partial^2 L}{\partial \beta_r \partial \beta_s} \right] = \sum_i \frac{D_i \lambda_i}{\lambda_i^2} \cdot \frac{\partial \lambda_i}{\partial \beta_r} \cdot \frac{\partial \lambda_i}{\partial \beta_s} \qquad (A6.1)$$

By applying the chain rule, we can obtain a more convenient form for the partial derivative of λ_i,

$$\frac{\partial \lambda_i}{\partial \beta_r} = \frac{\partial \lambda_i}{\partial \eta_i} \cdot \frac{\partial \eta_i}{\partial \beta_r} = \frac{\partial \lambda_i}{\partial \eta_i} \cdot X_{ir} \qquad (A6.2)$$

For the log-linear hazard, we have $\lambda_i = \exp\{\eta_i\}$ and

$$\frac{\partial \lambda_i}{\partial \eta_i} = \exp\{\eta_i\} = \lambda_i$$

Thus, the elements of the information matrix reduce to

$$I(\beta_r, \beta_s) = \sum_i D_i \, \lambda_i \, X_{ir} \, X_{is}$$

Weibull Hazards

In Chapter 2, we saw that the Weibull distribution offered a potentially interesting parametric alternative to the constant hazard model. A log-linear hazard in this instance can be expressed as $\lambda(\mathbf{t},\mathbf{X}) = \alpha \, t^{\alpha-1} \exp\{\mathbf{X}\boldsymbol{\beta}\}$, where α represents the shape parameter. The corresponding cumulative hazard is obtained by integrating over t:

$$\Lambda(t,\mathbf{X}) = \int_0^t \lambda(u,\mathbf{X}) \, du = t^\alpha \exp\{\mathbf{X}\boldsymbol{\beta}\}$$

Contributions to the likelihood by complete or uncensored observations are given by the probability density function for failure time, t, $f(t;\mathbf{X}) = \lambda(t;\mathbf{X}) \exp\{-\Lambda(t;\mathbf{X})\}$, and for a censored observation it is the survival function $\mathscr{F}(t;\mathbf{X}) = \exp\{-\Lambda(t;\mathbf{X})\}$.

The response, in this instance, must be represented by a pair of values, (δ_i, t_i), where t_i represents the length of follow-up for the ith observation, and δ_i is 0 if it is censored and 1 otherwise. We can now form the likelihood by

$$\ell \propto \prod_i [f(t_i;\mathbf{X})]^{\delta_i} \cdot [\mathscr{F}(t_i;\mathbf{X})]^{1-\delta_i}$$

$$= \prod_i \lambda(t_i;\mathbf{X})^{\delta_i} \cdot \exp\{-\Lambda(t_i;\mathbf{X})\}$$

Introducing covariates in the form of a log-linear hazard model, we can re-arrange this expression as a log likelihood:

$$L = \delta_+ \log \alpha + (\alpha - 1)\sum_i \delta_i \log t_i + \sum_i \delta_i \mathbf{X_i}\boldsymbol{\beta} - \sum_i \exp\{\mathbf{X_i}\boldsymbol{\beta} + \alpha \log t_i\}$$

(A6.3)

where δ_+ represents the total number of failures. Aitkin and Clayton (3) point out that when the shape constant, α, is known, then the first two components of the log likelihood can be ignored, as they are independent of the covariates. The remaining terms, once again, have the same kernel as a Poisson distribution with response δ_i, only now we would employ an offset of $\alpha \log t_i$.

In practice, we would generally estimate α from the data by solving the normal equation, found by setting

$$\frac{\partial L}{\partial \alpha} = (\delta_+/\alpha) + \sum_i (\delta_i - \hat{\Lambda}_i) \log t_i$$

to zero, where $\hat{\Lambda}_i$ is the estimate of the cumulative hazard using the maximum likelihood estimates of $\boldsymbol{\beta}$. This yields

$$\hat{\alpha} = \frac{\delta_+}{\sum_i (\hat{\Lambda}_i - \delta_i) \log t_i}$$

(A6.4)

Estimates of both α and $\boldsymbol{\beta}$ can be obtained by the successive relaxation method, in which we start the process by introducing an initial estimate, $\alpha_0 = 1$, and find the first maximum likelihood estimate for the regression parameters, $\boldsymbol{\beta}_1$. This is then used to update the estimate of α using equation A6.4, and the process is repeated until convergence in achieved. Aitken et al. (1) suggest a refinement to this technique in order to reduce oscillations between cycles by moving only halfway toward the next value for the shape parameter—thus, $\alpha_{j+1} = (\alpha_j + \alpha_j')/2$, where α_j' is obtained from equation A6.4.

To calculate an estimate of the covariance matrix for the model parameters, we can use the information matrix

$$I(\alpha,\boldsymbol{\beta}) = \left[\begin{array}{cc} \left(\dfrac{\partial^2 L}{\partial\beta_j\partial\beta_k}\right)_{(p+1)\times(p+1)} & \left(\dfrac{\partial^2 L}{\partial\beta_j\partial\alpha}\right)_{(p+1)\times 1} \\[2em] \left(\dfrac{\partial^2 L}{\partial\alpha\partial\beta_k}\right)_{1\times(p+1)} & \left(\dfrac{\partial^2 L}{\partial\alpha^2}\right)_{1\times 1} \end{array}\right]$$

The inverse of the upper left portion of the matrix is the nominal covariance matrix for the regression parameters given by a Poisson regression program, $\mathbf{V}(\boldsymbol{\beta})$. The remaining elements are given by

$$\frac{\partial^2 L}{\partial \alpha^2} = -\frac{\delta_+}{\alpha^2} - \sum_i (\log t_i)^2 \, \Lambda_i$$

and

$$\frac{\partial^2 L}{\partial \alpha \partial \beta_j} = -\sum_i X_{ij} \, (\log t_i) \, \Lambda_i$$

We can adjust the nominal covariance matrix obtained from Poisson regression software by using

$$\mathbf{V}^*(\boldsymbol{\beta}) = \left[\mathbf{V}(\boldsymbol{\beta})^{-1} - \left(\frac{\partial^2 L}{\partial \beta_j \partial \alpha} \right) \left(\frac{\partial^2 L}{\partial \alpha^2} \right) \left(\frac{\partial^2 L}{\partial \alpha \partial \beta_k} \right) \right]^{-1}$$

which is always somewhat larger than the variance provided by generalized linear model software that effectively ignores the fact that the shape parameter was estimated from the data.

Example A6–1 Consider once again the data from Table 5–1, which were from a study of the effect of 6-MP treatment on leukemia remission times. Maximum likelihood estimates of the regression parameters can be obtained when α is fixed by employing Poisson regression with an offset of $\alpha \log(t_i)$. Because we do not actually know α, we can estimate it, either by finding the value that maximizes the likelihood or, equivalently, by minimizing the scaled deviance. For the latter, however, the first term on the righthand side of equation A6.3 is not included in the Poisson scaled deviance, so we must obtain a corrected value by subtracting $2\delta_+ \log(\alpha)$. A plot of this corrected scaled deviance is shown in Figure A6–1, the minimum being $\hat{\alpha} = 1.366 = 1/0.7321$, and this result is identical to what we found in Example 8–3. Results from fitting this model using PROC GENMOD and the maximum likelihood estimate of our shape parameter are shown in Figure A6–2, and it is interesting to note that the parameter estimate is identical to what was obtained in Example 8–3. However, the comparable standard error for the treatment effect obtained using the approach in Example 8–3 is $0.31064/0.73219 = 0.4243$, which is greater than the value just obtained from PROC GENMOD, 0.3984. The reason for the discrepancy is because the current calculation treated the shape parameter as a known constant instead of as an estimator of it. When we appropriately allow for the fact that it is estimated, we obtain the correct standard error, which is greater than what is shown in Figure A6–2.

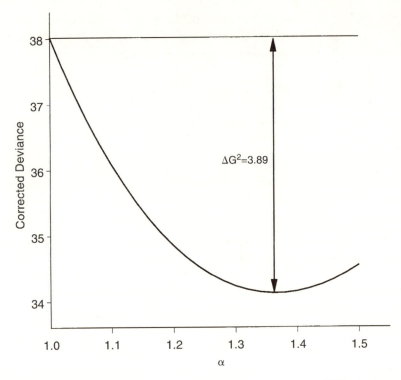

Figure A6–1 Plot of the corrected scales deviance against the Weibull shape parameter for the data in Table 5–1.

Alternatives to Log-Linear Hazard Models

An alternative to the log-linear model that we already considered in some detail makes use of the power transformation for the link function, as shown in equations 8.4 and 8.5. Once the power parameter, ρ, has been identified, we have specified the link function, and the problem reduces to a standard generalized linear model. However, we generally need to estimate ρ along with the other regression parameters, and this is readily accomplished using a grid search to find the ρ that either maximizes the log likelihood or, equivalently, minimizes the scaled deviance. To find estimates of the variance for this case we require the derivatives

$$\frac{\partial \lambda_i}{\partial \eta_i} = \frac{\eta_i^{(1-\rho)/\rho}}{\rho} = \frac{\lambda_i^{1-\rho}}{\rho}$$

```
The GENMOD Procedure

      Model Information
Distribution              Poisson
Link Function                 Log
Offset Variable             alpha
Observations Used              42

       Criteria For Assessing Goodness Of Fit

Criterion                 DF         Value        Value/DF
Scaled Deviance           40       52.8308          1.3208
Pearson Chi-Square        40      110.9060          2.7727
Log Likelihood                    -56.4154

             Analysis Of Parameter Estimates

                        Standard    Wald 95% Confidence     Chi-
Parameter   DF  Estimate   Error        Limits            Square   Pr > ChiSq
Intercept    1   -1.3398   0.5492   -2.4162   -0.2635      5.95       0.0147
treat        1   -1.7309   0.3984   -2.5117   -0.9500     18.87      <.0001
Scale        0    1.0000   0.0000    1.0000    1.0000

NOTE: The scale parameter was held fixed.
```

Figure A6–2 Output from fitting data from Table 5–1 using a Weibull offset and setting $\alpha = 1.366$.

and

$$\frac{\partial \lambda_i}{\partial \rho} = \frac{\eta_i^{1/\rho} \log \eta_i}{\rho^2} = \frac{\lambda_i \log \lambda_i}{\rho}$$

The information matrix in this case takes a form that resembles the one we obtained for the Weibull model:

$$\mathbf{I}(\rho,\boldsymbol{\beta}) = \begin{bmatrix} E\left(\dfrac{\partial^2 L}{\partial \beta_j \partial \beta_k}\right)_{(p+1)\times(p+1)} & E\left(\dfrac{\partial^2 L}{\partial \beta_j \partial \rho}\right)_{(p+1)\times 1} \\[2ex] E\left(\dfrac{\partial^2 L}{\partial \rho \partial \beta_k}\right)_{1\times(p+1)} & E\left(\dfrac{\partial^2 L}{\partial \rho^2}\right)_{1\times 1} \end{bmatrix}$$

As before, the upper left portion of this matrix is identical to that obtained for a generalized linear model when the power is known—that is, the value produced by model fitting using generalized linear model software. Elements in the final row and column are given by

$$E\left[\frac{\partial^2 L}{\partial \rho^2}\right] = \sum_i \frac{D_i \lambda_i (\log \lambda_i)^2}{\rho^2}$$

and

$$E\left[\frac{\partial^2 L}{\partial\rho\partial\beta_r}\right] = \sum_i \frac{D_i\lambda_i\,(\log\lambda_i)}{\rho^2\,\lambda_i^\rho}\cdot X_{ir}$$

This allows us to correct for the fact that we are estimating ρ by using

$$\mathbf{V}^*(\boldsymbol{\beta}) = \left[\mathbf{V}(\boldsymbol{\beta})^{-1} - E\left(\frac{\partial^2 L}{\partial\beta_j\partial\rho}\right)E\left(\frac{\partial^2 L}{\partial\rho^2}\right)E\left(\frac{\partial^2 L}{\partial\rho\partial\beta_k}\right)\right]^{-1}$$

The fact that the correction involves taking the inverse after having subtracted something implies that uncorrected estimates of variance will be too small, in general.

References

1. Aitkin M, Anderson D, Francis B, Hinde J. *Statistical Modelling in GLIM*. Oxford: Clarendon Press, 1989.
2. McCullagh P, Nelder JA. *Generalized Linear Models*. London: Chapman and Hall, 1989.
3. Aitkin M, Clayton D. The fitting of exponential, Weibull, an extreme value distributions to complex censored survival data using GLIM. *Applied Statistics* 1980;29:156–163.

Appendix 7

Theory on Proportional Hazards Regression

In Chapter 9, our first step toward formulating a model that did not require a specific parametric form for the effect of time was the piecewise constant hazard or piecewise exponential model, shown in equation 9.2. By employing the proportional hazards form for the model, we can obtain the survival function for an individual with covariates $\mathbf{X_i}$:

$$\mathcal{F}(\mathbf{X_i};t_i) = \exp\left\{-\int_0^{t_i} \lambda_0(u)\ h(\mathbf{X_i})\ du\right\}$$

$$= \exp\left\{-\sum_j \lambda_j\ t_{ij}\ h(\mathbf{X_i})\right\}$$

where i and j are indices for the subject and the interval, respectively, and t_{ij} is the observed length of follow-up for the ith individual during the jth interval. The probability density function for the failure times follows directly:

$$f(\mathbf{X_i};t_i) = \lambda_j\, h(\mathbf{X_i})\, \exp\{-\sum_j \lambda_j\, t_{ij}\, h(\mathbf{X_i})\}$$

where λ_j is the hazard for the final interval of follow-up in which the individual actually failed.

Let δ_{ij} be an indicator that takes the value 1 if the ith individual fails during the jth interval, but is 0 otherwise. The sum of this indicator over all intervals, δ_{i+}, is 1 for a complete observation and 0 for one that is censored. We can obtain the likelihood from

$$\ell = \prod_i f(\mathbf{X_i};t_i)^{\delta_{i+}}\ \mathcal{F}(\mathbf{X_i};t_i)^{1-\delta_{i+}}$$

$$= \prod_i \left[\prod_j \left(\lambda_j\, h(\mathbf{X_i})\right)^{\delta_{ij}} \exp\{-\lambda_j\, h(\mathbf{X_i})\, t_{ij}\}\right] \tag{A7.1}$$

A further simplification can be realized if individuals with identical levels of the covariates are divided into groups. If $d_{kj} = \sum_{\{i \in \text{Group } k\}} \delta_{ij}$ represents the sum of the status indicators for individuals in the kth risk group, it is clear that this quantity represents the total number of failures for the group during interval j. Likewise, the sum of the observed follow-up times during interval j for subjects in group k is $T_{kj} = \sum t_{ij}$, and the likelihood simplifies to

$$\ell = \prod_{kj} [\lambda_j \, h(\mathbf{X_k})^{d_{kj}} \exp\{-\lambda_j \, T_{kj} \, h(\mathbf{X_k})\}$$

Notice that the kernel of the contribution to this likelihood by individuals in the kth group during the jth interval is identical to the Poisson, which allows us to make use of this distribution when finding maximum likelihood estimates of the model parameters. If the hazard is a log-linear function of the covariates, the log likelihood becomes

$$L = \sum_{kj} [d_{kj} \, (\log \lambda_j + \mathbf{X_k}\boldsymbol{\beta}) - \lambda_j \, T_{kj} \exp\{\mathbf{X_k}\boldsymbol{\beta}\}]$$

As we saw in our discussion of survival curve estimates in Chapter 5, a completely nonparametric model with respect to the time component could be realized by passing to the limit, letting the interval widths go to 0 and the number of intervals to infinity. A somewhat simpler representation of the method of analysis results from establishing a log likelihood that depends only on the regression parameters, $\boldsymbol{\beta}$. For each interval containing a failure, we have a nuisance parameter involving the product of the interval width and the hazard, $\Delta\lambda_j$. Intervals that do not include deaths drop out entirely, and the only relevant information is provided by intervals that include failure times, so that the likelihood given in equation A7.1 can be expressed in terms of a product over the intervals. For the jth interval, the individuals that are available—that is, have nonzero observed times during the interval—constitute a risk set, $\mathfrak{R}_j$. Thus, the log likelihood becomes

$$L = \sum_{j} \sum_{i \in \mathfrak{R}_j} [\delta_{+j} \log[\lambda_j\Delta] + \delta_{ij} \, \mathbf{X_i}\boldsymbol{\beta} - \lambda_j\Delta \, \exp\{\mathbf{X_i}\boldsymbol{\beta}\}] \qquad \text{(A7.2)}$$

We can find an expression for the maximum likelihood estimate for $\lambda_j\Delta$ by setting

$$\frac{\partial \mathrm{L}}{\partial(\lambda_j\Delta)} = \frac{\delta_{+j}}{\lambda_j\Delta} - \sum_{i \in \mathfrak{R}_j} \exp\{\mathbf{X_i}\boldsymbol{\beta}\}$$

to zero and solving, which yields

$$\lambda_j \Delta = \frac{\delta_{+j}}{\sum_{i \in \mathfrak{R}_j} \exp\{\mathbf{X}_i \boldsymbol{\beta}\}}$$

Substituting this expression into equation A7.2 results in

$$L(\boldsymbol{\beta}) = \sum_j \log \left[\frac{\exp\{\mathbf{X}_j \boldsymbol{\beta}\}}{\sum_{i \in \mathfrak{R}_j} \exp\{\mathbf{X}_i \boldsymbol{\beta}\}} \right]$$

as a kernel log likelihood function (1–3), which is essentially the expression given originally by Cox (4). This expression can also be derived by selecting intervals over which the hazard is constant at cutpoints identified by the observed follow-up times (5). However, a mathematically rigorous development of this expression involves some of the deepest issues in statistical inference. Kalbfleisch and Prentice (6) give conditions under which this can be considered to be a marginal likelihood, but in a more general setting this problem has lead to the development of the concept of partial likelihood (7, 8).

A further extension of this likelihood involves the inclusion of time-dependent covariates, **Z(t)**. The contribution of each failure to the overall likelihood once again involves a consideration of the risk set at each failure time—those individuals under active follow-up at a given failure time. The contribution of the jth failure becomes

$$\frac{\lambda_0(t_j) \exp\{\mathbf{X}_i \boldsymbol{\beta}_{\mathbf{X}} + \mathbf{Z}_i(t_j) \boldsymbol{\beta}_{\mathbf{Z}}\}}{\sum_{k \in \mathfrak{R}_j} \lambda_0(t_k) \exp\{\mathbf{X}_k \boldsymbol{\beta}_{\mathbf{X}} + \mathbf{Z}_k(t_j) \boldsymbol{\beta}_{\mathbf{Z}}\}} = \frac{\exp\{\mathbf{X}_i \boldsymbol{\beta}_{\mathbf{X}} + \mathbf{Z}_i(t_j) \boldsymbol{\beta}_{\mathbf{Z}}\}}{\sum_{k \in \mathfrak{R}_j} \exp\{\mathbf{X}_k \boldsymbol{\beta}_{\mathbf{X}} + \mathbf{Z}_k(t_j) \boldsymbol{\beta}_{\mathbf{Z}}\}}$$

$$(A7.3)$$

and the time-dependent covariates are essentially functions that are evaluated at each failure time, t_j. The overall likelihood is found by multiplying these elements over the entire set of observed failure times.

References

1. Holford TR. Life tables with concomitant information. *Biometrics* 1976;32: 587–597.
2. Holford TR. The analysis of rates and survivorship using log-linear models. *Biometrics* 1980;36:299–305.

3. Laird N, Olivier D. Covariance analysis of censored survival data using log-linear analysis techniques. *Journal of the American Statistical Association* 1981;76: 231–240.
4. Cox DR. Regression models and life-tables (with discussion). *Journal of the Royal Statistical Society, Series B* 1972;B34:187–220.
5. Breslow N. Covariance analysis of censored survival data. *Biometrics* 1974; 30:89–99.
6. Kalbfleisch JD, Prentice RL. Marginal likelihoods based on Cox's regression and life model. *Biometrika* 1973;60:267–278.
7. Cox DR. Partial likelihood. *Biometrika* 1975;62.
8. Cox DR, Oakes D. Analysis of Survival Data. London: Chapman and Hall, 1984.

Appendix 8

Theory on Analysis of Matched Studies

The fundamental statistical problem in matched studies is to deal effectively with the uniqueness of each matched set. We can express this when establishing our model by the introduction of a parameter for each matched set. However, when making inferences, this is a nuisance parameter because it obviously must be dealt with, but we are not particularly interested in saying anything about the individual matched sets. The methods of analysis that we have discussed adopted the use of conditional inference (1), which results in a likelihood function that no longer depends on the matching parameters (2).

Conditional Likelihood for Case-Control Study

In a matched case-control study, we can consider the matching criteria as effectively representing different strata from which we draw our subjects. Both cases and controls may be drawn after they have been exposed for the same length of time, which we can generally think of as indicating that they are the same age. Hence, we represent the underlying hazard for the ith stratum by $\lambda_i(t)$. The likelihood contribution for the ith stratum is the probability that $\mathbf{X_0}$ occurs for the case, given the selection of a set of individuals that includes $\mathcal{J}_i$ controls that were selected at random from those at risk—that is, the matched set, $\mathbf{X_0}, \mathbf{X_1}, \ldots, \mathbf{X_{J_i}}$.

To envision a case-control study, we assume we have a time window of length Δ for recruitment of subjects, so that the probability that a case occurs in the ith stratum is approximately, $\lambda_i(t,\mathbf{X})\Delta$. The complementary event, remaining disease free, occurs with probability $1 - \lambda_i(t,\mathbf{X})\Delta \simeq 1$ in most practical situations. One or more controls are selected from among those that are eligible, and we shall assume that $\mathcal{I}_i$ controls are chosen independently, each with probability p_i. Therefore, the probability of selecting the case and matching controls for the ith stratum is approximately $p_i^{\mathcal{I}_i}$ $\lambda(\mathbf{t}, \mathbf{X_i})\Delta$. The usual likelihood methods do not work well in this instance because they require the estimation of a parameter for each stratum. These are not well estimated because the strata are small; in fact, in the situation we are now considering, there is only a single case and a small number of controls. Hence, we should not be surprised that the usual large sample theory breaks down, because when we increase the sample size, we must also increase the number of poorly determined parameters being estimated. An alternative that does work well in this instance is to use conditional likelihood methods.

Under a conditional likelihood, the contribution of the ith pair is given by

$$\ell_i = \Pr\{\mathbf{X_0} \text{ for case and } \mathbf{X_1} \ldots \mathbf{X_{J_i}} \text{ for controls} \mid \text{matched set}$$
$$\text{contains } \mathbf{X_0 X_1} \ldots \mathbf{X_{J_i}}\}$$

$$= \frac{p_i^{\mathcal{I}_i} \lambda(t, \mathbf{X_0})}{\sum_{j=0}^{\mathcal{I}_i} p_i^{\mathcal{I}_i} \lambda(t, \mathbf{X_j})} = \frac{\lambda(t, \mathbf{X_0})}{\sum_{j=0}^{\mathcal{I}_i} \lambda(t, \mathbf{X_j})}$$

(A8.1)

For a proportional hazards models, this reduces to a contribution that is independent of time

$$\ell_i = \frac{\lambda_0(t) \exp\{\mathbf{X_0}\boldsymbol{\beta}\}}{\sum_{j=0}^{\mathcal{I}_i} \lambda_0(t) \exp\{\mathbf{X_j}\boldsymbol{\beta}\}} = \frac{\exp\{\mathbf{X_0}\boldsymbol{\beta}\}}{\sum_{j=0}^{\mathcal{I}_i} \exp\{\mathbf{X_j}\boldsymbol{\beta}\}}$$

(A8.2)

For the overall conditional likelihood, we assume that these sets are independent of each other, so the resulting likelihood function is found by multiplying these contributions over all matched sets.

Matched Pairs for Case-Control Studies

For matched pairs, a single control is selected at random from the members of a stratum that remain free from disease during the recruitment period. The contribution of the pair to the conditional likelihood becomes

$$\ell_i = \frac{\exp(\mathbf{X_0}\boldsymbol{\beta})}{\exp(\mathbf{X_0}\boldsymbol{\beta}) + \exp(\mathbf{X_1}\boldsymbol{\beta})}$$

$$= \frac{\exp([\mathbf{X_0} - \mathbf{X_1}]\boldsymbol{\beta})}{1 + \exp([\mathbf{X_0} - \mathbf{X_1}]\boldsymbol{\beta})}$$

(A8.3)

For model fitting, it is useful to recognize that the probability for the contribution of a pair to the conditional likelihood is strikingly similar to the equation for a linear logistic model (3–5). In fact, we can see that they are identical when (1) the model does not include an intercept; (2) the covariates are the differences between values for the case and the control; and (3) the response is a success, $Y_i = 1$, for each pair.

N-to-One Matching in Case-Control Studies

We have already derived a general expression for the contribution to the likelihood by a particular matched set, shown in equation A8.2. The overall conditional likelihood for an N-to-one design is given by

$$\ell = \prod_{i=1}^{I} \frac{\exp\{\mathbf{X}_{i0}\boldsymbol{\beta}\}}{\sum_{j=0}^{N} \exp\{\mathbf{X}_{ij}\boldsymbol{\beta}\}} \tag{A8.4}$$

This can be fitted using a general log-linear model (6), but it is also interesting to notice that the form for this expression strongly resembles the partial likelihood for the proportional hazards. In fact, this suggests another backdoor approach to the computations, one that employs the algorithms used for fitting proportional hazards models (7). The equivalence can be achieved by establishing a time variable, albeit an artificial one, in which the value for the case is less than that for the controls: that is, the response is observed before the controls. We also require a unique identifier for each matched set, or stratum. Finally, a case-control indicator is needed, in which the case is coded as a complete observation, and a control is censored.

This basic approach of using software for fitting the proportional hazards model also extends to N-to-M matching. With more than one case, the situation is analogous to the establishment of a likelihood for the analysis of survival times in which ties may occur. However, for ties, the solution is not unique (7, 8), so some care is needed in selecting the particular option for handling ties, e.g., in SAS the option "TIES=DISCRETE" in the "MODEL" statement yields the appropriate form for the likelihood of interest (9).

Conditional Likelihood for Cohort Studies

For a matched cohort design, the probability of observing the responses $Y_{ij}\ (= 0,1)$, for the jth $(j = 1, \ldots, \mathcal{J}_i)$ member of the ith $(i = 1, \ldots, I)$ matched set depends on the exposure, $E_{ij}(= 0,1)$, and the set of covariates,

$\mathbf{X}_{ij}$. For a linear logistic model, the contribution to the likelihood for the ith matched set is

$$\ell_i = \frac{\exp\{\sum_j Y_{ij}[\alpha_i + E_{ij}\delta + \mathbf{X}_{ij}\boldsymbol{\beta}]\}}{\prod_j(1 + \exp\{\alpha_i + E_{ij}\delta + \mathbf{X}_{ij}\boldsymbol{\beta}\})}$$

$$= \frac{\exp\{Y_{i+}\alpha_i + \sum_j Y_{ij}[E_{ij}\delta + \mathbf{X}_{ij}\boldsymbol{\beta}]\}}{\prod_j(1 + \exp\{\alpha_i + E_{ij}\delta + \mathbf{X}_{ij}\boldsymbol{\beta}\})}$$

While other matched sets clearly contribute information to the estimation of the exposure parameter, δ, and the covariate parameters, β, the intercept, α_i, is unique to the matched set. Because these are typically small strata, the set's nuisance parameter, α_i, is poorly determined, even though uninteresting in its own right. Notice that Y_{i+} is a minimal sufficient statistic for α_i, and the likelihood contribution to the likelihood that is conditional on Y_{i+} becomes

$$\ell_i = \frac{\dfrac{\exp\{Y_{i+}\alpha_i + \sum_j Y_{ij}[E_{ij}\delta + \mathbf{X}_{ij}\boldsymbol{\beta}]\}}{\prod_j(1 + \exp\{\alpha_i + E_{ij}\delta + \mathbf{X}_{ij}\boldsymbol{\beta}\})}}{\sum_{\forall \eta_{ij}:\eta_{i+}=Y_{i+}} \dfrac{\exp\{\eta_{i+}\alpha_i + \sum_j \eta_{ij}[E_{ij}\delta + \mathbf{X}_{ij}\boldsymbol{\beta}]\}}{\prod_j(1 + \exp\{\alpha_i + E_{ij}\delta + \mathbf{X}_{ij}\boldsymbol{\beta}\})}}$$

$$= \frac{\exp\{\sum_j Y_{ij}[E_{ij}\delta + \mathbf{X}_{ij}\boldsymbol{\beta}]\}}{\sum_{\forall \eta_{ij}:\eta_{i+}=Y_{i+}} \exp\{\sum_j \eta_{ij}[E_{ij}\delta + \mathbf{X}_{ij}\boldsymbol{\beta}]\}} \qquad \text{(A8.5)}$$

as shown by Prentice (10). Notation for the summation in the denominator represents all possible patterns of disease outcomes, such that their total equals the observed total. Concordant sets are those with the same response for all members who either did or did not respond—that is, $Y_{i+} = 0$ or $\mathcal{J}$. Because each of these combinations can only occur one way, the contribution of these pairs to the conditional likelihood is just one; thus, they contribute no information on the parameters of interest because the contribution is independent of their value.

For matched pairs, $\mathcal{J}_i = 2$ for all i, and for the exposure of interest there is just one subject in each group, $E_{i1} = 0$ and $E_{i2} = 1$. If $Y_{i+} = 0$ or 2, the pair is concordant on the response, and hence it contributes no information with respect to either exposure or the covariates. The only remaining possibility is that $Y_{i+} = 1$, which can happen if (a) $Y_{i1} = 0$ and $Y_{i2} = 1$ or if (b) $Y_{i1} = 1$ and $Y_{i2} = 0$. For (a), the contribution to the conditional likelihood is

$$\ell_i = \frac{\exp\{E_{i2}\delta + \mathbf{X}_{i2}\boldsymbol{\beta}\}}{\exp\{E_{i1}\delta + \mathbf{X}_{i1}\boldsymbol{\beta}\} + \exp\{E_{i2}\delta + \mathbf{X}_{i2}\boldsymbol{\beta}\}}$$

$$= \frac{\exp\{\delta + (\mathbf{X}_{i2} - \mathbf{X}_{i1})\boldsymbol{\beta}\}}{1 + \exp\{\delta + (\mathbf{X}_{i2} - \mathbf{X}_{i1})\boldsymbol{\beta}\}} \qquad \text{(A8.6)}$$

Similarly, the contribution for case (b) reduces to

$$\ell_i = \frac{1}{1 + \exp\{\delta + (\mathbf{X}_{i2} - \mathbf{X}_{i1})\boldsymbol{\beta}\}} \tag{A8.7}$$

which is the complement of equation A8.6. As in the case of the matched pairs case-control study, we can once again see that the basic structure of a linear logistic model has been retained, which we can take advantage of for model fitting by using the steps set out in the section "Cohort Studies with Matched Pairs" in Chapter 10.

For more complex matching schemes, methods of analysis can be established using the conditional likelihood shown in equation A8.5. The likelihood contribution in these instances may be expressed in terms of a log-linear model (11), which is an extension of the linear logistic model to a more than two-level outcome (12).

References

1. Cox DR, Hinkley DV. *Theoretical Statistics*. London: Chapman and Hall, 1974.
2. Cox DR. *Analysis of Binary Data*. London: Methuen, 1970.
3. Holford TR, White C, Kelsey JL. Multivariate analysis for matched case-control studies. *American Journal of Epidemiology* 1978;107:245–256.
4. Holford TR. The analysis of pair-matched case-control studies, a multivariate approach. *Biometrics* 1978;34:665–672.
5. Breslow NE, Day NE, Halvorsen KT, Prentice RL, Sabai C. Estimation of multiple relative risk functions in matched case-control studies. *American Journal of Epidemiology* 1978;108:299–307.
6. Holford TR. Covariance analysis for case-control studies with small blocks. *Biometrics* 1982;38:673–683.
7. Gail MH, Lubin JH, Rubinstein LV. Likelihood calculations for matched case-control studies and survival studies with tied death times. *Biometrika* 1981;68: 703–707.
8. Peto R. Permutational significance testing. *Applied Statistics* 1973:112–118.
9. SAS Institute. *SAS/STAT User's Guide* (Version 6). Cary, NC: SAS Institute, 1989.
10. Prentice R. Use of the logistic model in retrospective studies. *Biometrics* 1976; 32:599–606.
11. Holford TR, Bracken MB, Eskenazi B. Log-linear models for the analysis of matched cohort studies. *American Journal of Epidemiology* 1989;130:1247–1253.
12. Haberman SJ. *Analysis of Qualitative Data*. New York: Academic Press, 1979.

Index

Actuarial method, 109, 110–113, 117, 135, 137, 369, 371
Acute herniated lumbar discs, 260–261, 262–265, 267–268
Adjusted survival curve, (*See* Survival curve, adjusted)
Age, 8, 179, 335
AIDS, 10
Alcohol, 161
Alternative hypothesis, 287, 288, 290, 293, 296, 298, 299, 306
Antagonism, 30
Asbestos, 152, 197
Aspirin, 5
Associations, 3
Augmented data, 332

B splines, (*See* Splines, B)
Bayesian methods, 258
Beta carotene, 5
Bias, 323, 324
Binary
    response, 147, 159
    risk factor, 43
Binomial distribution, 351, 371, 372, 377
Biological assay, 146
Biomarker, 5, 222, 254, 299
Birth order, 103
Blocking, 254
Blocks, 256
Bonferroni, 182
Boundary, 282, 284, 285
Box-Cox transformation, 196, 201, 213
Bradley-Terry model, 266
Breast
    adipose tissue, 7
    cancer, (*See* Cancer, breast)
    fluid, 190, 193

British Doctors Study, 213–215
Broken line, 326
Bulging rule, 197

Caliper matching, (*See* Matching, caliper)
Cancer, 5
    breast, 6, 81, 104, 337
    cervix, 136
    endometrial, 277
    esophageal, 161
    leukemia, 219, 389
    lung, 3, 152, 197, 230, 233, 237, 239–240
    malignant melanoma, 203–204
    ovarian, 53, 57, 76, 77, 161
    registry, 8
    vaginal, 255, 270-272
Canonical link function, 147
Cardiovascular death, 213
Case-control study, 39, 42, 45, 46, 257, 258–268, 268–272, 278, 305, 306, 310, 312, 397, 398, 401
Categorical variables, 163
Causes of disease, 3
Censored observations, 110, 119, 120, 311, 370, 372
Censoring
    interval, 135
    left, 134, 135
    right, 19, 133
    times, 116
Cervix cancer, (*See* Cancer, cervix)
Chi-square, 220, 223, 318, 353, 355, 366, 375, 379, 381, 382
    central, 295, 296
    noncentral, 296, 298, 304
Cholesterol, 202–203

Cigarette smoking, 3, 4, 46, 48, 58, 60, 62, 64, 90, 148, 179, 185, 213, 233
Classification and regression trees (CART), 316, 318, 324, 325, 339
Cochran's
    method, 367
    test, 65–67, 70, 75, 77, 95, 359
Coding
    0 1, 165–169, 171, 183, 187, 189, 190, 191, 193, 200, 206, 263, 273
    −1 0 1, 165, 169–172, 184, 185, 189, 191, 194, 200
Coffee, 76
Cohort, 8, 335
    study, 39, 41, 109, 272–276, 285, 310, 399
Collinearity, 316, 335–339, 340
Complementary log-log, 379
    model, 33, 146, 161
Complete symmetry, 265, 266, 268
Concordant, 270
    pairs, 259, 274
    sets, 400
Conditional, 257, 263, 264, 274, 277
    inference, 258, 292, 356, 357, 397
    likelihood, 49, 257, 262, 266, 356, 357, 398, 399, 400, 401
    logistic, 262, 267, 275
    score statistic, 357
    test, 62, 63
Conditionally linear model, 383
Confidence interval, 54, 281, 282, 310, 381
Confounding factor, 64
Congeners, 336–339
Congenital malformations, 41, 46, 48, 58, 60, 62, 64, 66, 143, 148
Connecticut Tumor Registry, 8, 230, 234
Consistency relationship, 266, 268
Constant
    hazard, 34, 109, 119, 121, 137, 206, 218, 224, 227, 228, 229, 230, 345, 346, 347, 361, 363, 385, 387
    rate, 21
Continuous variables, 186, 195, 201
Contrast, 189
    matrix, 187
Cornfield's method, 54, 55, 76
Coronary Artery Bypass Surgery Study, 234
Covariance matrix, 353
Covariate adjustment, 305, 311
Cox model, 24
Crossover effects, 234
Cross-sectional study, 39, 40, 45

Cross-validation, 323, 324
Crude rate, 97, 101, 103
Cubic splines, (See Splines, cubic)
Cumulative hazard, 33, 114, 218

Departure from trend, 180–182
DES, 255
Descriptive epidemiology, 82
Design matrix, 187
Deviance, 300, 378
Diabetes, 161, 202
Direct adjusted rate, 98, 99, 101, 104, 115
Discordant pairs, 274, 293, 294, 312
Discriminant analysis, 324
Disease
    density function, 345
    mapping, 333
    process, 15
Diseased, 19
Dose–response relationship, 58, 204, 211, 328, 340
Down syndrome, 100, 101, 103

Effect, 22–34
    modification, 10, 28, 182
Effective number at risk, 110
EM algorithm, 332
Endometrial cancer, (See Cancer, endometrial)
Entropy criterion, 321
Epidemiology, 3
Errors in variables, 333–335
Esophageal cancer, (See Cancer, esophageal)
Estimation, 47, 310, 324
Exact
    method, 54, 56
    test, 51, 54, 75
Exogenous estrogens, 277
Expected
    failures, 215, 218, 229, 373
    frequency, 206, 207
Exponential
    distribution, 119, 135, 219, 345
    random variable, 221
Exposure-response, 10, 13, 19, 195, 201
Extra Poisson variation, 223
Extreme-value distribution, 222, 224

F distribution, 224
Failure
    rate, 84, 224, 284
    time, 385, 393
    time density function, 34

Fisher, RA, 47
Fluid secretion, 167
Framingham Study, 202
Frequency matching, (*See* Matching, frequency)

Gamma distribution, 220, 221, 224
Gene–exposure interaction, 313
General linear hypothesis, 163
Generalized additive model (GAM), 329
Generalized linear model, viii, 142, 143, 147, 159, 201, 207, 211, 224, 298, 299, 304, 305, 311, 315, 337, 377, 383, 385, 389, 390, 391
Generational effects, 9
Gini diversity index, 321
Gompertz-Makeham model, 222, 224
Goodness of fit, 23, 143, 173, 209, 217, 223, 267, 268, 379, 382
Graunt, John, 109
Greenwood's formula, 111, 371
Gumbel distribution, (*See* Extreme-value distribution)
Guy's Hospital, 81, 104

Harvard, 225
Hazard
  function, 21, 33, 34, 126, 206, 344, 345, 366
  ratio, 24, 89, 349
  step function, 126, 343
Healthy, 19
  worker effect, 86
Heart
  attack, 225
  disease, 5, 202–203, 233
Hepatitis B, 134
Hierarchical model, 333
Histology, 230, 233, 235
HIV, 10
Hodgkin's disease, 106
Homogeneity of odds ratio, 70–73
Human mortality, 347
Hypernephroma, 105, 137
Hypertension Detection and Follow-up Program, 128
Hypothesis testing, 286, 310

Impurity, 318, 321, 323
Imputation, 331
Incidence rate, 21, 312
Indirect adjusted rate, 99, 100, 102, 104, 224
Information matrix, 353, 355, 358, 365, 367, 374, 380, 386, 388

Interaction, 28, 30, 183, 186, 234, 308, 309, 311
Invariance property of MLE, 189
Inverse link, 213, 300, 380

Kaplan-Meier estimator, 117
Knots, 326, 328

Large-sample approximation, 295
Latitude, geographic, 59
Lehman alternative, 375
Leukemia, (*See* Cancer, leukemia)
Leukocyte count, 90, 208–211
Lexis diagram, 86
Likelihood
  based inference, 47
  function, 351
  ratio statistic, (*See* Likelihood ratio test)
  ratio test, 48, 51, 53, 61, 76, 90, 161, 192, 201, 202, 203, 225, 226, 249, 277, 295, 300, 306, 354, 365
Linear
  constraint, 188
  contrast, 188
  function, variance of, 167
  hypothesis, 186, 192, 201
  logistic model, 31, 75, 142, 144, 146, 147, 148, 153, 159, 197, 257, 258, 262, 263, 264, 267, 269, 273, 274, 277, 299, 304, 306, 337, 348, 351, 355, 357, 382, 399, 400, 401
  model, 214
  odds model, 151, 153, 160, 379, 382
  splines, (*See* Splines, linear)
  predictor, 143, 178, 193, 378, 379, 382, 386
  trend, 300, 303, 304, 313, 355, 356
Link function, 143, 144, 208, 213, 300, 379, 380, 390
Log
  hazard ratio, 146, 235, 242, 373
  likelihood, 321, 352
  link, 207, 211–212
  normal distribution, 221, 224
  odds, 145
  odds ratio, 44, 70, 145
  rate, 284
  rate ratio, 286
Logistic regression, (*See* Linear logistic model)
Logit, 379
  link function, 144
  method, 54, 76

Log-linear
  hazards, 25, 145, 160, 207, 215, 239, 242, 347, 348, 387, 388, 394
  model, 89, 97, 206, 207, 208, 213, 214, 218, 224, 230, 233, 247, 299, 366, 390, 401
Log-log survival curve, (*See* Survival curve, log-log)
Log-rank test, 129, 131, 132, 133, 136, 137, 291, 317, 320, 374
LogXact, 75
Lost to follow-up, 42, 81, 83, 110, 371
Low birth weight, 4
Lung
  cancer, (*See* Cancer, lung)
  disease, 179

Malignant melanoma, (*See* Cancer, malignant melanoma)
Mantel-Haenszel methods, viii, 49, 65–67, 68–70, 72, 73, 75, 77, 95, 130, 142, 161, 259, 260, 277, 317, 320, 324, 359, 375
Many-to-one matching, (*See* Matching, many-to-one)
Marginal
  homogeneity, 261
  likelihood, 375, 395
Markov Chain Monte Carlo (MCMC), 332, 340
Mastectomy, 81
Matched
  pairs, 66, 254, 258–268, 272–276, 278, 292, 312, 398, 400, 401
  set, 397, 399, 400
Matching, 253, 310, 311, 312, 397
  caliper, 256–257
  frequency, 256
  many-to-one, 255, 268–272, 399
Maternal age, 101, 103
Maximum likelihood, 45, 47, 49, 84, 87, 89, 100, 148, 161, 178, 208, 218, 236, 332, 337, 352, 356, 358, 364, 365, 370, 371, 372, 373, 377, 378, 380, 382, 383, 384, 385, 386, 388, 394
McNemar's test, 66, 258, 261, 292
Measurement error, 334
Meta analysis, 333
Minimal sufficient statistic, 356
Missing
  at random (MAR), 331
  completely at random (MCAR), 330
  not at random (MNAR), 332
  observations, 331, 332

Model fitting, problems, 156–159
Moles, 203–204
Monitor, 5
Montana smelter, 86, 88, 93, 215–217
Monte Carlo simulation, 291
Mortality rate, 21, 347
Multi-level model, 334
Multinomial distribution, 371
Multiplicative model, 97
Multistage model for carcinogenesis, 346
Multivariate
  adaptive regression splines (MARS), 330
  confounder score, 324
  method, vii, 10
  normal distribution, 189
Myocardial infarction (MI), 76, 90, 208–211

Natural ordering, 164
Nephrectomy, 226, 249
Nested case-control study, 253
Nominal
  categories, 58, 163, 164, 172
  variables, 186
Noncentrality parameter, 296, 297, 298, 300, 303, 304, 305, 306, 307
Nonparametric
  methods, 109, 135, 347
  model, 200
Normal distribution, 221, 222
Nuisance parameter, 356, 397
Null hypothesis, 290, 293
Number of failures needed, 291

Obesity, 77
Observed failures, 215
Odds
  for disease, 43
  power family, 154–155, 160
  ratio, 32, 43, 44, 45, 75, 77, 299, 313, 323, 349
Offset, 207, 208, 219, 382, 386
Oral contraceptives, 77, 161
Ordered categories, 62, 172
Organic solvents, 274–276
Ovarian cancer, (*See* Cancer, ovarian)
Over dispersion, 223

Parallelism, 182
Paris Prospective Study, 85, 90–93, 94, 95, 208–211, 212

PCBs, 6, 7, 336
Pearson chi-square, 48, 49, 60, 61, 72, 75, 76, 150, 154, 321, 356, 366, 382
Period, 8, 335
Physician's Health Study, 5, 6
Piecewise
  constant hazard, 109, 114, 127, 135, 228, 249, 372, 374, 393
  exponential model, 113, 137, 228, 229, 230, 236, 369, 393
Poisson
  distribution, 207, 208, 212, 213, 215, 218, 219, 223, 230, 283, 362, 385, 388
  likelihood, 229, 386
  mean, 386
  regression, 224, 225, 389
Polynomial
  model, 174, 175, 195, 200, 326
  regression, 201
  splines, (*See* Splines, polynomial)
Postal survey, 179, 185
Power, 281, 288, 295, 297, 298, 299, 300, 301, 302, 303, 305, 307, 308, 309, 310, 311, 312
  family, 195, 201, 213
  odds model, 379
  transformation, 198, 199, 390
Preeclampsia, 274–276
Principal components, 336
Probability density function, 344, 361, 387, 393
Probit, 379
  model, 146, 160
Product limit
  estimate, 236, 372
  method, 109, 115, 117, 119, 127, 135, 137
Profile likelihood, 149, 382
Proportional
  hazards, 24, 28, 126, 127, 129, 132, 133, 137, 215, 227, 228, 233, 235, 239, 240, 241, 247, 249, 257, 277, 291, 398, 399
  hazards, stratified, 269
  linear hazard, 28
Proportions, viii, 39, 281, 282, 310, 315
  difference, 288
Pruning trees, 319
Psittacosis, 57, 157

Quadratic splines, (*See* Splines, quadratic)
Quartile, 313
Quasi symmetry, 266, 267, 268

Quetelet's index, 77
Quintiles, 299, 300, 305

Random error, 143
Rate, xi, 20, 23, 205, 206, 212, 283, 289, 311, 315, 347, 361
  comparison, 289–290
  ratio, 285, 312
Recursive partitioning, 317
Reference group, 28
Regression calibration, 335
Relative risk, 285, 289
Repeated measurement, 334
Ridge
  regression, 336–339
  trace, 338–339
Risk, 20, 21, 347
  set, 394, 395

Sample size, 281, 288, 295, 298, 299, 300, 301, 305, 308, 309, 310, 311
SAS, viii, 208, 230, 232, 237, 238, 243, 244, 247, 248, 263, 264, 267, 268, 269, 271, 274, 300, 301, 302, 303, 306, 307, 308, 309, 338, 399
Savage test, 375
Scaled deviance, 150, 154, 192, 209, 216, 267, 389, 390
Schistosoma haematobium, 328
Schistosoma mansoni, *17*, *22*
Score
  function, 356
  statistics, viii, 47, 48, 60, 74, 77, 88, 90, 94, 95, 126, 129, 161, 260, 295, 355, 358, 365, 367, 372, 373
Screening test, 167
Sex, 179, 226
Shape parameter, 220, 221, 387
Significance
  level, 297
  test, 47
Simulation, 309
SMR, 86, 87, 93, 99, 106, 215, 224, 361, 363, 364
Splines, 200, 316, 326, 329, 340
  B, 328
  cubic, 327, 328
  linear, 326, 328
  polynomial, 327, 328
  quadratic, 327
Spontaneous abortion, 322
Square tables, 266
Stage, 230, 233, 235
Standard normal distribution, 146

Standardized Mortality/Morbidity Ratio, (*See* SMR)
Stanford Heart Transplant Study, 245
StatXact, 75
Stilbesterol, 270–272
Stochastic model, 17
Stratification, 63, 73, 95, 132, 133, 137, 205, 239, 254, 256, 269, 277, 305, 315, 317, 320, 325, 357, 366, 397, 398, 399
Stratified proportional hazards, (*See* Proportional hazards, stratified)
Study design, vii, 253, 310
Summary rates, 85, 97
Survival
  analysis, 320
  curve, (*See* Survival function)
  curve, adjusted, 239
  curve, log-log, 242
  function, 34, 109, 110, 112, 114, 115, 116, 118, 119, 122, 123, 124, 125, 135, 137, 236, 291, 311, 343, 345, 347, 361, 369, 374, 387
  study, 20, 325
  time, 205
Synergy, 30
Systematic component, 143
Systolic blood pressure, 202–203

Talc, 53, 57
Threshold, 201
  dose, 176
Ties, 375
Time to failure, xi, 20, 21, 315, 361
Time-dependent covariate, 240–241, 242, 395
Time-varying effects, 241, 245–247
Tobacco, 161
Tobit regression, 222

Tolerance, 147
Total person-years, 206
Tranquilizers, 64, 66, 71
Trend test, 73, 76, 94, 103
Truncate follow-up, 284
Type I
  censoring, 133
  error, 287, 288
Type II
  censoring, 134
  error, 287, 288, 296, 310

Vaginal cancer, (*See* Cancer, vaginal)
VA Lung Cancer Trial, 242–245
Variable reduction, 336
Variance
  components, 332–333
  of linear function, (*See* Linear function, variance of)
Variate, vii,
Vital
  registries, 82
  statistics, 8

Wald test, 47, 48, 53, 54, 76, 89, 161, 189, 190, 192, 201, 202, 203, 225, 226, 249, 295, 353, 381
Weibull
  distribution, 135, 219, 220, 224, 386, 387
  hazard, 34, 121, 122, 137, 218, 222, 347, 385
  model, 226, 227, 346, 390, 391
Wilcoxon test, 136, 375
Withdrawn alive, 83, 110

Yates correction, 50, 53, 56, 76

z test, 47